# Tardive Dyskinesia: A Task Force Report of the American Psychiatric Association

# The American Psychiatric Association Task Force on Tardive Dyskinesia

John M. Kane, M.D. (Chairman)

Dilip V. Jeste, M.D. (Co-Chairman)

Thomas R. E. Barnes, M.D. (Consultant)

Daniel E. Casey, M.D.

Jonathan O. Cole, M.D.

John M. Davis, M.D.

C. Thomas Gualtieri, M.D.

Nina R. Schooler, Ph.D. (Consultant)

Robert L. Sprague, Ph.D. (Consultant)

Robert M. Wettstein, M.D. (Consultant)

# Tardive Dyskinesia: A Task Force Report of the American Psychiatric Association

Published by the American Psychiatric Association
Washington, DC

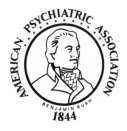

Note: The contributors have worked to ensure that all information in this book concerning drug dosages, schedules, and routes of administration is accurate as of the time of publication and consistent with standards set by the U.S. Food and Drug Administration and the general medical community. As medical research and practice advance, however, therapeutic standards may change. For this reason and because human and mechanical errors sometimes occur, we recommend that readers follow the advice of a physician who is directly involved in their care or the care of a member of their family.

The findings, opinions, and conclusions of the report do not necessarily represent the views of the officers, trustees, or all members of the American Psychiatric Association. Each report, however, does represent the thoughtful judgment and findings of the task force of experts who composed it. These reports are considered a substantive contribution to the ongoing analysis and evaluation of problems, programs, issues, and practices in a given area of concern.

Copyright © 1992 American Psychiatric Association, Washington, DC.
ALL RIGHTS RESERVED
Manufactured in the United States of America on acid-free paper.
95 94 93 92 4 3 2 1


American Psychiatric Association
1400 K Street, N.W., Washington, DC 20005


**Library of Congress Cataloging-in-Publication Data**
American Psychiatric Association.   Task Force on Tardive Dyskinesia.
    Tardive Dyskinesia: A Task Force Report of the American Psychiatric
  Association.
      p.  cm.
    The findings, opinions, and conclusions of the American Psychiatric
  Association, Task Force on Tardive Dyskinesia.
      Includes index.
      ISBN 0-89042-230-3
      1.  Tardive dyskinesia.    I. Title.
      [DNLM: 1. Diagnosis, Differential.  2. Dyskinesia, Drug-Induced–
    diagnosis.  3. Dyskinesia, Drug-Induced–prevention & control.
    4. Tranquilizing Agents, Major–adverse effects.    WL  390  A512r]
    RC394.T37A44    1991
    616.8'3—dc20
    DNLM/DLC
    for Library of Congress                                        91–22033
                                                                        CIP


**British Cataloguing in Publication Data**
A CIP record is available from the British Library.

# Contents

# Chapter 1

# Introduction

In 1979 the American Psychiatric Association published the report of its Task Force on Late Neurologic Side Effects of Antipsychotic Drugs, entitled "Tardive Dyskinesia." In the subsequent decade considerable research has been conducted on the prevalence, incidence, and risk factors associated with the development of late-occurring neurologic side effects, as well as factors influencing their course and outcome. In addition, these adverse effects have been further characterized phenomenologically into subtypes, including tardive dystonia and tardive akathisia. Although no proven safe and effective treatments for tardive dyskinesia have emerged, improvements in research design and methodology have been applied to clinical trials involving movement disorders, setting the stage for further advances.

Continued concern regarding tardive dyskinesia has also served as an impetus to explore alternative neuroleptic maintenance treatment strategies, such as low-dose or microdose and intermittent or targeted treatments. In general, there has been a reevaluation of minimum dosage requirements in the acute and long-term uses of neuroleptics in the treatment of schizophrenia. In addition, there is increased awareness of the various ways in which drug-induced neurologic adverse effects may manifest themselves and the extent to which they may influence compliance and impede optimal vocational and psychosocial rehabilitation.

Disabilities associated with tardive dyskinesia may be directly related to the specific movements involved. For example, severe dyskinesia of the trunk and limbs can cause impairment of mobility. More common, orofacial movements interfere with speech and eating, with difficulty in swallowing and possibly an increased risk of choking (Casey and Rabins 1978; Schmidt and Jarcho 1966). The condition may also be associated with respiratory irregularity, including such symptoms as shortness of breath and involuntary grunting or gasping noises (Weiner et al. 1978; Yassa and Lal 1986), and dyspnea and cyanosis (Hunter et al. 1964). More generally, patients with severe dyskinesia may carry an excess burden of mortality, although studies addressing this issue have not yielded consistent findings

1

(Kucharski et al. 1978; McClelland et al. 1986; Metha et al. 1978; Yassa et al. 1984). In a 32-month follow-up of 101 chronic schizophrenic inpatients, Youssef and Waddington (1987) found not only an increased mortality in those patients with tardive dyskinesia compared with their nondyskinetic control subjects, but also a higher morbidity related to respiratory tract infections and cardiovascular disorders.

Much of the disability related to tardive dyskinesia is of a more subtle nature. The population in which the condition is most prevalent is that of chronic schizophrenic patients, many of whom are already socially crippled by the negative and deficit symptoms associated with the illness. The constant, and often grotesque, movements of the lips, cheeks, jaw, and tongue constitute a severe social handicap. The presence of these obvious and odd movements stigmatize the patients. By causing embarrassment to family and friends and apprehension on the part of potential employers and coworkers, these movements can hinder the efforts being made to improve the ability of patients to function successfully within the community (Barnes and Kidger 1979).

Given that in some cases tardive dyskinesia can be extremely severe and disabling, considerable attention has been focused on medicolegal issues relating to this disorder, and the report reviews this area. In general, it is the consensus of the Task Force on Tardive Dyskinesia that the potential benefits of neuroleptics, when used appropriately, continue to outweigh the potential risks; however, this assessment must be made on an individual basis. At the same time, it is important that patients and families understand the nature of the illness being treated, the options for treatment that do exist, and their respective benefits and risks. Fortunately, during the past decade we have seen a move toward increased psychoeducation, thereby facilitating a more open discussion about the nature of schizophrenia with patients and their families.

The task force has chosen not to review extensively the literature regarding the role of long-term neuroleptic treatment in the management of schizophrenia. This topic was covered in considerable depth in the previous task force report, and recent comprehensive reviews have appeared (Davis et al. 1989; Kane and Lieberman 1987). We have reviewed recent developments in alternative maintenance strategies, particularly as they relate to a potential reduction in the risk of tardive dyskinesia development, and we provide a review of the indications for neuroleptic use in general.

We have also chosen not to review current hypotheses regarding the pathophysiology of tardive dyskinesia. This decision was based on the fact that there have been no major advances in this area with direct clinical application, and the animal models on which many of these hypotheses are based are fraught with potential pitfalls. We also believe that tardive dyskinesia may be a syndrome that includes a heterogeneous group of conditions, the development of which may be influenced by various different factors, not simply a specific drug-receptor interaction.

A related issue is the putative site specificity of individual compounds and their consequent propensity or lack of propensity to produce neurologic adverse effects. Given the current limitations of our preclinical models, such hypotheses are heuristic at best and any conclusions regarding the risk of tardive dyskinesia associated with particular compounds should be based on appropriately designed clinical studies. Preclinical models may help to identify which compounds should be tested in that context, but even here there is a risk of putting too much emphasis on unvalidated assumptions about the relevance of these models to the clinical condition.

As we reviewed the two topics—the extent of the utilization of neuroleptic drugs in general and the prevention of tardive dyskinesia—some major gaps in our knowledge base were highlighted. It is clear that neuroleptic drugs are used in treating various conditions other than schizophrenia and that many cases of tardive dyskinesia occur in that context. For example, neuroleptics are widely used in the treatment of bipolar disorder. If such usage occurs when patients fail to benefit adequately from lithium, it may be justified; however, the research data on which to base benefit-to-risk assessments of this indication are almost nonexistent. Many questions remain, for example, about the indications for neuroleptic treatment in the elderly, children, and borderline or schizotypal personality disorders. Clearly, further research directed toward establishing appropriate indications for short-term and long-term neuroleptic utilization in any of these patient populations would, in all likelihood, contribute to our preventive efforts. It is also evident that, given our present state of knowledge, even the most appropriate and judicious use of neuroleptic drugs will not necessarily prevent the development of tardive dyskinesia in many cases.

For further introduction to the body of the report, what follows is a brief summary or description of each chapter.

In Chapter 2, we provide an overview of the differential diagnosis of tardive dyskinesia. It is important to emphasize that abnormal involuntary movements occurring in patients receiving neuroleptic drugs are not necessarily manifestations of tardive dyskinesia. Various neuromedical conditions may cause movement disorders, and clinicians must consider these in the differential diagnosis. It is also important to recognize that tardive dyskinesia and other movement disorders may coexist and that motoric disorder may in some cases be a feature of schizophrenia. This chapter includes specific criteria for the diagnosis of tardive dyskinesia and a schema for diagnostic steps in clinical practice. We also discuss new data with regard to subsyndromes of tardive dyskinesia and related syndromes, such as tardive akathisia and tardive dystonia.

In Chapter 3 we discuss the assessment of tardive dyskinesia. Various problems relating to assessment are reviewed (e.g., intrapatient variation and changes related to medication status). In addition, different rating methods, ranging from instrumentation to multi-item clinical rating scales, are reviewed. This chapter also includes a discussion of some problems encountered in the assessment of specific clinical populations, such as children and individuals with mental retardation. It is important to emphasize that scores on a rating scale cannot be used to make a diagnosis. Assessment techniques are important for identifying possible cases as well as for documenting severity and measuring treatment response or long-term outcome, but a process of clinical evaluation and differential diagnosis is necessary to establish the presence of tardive dyskinesia.

In Chapter 4 we review current knowledge with regard to epidemiology, risk factors, and outcome of tardive dyskinesia. The available epidemiologic data suggest that neuroleptic drugs play an important role in producing or evoking abnormal involuntary movements in some patients while there are individuals with schizophrenia and other psychotic disorders who may have or develop abnormal involuntary movements unassociated with long-term drug treatment. In this chapter we review data from recent prospective studies that have provided better estimates of incidence and more meaningful information with regard to risk factors. New data on the long-term outcome of tardive dyskinesia provide some reassurance that the disorder in most cases is nonprogressive and that even with continued neuroleptic administration (when indicated), there may be improvement over time, particularly if the lowest effective dosage can be employed. The problem remains, however, that a subgroup of patients does develop a severe and disabling form of the condition; without means to reliably identify such individuals, preventive efforts remain very important.

In Chapter 5 we summarize studies of various treatments for tardive dyskinesia. There remains no proven safe and effective treatment for this condition. The most logical "treatment" remains neuroleptic withdrawal; however, this is frequently not feasible when there is a risk of worsening or relapse of psychotic symptoms. If continued neuroleptic treatment is indicated, an attempt at dose reduction should be considered. Noradrenergic antagonists and "GABAergic" (γ-aminobutyric acid) drugs may be helpful in subsets of patients, at least on a temporary basis. Anticholinergic drugs deserve a trial in patients with tardive dystonia. Various other compounds may be tried in patients with moderate to severe tardive dyskinesia, bearing in mind that each of these treatments must be evaluated on an individual basis in terms of benefit and risk. It is important to emphasize that in most cases tardive dyskinesia is mild and may not require any specific treatment apart from neuroleptic withdrawal or dosage reduction when feasible.

In Chapter 6 we summarize the indications for and efficacy of neuroleptic drugs in the treatment of various psychiatric and neuropsychiatric conditions. This review was felt to be necessary to help to establish a framework for developing benefit and risk assessments of neuroleptic treatment in various conditions. The use of antipsychotic or neuroleptic drugs remains a matter of clinical judgment that must be made on an individual basis; however, it is critical that clinicians weigh the relative indications for alternative treatments when neuroleptics are not the only available treatment.

The overall indications for short-term and long-term utilization of neuroleptics have not changed appreciably in the past decade. The primary indications for short-term use include 1) the treatment of an acute episode or exacerbation of a schizophrenic illness, 2) delusional disorder and other psychotic disorders, 3) the manic phase of bipolar disorder when very rapid control is necessary in a highly agitated patient or when lithium treatment is inadequate, 4) the treatment of agitation or psychosis in some organic mental disorders, 5) major depressive episodes with psychotic features, and 6) neurologic or psychiatric manifestations of certain neuropsychiatric conditions such as Huntington's disease and Tourette's disorder. In addition, a brief therapeutic trial of neuroleptics may be indicated in some severe personality disorders. In children or adolescents, neuroleptics may be indicated in schizophrenia, autism, pervasive developmental disorder, Tourette's disorder, attention-deficit hyperactivity disorder, conduct disorder, and in some cases of aggressive and nonspecific behavioral symptoms associated with mental retardation.

In Chapter 7 we summarize the results of studies conducted during the past 10 years involving alternative maintenance medication strategies in the treatment of schizophrenia. The risk of tardive dyskinesia associated with long-term neuroleptic treatment has served as an impetus to explore means of reducing cumulative neuroleptic exposure either through substantial dosage reduction (i.e., the low-dose strategy) or through lengthy periods of complete drug discontinuation (i.e., the intermittent or targeted medication strategy). Although these strategies have proven to be clinically feasible for some patients, there is an increase in the risk of relapse, and the impact of these strategies on the development of tardive dyskinesia has not been striking or consistent. Indeed, if medication must be started and stopped frequently in order to prevent an exacerbation in psychopathology, the effects on tardive dyskinesia may be worse than simply maintaining the patient on continuous medication.

In Chapter 8 we provide a review of alternatives to neuroleptic pharmacotherapy. Although (as reviewed in Chapter 6) neuroleptic drugs play an important role in the treatment of various conditions, their association with tardive dyskinesia and other neurologic side effects remains a limiting factor in their use. As a result, there have been continued efforts to develop alternatives to neuroleptic treatment. It appears that, at present, proven safe and effective alternatives for neuroleptic treatment in the acute and long-term treatment of schizophrenia have not emerged. Although subgroups of patients may benefit at times from nonneuroleptic medications, we are unable to identify these individuals before appropriate treatment trials. Therefore, neuroleptic drugs continue to remain the treatment of choice for patients with schizophrenia unless there are specific contraindications or clear evidence that such agents are not helpful. The treatment of those patients who fail to benefit adequately from available neuroleptics continues to present a challenge to clinicians, and in this context, various "unproven" or experimental treatments might be indicated. Alternatives to neuroleptic treatment are, however, well established in various conditions other than schizophrenia, and the use of neuroleptics in that context must be weighed carefully and justified fully.

In Chapter 9 we review the issue of whether prolonged neuroleptic administration might result in neuropharmacological changes, producing alterations in behavior in a fashion analogous to tardive dyskinesia. Such syndromes as supersensitivity psychosis, tardive dysmentia, and tardive dysbehavior have been proposed. There is currently no methodologically acceptable basis on which to prove that these syndromes do or do not exist. Clearly, some psychotic patients relapse rapidly or severely when neuroleptic drugs are reduced or discontinued, and some psychotic (and nonpsychotic) patients may show different behavior patterns over time as well as different degrees of neuroleptic responsiveness. It is difficult to determine, however, what (if any) role neuroleptic treatment has in changing these patterns in specific patients without comparable longitudinal data in untreated patients. It is difficult to avoid the conclusion that if these syndromes exist, they are relatively rare or hard to identify compared with the varied symptom course and clinical response of patients who receive neuroleptic treatment.

In Chapter 10 we summarize the clinical-legal issues related to tardive dyskinesia, including examples of litigation cases involving tardive dyskinesia, a discussion of informed consent (with case examples), and recommendations for monitoring and documentation. It is clear that even the most appropriate and judicious use of neuroleptic treatment is associated with a risk of untoward effects, including tardive dyskinesia. Litigation is a pervasive concern in contemporary American society, both within and outside medicine. Therefore, the task force felt it was important to address general issues of liability for the prescribing physician and the treatment team. The physician's prescription liability pertains largely to two areas, negligence and informed consent. We discuss these issues in detail. The task force felt it was necessary to carefully review the elements of informed consent, clinical concerns surrounding the process, and areas of possible exception. The task force does not, however, recommend routine written consent forms for neuroleptic medication.

In Chapter 11 we summarize the task force's recommendations about what lines of investigation could be particularly helpful in addressing the problem of tardive dyskinesia. Although we have an enormous data base from prevalence surveys, additional surveys in special populations could be helpful. Certainly, additional prospective studies would be valuable, particularly those comparing treatments with different putative risk profiles (e.g., clozapine or sulpiride). In exploring preventive strategies it will be important to address not only incidence, but also severity, course, and associated disability. Much remains to be learned regarding the pathophysiology of tardive dyskinesia, and the increasing availability of compounds with more specific and relatively pure effects on particular neurotransmitter receptors may be helpful in providing new knowledge of receptor mechanisms. In terms of treatment, although no proven safe and effective treatments have emerged, we hope that further advances in our understanding of pathophysiology might lead to more effective treatments. In addition, our continued efforts to subtype tardive dyskinesia may provide a basis for applying specific treatments to particular patients. Perhaps the most striking reminder resulting from the task force's efforts is that a considerable amount of basic clinical research is still necessary to better establish the appropriate indications and relative efficacy of neuroleptic treatment in various nonschizophrenic conditions.

In Chapter 12 we provide an overview of the report and recommendations for the prevention and management of tardive dyskinesia.

# References

Barnes TRE, Kidger T: Tardive dyskinesia and problems of assessment, in Current Themes in Psychiatry, Vol 2. Edited by Caind RN, Hudson BL. London, Macmillan, 1979, pp 145–162

Casey DE, Rabins P: Tardive dyskinesia as a life-threatening illness. Am J Psychiatry 135:486–488, 1978

Davis JM, Barter JT, Kane JM: Antipsychotic drugs, in Comprehensive Textbook of Psychiatry. Edited by Kaplan HI, Sadock BJ. Baltimore, MD, Williams & Wilkins, 1989, pp 1591–1626

Hunter R, Earl CJ, Thornicroft S: An apparently irreversible syndrome of chronic movements following phenothiazine medication. Proc R Soc Med 57:758–762, 1964

Kane J, Lieberman J: Maintenance pharmacotherapy in schizophrenia, in Psychopharmacology: The Third Generation of Progress. Edited by Meltzer HY. New York, Raven, 1987, pp 1103–1109

Kucharski LT, Smith JW, Dunn DD: Mortality and tardive dyskinesia. Am J Psychiatry 136:1228, 1978

McClelland HA, Dutta D, Metcalfe A, et al: Mortality and facial dyskinesia. Br J Psychiatry 148:310–316, 1986

Metha D, Mallya A, Volavka J, et al: Mortality of patients with tardive dyskinesia. Am J Psychiatry 135:371–372, 1978

Schmidt WR, Jarcho LW: Persistent dyskinesias following phenothiazine therapy. Arch Neurol 14:369–377, 1966

Weiner WJ, Goetz CG, Nausieda PA, et al: Respiratory dyskinesias: extrapyramidal dysfunction and dyspnoea. Ann Intern Med 88:327–331, 1978

Yassa R, Lal S: Respiratory irregularity and tardive dyskinesia. Acta Psychiatr Scand 73:506–510, 1986

Yassa R, Mohelsky H, Dimitri R: Mortality rate in tardive dyskinesia. Am J Psychiatry 141:1018–1019, 1984

Youssef HA, Waddington JL: Morbidity and mortality in tardive dyskinesia: associations in chronic schizophrenia. Acta Psychiatr Scand 75:74–77, 1987

Chapter 2

# Differential Diagnosis of Tardive Dyskinesia

$\mathbf{A}$ny and all abnormal involuntary movements in a patient taking neuro-leptics do not constitute tardive dyskinesia. In this chapter we review the various clinical entities that may appear in the differential diagnosis of a movement disorder, specific criteria for the diagnosis of tardive dyskinesia, and a schema for diagnostic steps in clinical practice.

## Differential Diagnosis

The conditions in the differential diagnosis of tardive dyskinesia can be considered under the following categories:

1. Nondyskinetic abnormal involuntary movements
2. Other neuroleptic-induced nontardive dyskinesias
3. Dyskinesias due to other drugs
4. Disorders of basal ganglia
5. Other identifiable movement disorders
6. Miscellaneous "spontaneous" dyskinesias

### Nondyskinetic Abnormal Involuntary Movements

The term *dyskinesia* is not a well-defined movement disorder but a broad term that includes several types of abnormal involuntary movements. There is no universal agreement on what constitutes dyskinesia; however, the following kinds of abnormal movements are generally included: cho-rea (rapid, jerky, quasi-purposive, nonrhythmic movements, especially of proximal body parts), athetosis (slow, sinuous, or writhing movements of distal parts of extremities), and dystonia (slow, sustained muscular contrac-tions or spasms that may produce involuntary movements). Dyskinesia does not include akathisia, compulsions, continuous partial seizures, man-nerisms, myoclonus, stereotypy (repetitive uniform purposeless move-ments), tics, or tremors. Table 2–1 compares the main features of the

9

different types of abnormal movements.

*Akathisia* is a term coined by Haskovec (1903) to describe an inability to sit still, which he observed in two apparently psychoneurotic patients. Following the introduction of antipsychotic drugs, Steck (1954) observed jittery, restless or rhythmic movements frequently occurring in the lower extremities among patients receiving these medications. The patterns of restless movements observed with neuroleptic-induced acute akathisia include rocking from foot to foot, walking in place, shuffling of feet while sitting, and repeated leg crossing or leg swinging. In its most severe form, those affected are unable to maintain any position for more than a few minutes. The extreme distress associated with this experience may have contributed to suicide attempts (Drake and Erlich 1985). Patients also experience a subjective sense of discomfort, inner restlessness, or anxiety. As

**Table 2–1.**  Types of abnormal involuntary movements

| Type | Rhythmicity | Speed | Localization | Causes |
|---|---|---|---|---|
| Akathisia | Absent | Variable | Limbs, axial muscles | Usually neuroleptics |
| Athetosis | Present | Slow | Distal parts of limbs | Lesions of putamen |
| Chorea | Absent | Rapid, jerky | Proximal parts of limbs, orofacial regions | Huntington's disease, rheumatic fever, drugs |
| Compulsion | Usually absent | Usually slow | Limbs, occasionally other areas | Psychological, encephalitis (?) |
| Dystonia | Absent | Slow | Axial muscles | Genetic disorders, encephalopathies, drugs, tetanus |
| Mannerism | Absent | Slow | Limbs, orofacial region, axial muscles | Psychological |
| Myoclonus | Absent | Rapid, jerky | Limbs | Certain genetic and acquired disorders, epilepsy |
| Stereotypies | Present | Slow | Limbs, occasionally other areas | Mental retardation, schizophrenia |
| Tic | Present or absent | Variable | Limbs, orofacial region; may be generalized | Psychological, Tourette's disorder, encephalitis |
| Tremor | Present | Usually 3–12 seconds | Fingers, toes, head, tongue | Psychological, drugs, parkinsonism, alcohol, encephalopathies, hyperthyroidism |

*Source.*  Modified from Jeste and Wyatt 1982.

a result of this pattern of presentation and the patient population receiving neuroleptic medication, akathisia is frequently misdiagnosed as psychotic agitation or increased anxiety and, therefore, treated with increasing doses of neuroleptic medication leading to an aggravation of the akathisia.

The incidence of this adverse effect varies depending on methodology, but 20% is probably a reasonably conservative estimate (Ayd 1961). Van Putten (1974) emphasized that this adverse effect may contribute to subsequent noncompliance in medication taking. Acute akathisia usually responds well to neuroleptic dosage reduction, anticholinergic drugs, or β-adrenergic antagonists. Although akathisia is usually most evident during the early phases of neuroleptic treatment (and particularly with rapid dosage escalation of high-potency neuroleptics), it may continue to be present even during long-term maintenance treatment (Barnes and Braude 1985; Barnes et al. 1990; Rifkin et al. 1978). Chronic or tardive akathisia has also been described and is discussed separately later in this chapter.

*Compulsions* are irresistible, sometimes complex, motor acts that occur in spite of a conscious effort to suppress them. Compulsions are a characteristic feature of obsessive-compulsive disorder, but they may also occur in normal individuals.

*Epilepsia partialis continua* may cause repetitive abnormal involuntary movements of one or more limbs without loss of consciousness. This may be secondary to a structural (e.g., brain tumor) or metabolic (e.g., nonketotic hyperglycemia) lesion. Similar to palatal myoclonus, but unlike tardive dyskinesia, epilepsia partialis continua is present during sleep.

*Mannerisms* refer to irregularly repetitive, somewhat purposeful movements that are often peculiar to an individual. Mannerisms are seen in normal people, although bizarre mannerisms are more common in schizophrenic and other psychotic patients. The terms *mannerism* and *stereotypy* are easily confused; the latter is intended to describe movements that are more regular than the former.

*Myoclonus* refers to an abrupt, irregular contraction of muscles producing sudden, jerky movements. Pathological conditions that produce myoclonus include seizure disorder, encephalitis (especially Dawson's inclusion body encephalitis), and certain structural lesions (particularly palatal myoclonus secondary to tumors or strokes affecting Mollaret's triangle, formed by the inferior olivary nucleus, red nucleus, and cerebellar dentate nucleus).

*Stereotypies* are repetitive, uniform purposeless movements frequently seen among the developmentally disabled and chronic schizophrenic patients (even prior to the administration of neuroleptic medication).

*Tics* are brief, sudden, recurrent contractions of related muscles producing apparently purposeless movements. Tics often occur in normal persons, especially when anxious. In children, multiple motor and vocal tics may suggest Tourette's syndrome.

*Tremors* are rhythmic, regular, oscillatory movements varying in frequency from 3 to 20 per second. Tremors may occur at rest (as in Parkinson's disease) or only when certain muscles are activated (as in cerebellar disorders). Other common causes of tremors include anxiety, hyperthyroidism, neuroleptics, alcoholism, lithium, and numerous other substances, such as mercury.

The aforementioned nondyskinetic movement disorders can generally be distinguished from tardive dyskinesia on clinical, phenomenological grounds. Sometimes, however, the differentiation can be difficult. Moreover, coexistence of certain nondyskinetic movements (e.g., mannerisms or parkinsonian tremor) and tardive dyskinesia is not rare. Furthermore, there is some recent literature on other "tardive" syndromes, such as tardive akathisia and tardive Tourette-like syndrome (Barnes, in press; Jeste et al. 1986; Klawans et al. 1981). Tardive akathisia and tardive dystonia will be discussed subsequently.

### Other Neuroleptic-Induced Nontardive Dyskinesias

**Acute dyskinesia.** Dyskinesias may occur early in the course of neuroleptic treatment. Their prevalence has been reported to be about 2.3% (Ayd 1961). They typically remit quickly after a dose reduction or discontinuation of neuroleptics. Anticholinergic or antihistaminic drugs are also effective treatments. Acute dyskinesia may be associated with dystonia, that is, intermittent and/or sustained muscular contractions of the eye, neck, and throat. These may lead to oculogyric crisis, dysarthria, dysphagia, and difficulty breathing. There may be opisthotonos, torticollis, and tortipelvis. The dystonia may only be manifested by cramps, tightening of the jaw, or difficulty speaking. They are often disturbing and painful. They too respond well to anticholinergic or antihistaminic agents.

**Withdrawal-emergent dyskinesia.** Discontinuation of neuroleptics produces dyskinesia in some patients. The reported incidence of withdrawal-induced dyskinesia in children may be as high as 45%–50%; (Engelhardt et al. 1975; Winsberg et al. 1977). The incidence in adults is not known. Withdrawal-emergent dyskinesia remits within a month of discontinuation of oral neuroleptics or is suppressed by readministration of neuroleptics. Sometimes, however, the symptoms persist, warranting a diagnosis of tardive dyskinesia. The extent to which the occurrence of withdrawal dyskinesia might indicate vulnerability to the subsequent development of tardive dyskinesia has not been determined.

## Dyskinesias Due to Other Drugs

Numerous drugs—such as caffeine, phenytoin, estrogens, lithium, and chloroquine—induce acute dyskinesias. These acute dyskinesias are accompanied by other signs of toxicity associated with those drugs and are rapidly reversible when the offending agents are discontinued (Baldessarini et al. 1980; Jeste and Wyatt 1982).

Tardive dyskinesias occur with L-dopa, amphetamines, and metoclopramide. There have been isolated case reports of tardive dyskinesia associated with tricyclic antidepressants, anticholinergic drugs, and antihistamines. The number of reported cases of tardive dyskinesia with these latter groups of drugs is, however, too small to establish a causal relationship between those agents and tardive dyskinesia.

The most frequently encountered tardive dyskinesia induced by nonneuroleptics is L-dopa-induced tardive dyskinesia in patients with

**Table 2–2.** Comparison of tardive dyskinesias induced by L-dopa and neuroleptics

| Variable | L-dopa | Neuroleptics |
|---|---|---|
| Prevalence | 40%–80% | 5%–40% |
| Manifestations | | |
|   Oral manifestations | Common | More common |
|   Limb dyskinesias | Common | Less common |
|   Intermittent dyskinesias | Frequent | Uncommon |
|   Unilateral dyskinesias | Frequent | Rare |
|   Drug-withdrawal dyskinesias | Rare | Frequent |
| Etiologic factors | | |
|   Daily high doses | Important | Less important |
|   Length of treatment | Less important | More important |
|   Primary illness | Parkinson's disease | Unimportant |
|   Need for predisposing brain damage | Present | Nonapparent |
|   Aging as predisposition | Less important | Important |
| Course | | |
|   Relationship between duration and severity of dyskinesia | Positive | Variable |
|   On-off phenomena | Sometimes | Not reported |
|   Persistence on drug withdrawal | Not reported | In 67% of patients |
| Treatment | | |
|   Dose reduction | Effective | Sometimes effective |
|   Dose increase | Dyskinesia worsens | Dyskinesia may be masked |

*Source.* Modified from Jeste and Wyatt 1982.

Parkinson's disease. In Table 2–2 we compare the salient clinical features of dyskinesias induced by L-dopa and neuroleptics.

### Disorders of Basal Ganglia

**Huntington's disease.** Huntington's disease is an autosomal dominant neurodegenerative disorder that usually appears in mid-adulthood. A DNA segment mapped to chromosome 4 was demonstrated to be closely linked to the gene for Huntington's disease (Gusella et al. 1983). The prevalence of Huntington's disease varies between 5 and 10 per 100,000 (Wexler 1984).

The cardinal manifestations of Huntington's disease include choreic movement abnormalities, psychopathological disturbances, and other neuropsychiatric symptoms (Hayden 1981). The choreic movements usually involve the face, fingers, and toes. The patients have abnormal eye movements, motor impersistence, and stuttering gait pattern. As the disease progresses, there are impairments of memory, inattention to activities of daily living, and deterioration of intellectual capacity. There may be associated depression, frank psychotic episodes, and occasional violent outbursts (Jeste et al. 1984; Wexler 1984). Except for the childhood-onset, akinetic rigid type (Westphal variant), the patients show marked hypotonia (Hayden 1981).

One clinical difficulty in differentiating tardive dyskinesia from Huntington's disease has to do with the fact that some patients with Huntington's disease might present initially with neuropsychiatric symptoms (Cummings 1985). When, in the course of their illness, after having been treated with antipsychotic drugs, patients with Huntington's disease develop chorea, it might be difficult to attempt to differentiate the two conditions. Huntington's disease patients often exhibit pronounced postural instability, which is uncommon in tardive dyskinesia. A computed tomography (CT) or magnetic resonance imaging (MRI) scan of the head might also be helpful because patients with Huntington's disease tend to show atrophy of the caudate nucleus, which is rare in tardive dyskinesia.

**Wilson's disease.** Wilson's disease is an autosomal recessive disorder characterized by a marked deficiency of ceruloplasmin. It has a prevalence rate of 30 per million (Scheinberg and Sternlieb 1984). Its neurologic presentation includes choreiform movements, tremors, diminished dexterity, marked rigidity, dystonia, and dysarthria. Other neuropsychiatric manifestations are manic-depressive illness or schizophrenialike psychosis, marked impulsivity, and other complaints that are difficult to characterize (Goldstein et al. 1968; Jeste et al. 1984). The disorder appears in early adulthood and may present initially as a psychosis. Other clinical signs include jaundice, Kayser-Fleischer rings in the cornea, and "blue moons" on the finger-nails. The subtlety of the movement disorder, when associated with an overt psychiatric disease, may prompt the clinician to make a diagnosis of stereotypic complex motor behavior. All such patients should have a serum ceruloplasmin level determined because of the treatability of Wilson's disease. Untreated patients with this disease show a progressive degenerative course that is fatal. The mainstay of treatment involves lifelong therapy with penicillamine. Patients who do not tolerate it may be treated with triethylenetetramine dihydrochloride (Scheinberg and Sternlieb 1984).

**Sydenham's chorea.**   Sydenham's chorea (rheumatic chorea, chorea minor, Saint Vitus's dance) occurs in childhood and is characterized by a relatively sudden onset of rapid, aimless, involuntary movements of the face, limbs, and trunk. Patients may have weakness of voluntary muscles, incoordination, and an abnormal gait. The neurologic examination shows flexion at the wrist and hyperextension of distal and proximal phalanges on extension of the arms (Warner hand sign). Reflexes may be pendular or held up in extension for a brief period of time (hung up). Some minor choreic movements may last for as long as 10 years (Thiebaut 1968). There may be emotional lability and, in severe cases, agitation, confusion, delusions, and hallucinations (Schwartzman 1950). Some of these patients may present with chorea gravidarum or contraceptive-induced chorea. There have been several reports of an association between Sydenham's chorea and schizophrenia (see Jeste et al. 1984). Rheumatic chorea can be distinguished from tardive dyskinesia by its association with a history of rheumatic polyarthritis and its clinical course. Husby et al. (1977) identified an antineuronal antibody directed against cells in the basal ganglia in Sydenham's chorea patients. Nausieda et al. (1980) suggested that the end of the attack might be related to cessation of the immunologic disturbance and functional recovery of the motor system.

**Fahr's syndrome.**   Fahr's syndrome is a rare hereditary disorder characterized by movement disorder, neuropsychiatric symptoms, and abnormal calcification in the brain, especially basal ganglia. The differential diagnosis for basal ganglionic calcification includes parathyroid disorders, infectious conditions, toxic disorders, and other hereditary movement disorders (Cummings and Benson 1983). The motor symptoms consist of a Parkinson-like syndrome, choreoathetosis, cerebellar ataxia, and paralysis. Neuropsychiatric symptoms include dementia, schizophrenialike psychoses, and depression (Cummings and Benson 1983).

**Hallervorden-Spatz disease.**   Hallervorden-Spatz disease is a rare hereditary (autosomal recessive) condition associated with pathological deposition of iron pigment in the globus pallidus, pars reticulata of the substantia nigra, and red nucleus (Adams and Victor 1977). The symptoms usually begin at age 10–15, and the early signs include rigidity, dystonia, choreoathetosis, spasticity, and hyperreflexia. The movement disorder progresses along with dementia for an approximately 20-year period before death usually occurs. There is no known effective treatment.

**Other disorders of basal ganglia.**    Chorea is a well-recognized complication of systemic lupus erythematosus (SLE; Nadeau and Watson 1983). The onset is typically in childhood. Other clinical symptoms, including schizophreniform psychosis and affective disturbance, may also be present (Feinglass et al. 1976). The diagnosis is based on a demonstration of hematologic and serological findings and the involvement of other organ systems by SLE. Polycythemia vera may also be complicated by chorea (Gauthier et al. 1966).

### Other Identifiable Movement Disorders

**Hyperthyroidism.**    Hyperthyroidism may present with choreiform movements of limbs. The patient is likely to have signs of thyrotoxicosis, such as fine tremor of the hands, excessive sweating, and exophthalmos. The thyroid is often enlarged, and thyroid function tests (e.g., $T_3$ and $T_4$ levels) are abnormal (Klawans 1973).

**Hypoparathyroidism.**    Hypoparathyroidism is an uncommon cause of dyskinesia. Its manifestations include carpopedal spasm, numbness and cramps in the limbs, laryngeal stridor, and seizures, with laboratory evidence of hypocalcemia, hyperphosphatemia, absence of calcium in the urine, and increased calcifications in the brain.

**Tourette's disorder.**    Tourette's disorder is an uncommon chronic disease with onset in childhood (Robertson 1989; Shapiro et al. 1978). It is more frequent in boys, especially those with a family history of tics. The syndrome consists of motor tics, vocal tics, and coprolalia (compulsive utterances of obscenities). Pharmacotherapy for Tourette's disorder consists of haloperidol or clonidine (Cohen et al. 1984). There have been case reports of tardive dyskinesia due to long-term use of haloperidol for Tourette's disorder (Mizrahi et al. 1980). Detailed documentation of abnormal movements before and during the course of neuroleptic use is needed to diagnose tardive dyskinesia in Tourette's disorder patients.

**Torsion dystonia.**    Usually transmitted as an autosomal recessive disorder, torsion dystonia is characterized by twisting and sustained contraction of muscles producing rapid, repetitive, and distressful movements. Torsion dystonia occurs most commonly among Ashkenazi Jews and begins in childhood (Eldridge and Gottlieb 1976). The first symptoms usually consist of dystonic inversion of the foot and spasms of proximal muscles of lower limbs leading to gait abnormalities. Later signs include scoliosis, torticollis, and tortipelvis, which limit the patient's daily activities (Fahn 1982). The symptoms are variable, somewhat bizarre, and exacerbated by stressful situations, thereby suggesting a possible diagnosis of hysterical conversion reaction.

Less commonly, torsion dystonia follows an autosomal dominant pattern of inheritance without any racial predilection (Eldridge and Gottlieb 1976). It is also milder, and it may remain localized to one body part. Although there is no consistently effective treatment, Fahn (1983) reported some success with high-dose anticholinergic therapy.

Tardive dystonia is a condition that may present a clinical picture similar to that of torsion dystonia, but it is believed to be associated with long-term neuroleptic treatment and will be discussed subsequently.

**Meige syndrome.**    Meige syndrome is characterized by dystonic movements of the face, blepharospasm, and spasms of jaw and neck muscles. Marsden (1976) named it Breughel's syndrome after the Flemish artist. Some patients may have only blepharospasm or orofacial-cervical dystonia; in some, it is associated with essential tremor, parkinsonian symptoms, palatal myoclonus, mild chorea, and akathisia (Jankovic and Ford 1983).

These symptoms have also been reported as complications of neuroleptics (Weiner et al. 1981). Jankovic and Ford (1983) suggested, however, that the term *Meige syndrome* should be reserved for the idiopathic variety and the term *tardive facial dystonia* should be used for the neuroleptic-induced syndrome.

The treatment of Meige syndrome is also disappointing, although there have been reports of successful treatment with high-dose anticholinergic medication (Duvoisin 1983), a combination of haloperidol and benztropine (Ortiz 1983), and botulinus toxin (National Institutes of Health 1990).

**Spasmodic torticollis.**    Spasmodic torticollis, an adult-onset dystonia, consists of spasms of the scalenus, sternocleidomastoid, and trapezius muscles, producing torticollis, anterocollis, or retrocollis. Gilbert (1977) and others have reported it to be familial in some cases. Jayne et al. (1984) reported spontaneous remission in 6 of 26 patients, maintained for more than 6 years. Recently, botulinus toxin has proven to be of some value in treating this condition as well (National Institutes of Health 1990).

### Miscellaneous "Spontaneous" Dyskinesias

Dyskinesias are occasionally present in patients who have not been treated with neuroleptics or other dyskinesia-producing drugs and who do not have any of the other disorders considered in this chapter. These types of abnormal movements are relatively more common in patients with certain psychiatric illnesses (mainly chronic schizophrenia), elderly subjects, and patients subjected to long-term institutionalization. Patients with ill-fitting dentures often have mild oral dyskinesia.

Psychogenic spontaneous dyskinesias include hysterical conversion reaction and malingering. Hysterical conversion reaction, more common in the young, generally involves multiple parts of the body, tends to be more severe when the patient is attended to, and disappears when the subject is alone. The movements may be dramatic and bizarre, yet the patient rarely falls or gets injured from the abnormal movements. A careful history usually reveals an unconscious motivation (the so-called "primary" gain) for the symptoms. Premorbid personality may be histrionic—that is, characterized by labile moods, self-centered attitude, attention-seeking tendency, low frustration tolerance, and excessive dependence. The onset of dyskinesia follows environmental stress, and removal of the stressful situation is likely to produce remission. Malingering differs from hysteria in that it has a conscious motivation. In practice, however, the difference between hysteria and malingering is not always apparent.

# Abnormal Involuntary Movements as a Feature of Schizophrenia

There is evidence that motor disorder is an inherent feature of the schizophrenic illness. Spontaneous movements associated with psychosis were recognized for many years before the introduction of antipsychotic drugs (Jones and Hunter 1969; Marsden et al. 1975). They range from simple ticlike disturbances to complex patterns of movement and activity, referred to as stereotypies and mannerisms, perseverative movements, tics, grimaces and general clumsiness, awkwardness, and lack of coordination. However, abnormal involuntary movements, such as choreiform and orofacial dyskinesia, are also clearly described (Farran-Ridge 1926; Jones and Hunter 1969; Kraepelin 1919).

Kraepelin (1919) described abnormal orofacial and limb movements under a number of headings. His descriptions of mannerisms accompanying speech include "wrinkling of the eyes, senseless shaking and nodding of the head and drawing of the muscles of expression" (Defendorf 1902, p. 181) and "loud hawking and grunting . . . with smacking movements of the lips, the face is distorted by spasmodic phenomena in the musculature of the face and of speech," some of which

> resemble movements of expression, wrinkling of the forehead, distortion of
> the corners of the mouth, irregular movements of the tongue and lips, twist-
> ing of the eyes, opening them wide and shutting them tight, in short, these
> movements which we bring together under the name of making faces or
> grimacing; they remind one of the corresponding disorders of chronic pa-
> tients. Nystagmus may also belong to this group. Connected with these are
> further, smacking and clicking of the tongue, sudden sighing, laughing and
> clearing the throat. But besides, we observe, specially in the lip muscles, fine
> lightning-like or rhythmical twitchings, which in no way bear the stamp of
> voluntary movements. The same is the case of the tremor in the muscles of
> the mouth which appears sometimes in speaking and which may completely
> resemble that of paralytics. (Kraepelin 1919)

He goes on to mention "peculiar, sprawling, irregular, choreiform, outspreading movements," which he labels "athetoid ataxia" (Kraepelin 1919,
p. 83).

Although some of the movements described resemble those of tardive
dyskinesia, for example, smacking of the lips and choreiform limb movements, MacKay (1981) considered that most are not recognizable as part of
the syndrome and may be differentiated from tardive dyskinesia by their
appearance, which is stereotyped and manneristic, in contrast to the non-
repetitive, irregular, jerky, quasi-purposive movements that characterize
tardive dyskinesia.

Kraepelin (1919) considered most of these abnormal movements under
a heading of "spasmodic phenomena," which hints at a dystonic rather
than dyskinetic appearance. Although he referred to some as "choreiform," it is not clear in this context how this description should be interpreted. Bleuler (1950) claimed that he had never seen true chorea in
schizophrenia and was skeptical of reports of a relatively high incidence,
attributing these to differences in the definition of the term. Choreiform
or choreoathetoid movements appear to have been relatively rare in
chronic psychiatric patients before the advent of antipsychotic drugs. Such
a conclusion is supported by the findings of Mettler and Crandell (1959),
who conducted a study of neurologic disorder in a population of chronic
psychiatric patients and found that only about 0.5% had evidence of chorea or athetosis.

Currently, most schizophrenic patients are treated at some time in the
course of their illness with antipsychotic drugs. The opportunity to study
abnormal, involuntary movements in chronic patients who have not
received medication rarely presents itself. Owens et al. (1982), however,
while assessing movement disorder in a sample of 411 hospitalized schizophrenic patients, identified 47 who, they claimed, had never been exposed

to antipsychotic drugs. Comparison of the drug-treated and non-drug-treated groups failed to reveal many significant differences with regard to prevalence, severity, and distribution of abnormal, involuntary movements. Although movements were recorded using the Abnormal Involuntary Movement Scale (AIMS) and the Rockland/Simpson Tardive Dyskinesia Rating Scale, the authors refrained from applying diagnostic categories or classifying the movements in terms of their nature of characteristics. Owens (1985) later analyzed the data further, examining clinically recognizable syndromes of abnormal movements, and this revealed a particular susceptibility to orofacial dyskinesia in drug-treated patients. He pointed out, however, that such movements were seen in 30% of those cases never treated with drugs.

One inescapable conclusion from their findings is that spontaneous, involuntary, orofacial movements can be a feature of chronic schizophrenia that has not been modified by the administration of antipsychotic drugs. A proportion of such movements may merely represent spontaneous orofacial dyskinesia of the elderly, but Owens et al. (1982) postulated that in some patients the syndrome reflects the pathological cerebral process underlying severe chronic schizophrenia. A similar notion has been put forward by Lidsky et al. (1979), who discussed the possibility that the repetitive motor acts displayed by patients with schizophrenia could be related to an underlying dysfunction of the basal ganglia associated with the condition.

Further evidence suggesting an intrinsic relationship between motor disturbance and psychotic phenomena is the occurrence of motor disturbance in amphetamine-induced psychosis. Chronic abuse of amphetamine can induce a paranoid state almost indistinguishable from paranoid schizophrenia (Snyder 1973). This mental state is accompanied by complex patterns of perseverative, stereotyped behavior and impulsive fidgety movements, as well as simpler phenomena such as grimacing, chewing, and twisting of the trunk and limbs (Segal and Janowsky 1978).

A major methodological problem facing researchers in this area is the difficulty distinguishing between the various types of movement disturbance. The descriptive categories of dyskinesia, such as choreiform and dystonic, may be useful, as may distinction between purposeful and purposeless or voluntary and involuntary, but none of these analyses guarantees differentiation between drug-related and illness-related motor anomalies. Indeed, if schizophrenic patients with motor disturbances inherent to their illnesses are more vulnerable to the neurologic side effects of antipsychotic drugs, then the two types of movement will tend to coexist in the same individuals. This seems a plausible hypothesis and is supported by the finding that both types of movement may share an association with similar clinical features.

## Clinical Associations of Schizophrenic and Drug-Related Abnormal Movements

Yarden and Discipio (1971) reported on a sample of young, drug-free schizophrenic patients presenting with a variety of abnormal movements, labeled as choreiform and athetoid, and including tics, stereotypies, and mannerisms. Their follow-up data, after 2.5 to 3.5 years, led them to conclude that schizophrenic patients distinguished by abnormal movements constituted a group with an early onset, a steadily progressive course, severe deterioration with marked thought disorder, and a resistance to pharmacological treatment. Studies by Manschrek et al. (1982) found that disturbed voluntary motor activity, which they claimed was unrelated to drug effects, occurred frequently among schizophrenic patients. They reported statistically significant associations between this apparently schizophrenic movement disturbance and neurologic "soft" signs, cognitive impairment, affective blunting, and formal thought disorder. One conclusion would be that schizophrenic patients with negative symptoms of the Type II syndrome are more likely to exhibit motor abnormalities, independent of drug treatment.

## Diagnostic Criteria for Tardive Dyskinesia

Diagnosis of tardive dyskinesia should not be made merely by excluding other conditions in the differential diagnosis. It should also be based on satisfying some "positive" criteria for tardive dyskinesia. The following list of diagnostic features is based on the criteria proposed by Jeste and Wyatt (1982) and Schooler and Kane (1982). (We stress again that tardive dyskinesia and other movement disorders may coexist.)

### Phenomenology

**Nature of the abnormal movements.**   Choreiform, athetoid, or rhythmic abnormal involuntary movements are reduced by voluntary movements of the affected parts and increased by voluntary movements of the unaffected parts.

**Other characteristics.**   The abnormal movements increase with emotional arousal and decrease with relaxation and volitional effort. The movements are absent during sleep.

**Specific localization of neuroleptic-induced tardive dyskinesia.**   The tongue, jaw, or extremities are involved in most cases. (Putative anatomical subsyndromes will be discussed subsequently.)

**Severity.**  At least "moderate" abnormal, involuntary movements in one or more body areas or "mild" movements in two or more body areas (face, lips, jaw, tongue, upper extremities, lower extremities, and trunk) are present. Because of the variability in the manifestation of movements associated with tardive dyskinesia, if the examination reveals movements that are only "minimal" or "mild" in only one body area, the examination should be repeated within 1 week to confirm their presence. Determination of the presence of these movements should be made using a standardized examination procedure and rating scale (e.g., the AIMS or the Rockland/Simpson Tardive Dyskinesia Rating Scale; see Chapter 3 and the Appendix).

### History

**Duration of dyskinesia.**  The abnormal movements should be present continually for at least 4 weeks.

**Neuroleptic treatment.**  There should be a history of at least 3 months of total cumulative neuroleptic exposure. Exposure may be continuous or discontinuous. Patients who fail to meet the criterion for duration of neuroleptic exposure should receive the appropriate diagnosis with the qualification "less than 3 months of neuroleptic exposure."

**Onset of dyskinesia.**  The onset of the dyskinesia should be either while the patient is on neuroleptics or within a few weeks of discontinuing neuroleptics.

### Treatment Response

**Antiparkinsonian agents.**  Antiparkinsonian agents usually have no effect or may even aggravate tardive dyskinesia (although they may improve tardive dystonia).

**Changes in neuroleptic doses.**  Increasing the dose of neuroleptics usually suppresses dyskinesia. Reduction or discontinuation of neuroleptics worsens the symptoms temporarily.

**Anatomical subsyndromes of tardive dyskinesia.**  Supportive evidence may be adduced from a number of sources to support the validity of distinct orofacial and trunk and limb subsyndromes of tardive dyskinesia. Particularly, the findings of the more recent studies of Glazer et al. (1988) and Gureje (1989) support the original notion of Barnes and Kidger (1979) that orofacial and trunk and limb dyskinesia should be considered as separate clinical subsyndromes that might be pathophysiologically distinct with different prognostic and etiologic determinants (Barnes et al. 1983; Kidger et al. 1980).

**Emergence of subsyndromes from multivariate statistical analysis.**   Four studies have reported on multivariate analysis of abnormal, involuntary movements in patients receiving long-term antipsychotic medication (Crane et al. 1971; Glazer et al. 1988; Kennedy et al. 1971; Kidger et al. 1980). Their results are relatively consistent. In three of the studies (Crane et al. 1971; Kennedy et al. 1971; Kidger et al. 1980), three general factors emerged: an orofacial movement factor, a trunk and limb movement factor, and a parkinsonian factor.

Comparing the factors identified by Kennedy et al. (1971) and Kidger et al. (1980), the main difference is in interpretation of the peripheral movement factor. Kennedy and his associates classified almost all limb movements observed as restlessness, although no confirmatory reports were sought from the patients. Having made the assumption of restlessness for most limb movements, their trunk and limb movement factor clearly appears to represent akathisia. Following drug withdrawal (Hershon et al. 1972), however, the parkinsonism and orofacial movement factor scores did not change, but the motor restlessness factor scores increased significantly. In this respect their restlessness factor proved to be unlike akathisia, which would be expected to persist without change or improve (Braude et al. 1983; Marsden et al. 1975), and resembled tardive dyskinesia, which is almost invariably exacerbated by reduction or withdrawal of antipsychotic drug therapy (Crane 1973; Crane et al. 1971; Marsden et al. 1975). Thus, the orofacial and trunk and limb movement factors extracted by Kennedy et al. (1971) also seem to describe two separate components of tardive dyskinesia.

Glazer et al. (1988) applied factor analysis to the seven anatomical variables of the AIMS in 228 psychiatric patients referred to a tardive dyskinesia clinic, all of whom had received a minimum of 3 months of treatment with antipsychotic drugs. The statistical techniques employed for data analysis by Glazer et al. (1988) were virtually the same as those used by Kidger et al. (1980), constituting a principal components analysis with the Varimax method of orthogonal rotation. Their findings were also similar—that is, three independent factors emerged that together accounted for nearly 54% of the total variance compared with 46% for the factors of Kidger et al. (1980); however, the factors did not entirely correspond to the three factors reported earlier. Glazer et al. (1988) confirmed the split between orofacial (factors 2 and 3) and trunk and limb (factor 1) dyskinesia, but the signs and symptoms of drug-induced parkinsonism had not been assessed in this study, so no factor representing this condition could emerge. Rather, the orofacial movement items loaded differently on factors 2 and

3, with high factor loadings on factor 2 found for jaw and tongue movements; facial and lip movements both loaded high on factor 3. The investigators decided to merge factors 2 and 3 because they acknowledged the difficulty of discriminating between jaw and lip movements during clinical examination and because of the relatively low correlation between face and lip movements (Pearson's $r = .09$), which suggested a "lack of internal consistency" for factor 3.

**Differentiation by pharmacological response.** Several pharmacological investigations have identified a discrepant response between orofacial and trunk and limb dyskinesia, reinforcing the notion that different pathophysiological mechanisms underlie the two subsyndromes (Bobruff et al. 1981; Casey and Denney 1977; Casey and Hammerstad 1979; Fann et al. 1974; Gardos et al. 1976; Greil et al. 1985; Simpson et al. 1977). Various drugs have exhibited this selective effect, including dopamine antagonists, cholinomimetic agents, sodium valproate (a putative $\gamma$-aminobutyric acid potentiator), phenobarbital, and clonazepam.

For example, Gardos et al. (1976) tested papaverine, a dopamine-blocking agent in tardive dyskinesia. They found, overall, a significant improvement in orofacial dyskinesia and a worsening of dyskinesia of the lower limbs. They concluded that "tardive dyskinesia is not a unitary syndrome, the results may indicate that certain abnormal movements in the leg are unrelated to orofacial dyskinesia or may even be negatively related to it." Bobruff et al. (1981) reported that clonazepam was more effective for orofacial dyskinesia, whereas phenobarbital had a stronger effect on peripheral dyskinesia. In a double-blind placebo-controlled study of anticholinergic withdrawal, Greil et al. (1985) found more improvement in orofacial dyskinesia compared with trunk and limb movements.

Unfortunately, the findings have not been sufficiently consistent between studies to allow predictive statements to be made regarding the nature of the response of the subsyndromes to specific classes or types of drugs. A possible interpretation of this discrepancy between drug effects on the two subsyndromes is that they reflect different neurochemical mechanisms. A similar differential drug effect has also been recorded for spontaneous dyskinesia in the elderly. Delwaide and Desseilles (1977) concluded that this condition should be considered as two separate syndromes, buccolinguofacial dyskinesia and "stereotyped movements of the limbs," on the basis of their differential sensitivity to antipsychotic drugs.

**Different clinical and demographic predictors.** Support for these subsyndromes is also provided by studies that have demonstrated different clinical and demographic predictors for the two subsyndromes. For example, the two phenomena are differentially associated with age. Limb dyskinesia is more common in younger patients (McAndrew et al. 1972; Polizos et al. 1973), whereas the reverse is found with orofacial dyskinesia.

The results of the follow-up study by Barnes et al. (1983) suggested that the presence and severity of orofacial dyskinesia was significantly associated with advancing age, but this relationship did not hold true for trunk and limb movements. In the cross-sectional study by Glazer et al. (1988) already discussed, the investigators adopted virtually the same statistical methods employed by Barnes et al. (1983) to identify clinical "predictors" of tardive dyskinesia. Using a logistic regression analysis, they identified different clinical associations for orofacial and trunk and limb dyskinesia. For example, they found that the severity of orofacial dyskinesia was positively associated with age and schizoaffective or affective disorder. Trunk and limb dyskinesia was not associated with advancing age, but there was a positive association with current antipsychotic drug dose and nonuse of psychiatric medication, principally anticholinergics.

Similarly, Gureje (1989) used multivariate statistical methods to explore the clinical associations of the same anatomical subsyndromes, which he referred to as orofacial and appendicular dyskinesia. He assessed 137 Nigerian psychiatric inpatients for abnormal movements, also using the AIMS, and investigated the relationship between the two subsyndromes and several demographic, treatment, and clinical variables. Only one variable, length of current hospitalization, was found to correlate significantly with orofacial dyskinesia. Seventy-two percent of the cases could be correctly classified on this variable, which also correctly identified 40% of patients with orofacial dyskinesia. Appendicular tardive dyskinesia was significantly associated with the cumulated duration of exposure to "high-potency" antipsychotic drugs and the number of electroconvulsive therapies received. Gureje (1989) concluded that the central findings of his study are that "different risk factors are associated with each of these subsyndromes."

Further evidence of a differentiation between the two subsyndromes in terms of clinical correlations was provided by a study by Waddington et al. (1987). They found a strong association between both cognitive dysfunction and negative symptoms and the presence and severity of orofacial dyskinesia in chronic schizophrenic patients; however, there was no such association with trunk and limb movements.

One explanation for the results of some of these studies might be a problem of differential diagnosis when assessing abnormal involuntary movements. Movements rated as trunk and limb tardive dyskinesia may include not only choreiform movements but also movements representing tardive dystonia or akathisia or other types of motor disturbance seen in psychotic patients. Such a mixture of types of trunk and limb movement might not be expected to show consistent associations with clinical variables or a consistent pattern of drug response, compared with the relatively discrete syndrome of choreiform orofacial dyskinesia. Nevertheless, overall these findings seem to provide evidence that these two regional distributions of dyskinesia do not constitute a unitary syndrome and should be examined separately in future studies.

# Tardive Dystonia

Tardive dystonia is considered to be a particular form of involuntary movement associated with long-term neuroleptics. The extent to which this condition should be viewed as a distinct entity or a subtype of tardive dyskinesia remains controversial. As Burke and Kang (1988) suggested, tardive dystonia is distinguished from the classic oral-buccal-lingual choreic form of tardive dyskinesia not only by the dystonic nature of the involuntary movements, but also by the frequency with which it causes significant neurologic disability. Keegan and Rajput (1973) used the term "dystonia tarda" to refer to dystonic phenomena occurring as a discrete side effect of chronic antipsychotic drug treatment. General attention was brought to this condition when Burke et al. (1982) noted a frequent association between dopamine antagonist use and dystonia in patients who had no other known cause of dystonia; they termed the disorder "tardive dystonia." There have now been more than 20 reports describing in excess of 100 patients with persistent dystonia developing in the context of such treatment (Burke and Kang 1988).

The movements evident in tardive dystonia are not dissimilar to those observed in primary torsion dystonia. The face and neck are the most frequently involved body regions. It is important to recognize, however, that some patients with tardive dystonia may have classic orofacial dyskinetic movements at some time during the course of their dystonia or at some time prior to its development. The distinction between dyskinetic and dystonic movements does not influence one aspect of management in terms of the desirability, if possible, of discontinuing the neuroleptic involved. Since the dystonia may in general be more severe and more disabling, the rationale for drug discontinuation may be even greater. The distinction may also have an impact on considerations of treatment for the movement disorder in that tardive dystonia has been reported to benefit from anticholinergic medications, whereas in general tardive dyskinesia does not respond to this class of pharmacologic agents (Burke and Kang 1988).

Acute dystonic reactions tend to occur in the first 24–48 hours of dopamine antagonist treatment; tardive dystonia, as a rule, occurs much later. In a series of 67 patients, Kang et al. (1986) reported that the tardive dystonia occurred after a median of 5 years of exposure, with the shortest exposure being 3 weeks. Given the evidence suggesting that tardive dystonia differs to some extent from tardive dyskinesia phenomenologically, epidemiologically, and pharmacologically, this should be an important distinction to make both clinically and heuristically.

## Tardive Akathisia

Although akathisia usually occurs during the early stages of neuroleptic treatment, it can also be a persistent problem (Barnes and Braude 1984, 1985), even after discontinuation of dopamine antagonists (Weiner and Luby 1983). Burke et al. (1989) described 27 patients withdrawn from medication in whom akathisia persisted for a mean of 2.7 years (range 0.3–7). Barnes et al. (1983) reported that akathisia and orofacial dyskinesias tend to coexist in patients on maintenance antipsychotic medication. Barnes and Braude (1984) described two patients in whom persistent akathisia seemed to be a precursor of tardive dyskinesia. Saltz et al. (1991) reported that those patients who developed parkinsonian signs early in their course of antipsychotic treatment were at significantly greater risk of developing tardive dyskinesia faster than those without such signs. Therefore, akathisia may be a precursor or a concomitant feature of some cases of tardive dyskinesia. In addition, akathisia may emerge or become more severe following a dosage reduction or withdrawal of neuroleptic medication (Barnes et al. 1990).

Braude et al. (1983) reported that tardive akathisia shares some of the pharmacological characteristics of tardive dyskinesia in that it is exacerbated or provoked by drug reduction or withdrawal and improves at least temporarily when the dose is increased.

As Barnes (in press) has suggested, it would appear that the motor phenomena of akathisia can be differentiated from orofacial dyskinesias and that persistent akathisia can occur in the absence of orofacial dyskinesia and tardive dystonia. This suggests that persistent or chronic akathisia might be viewed as a distinct syndrome; however, further research will be necessary to clarify its relationship with tardive dyskinesia. As Burke et al. (1989) emphasized, assessment is not confounded by the presence of "spontaneous" or idiopathic cases, as may occur with tardive dystonia and tardive dyskinesia.

## Tardive Tourette-like Syndrome

There have been numerous cases of Tourette-like syndrome in adults following prolonged neuroleptic treatment (Jeste et al. 1986). These are characterized by the emergence of motor and vocal tics, and occasionally coprolalia, during the course of neuroleptic treatment or following neuroleptic discontinuation. Management of such patients includes keeping

them off neuroleptics or using clonidine. Increasing the dose of a neuroleptic may temporarily suppress the tics, just as in the case of tardive dyskinesia. Since there have been no large-scale epidemiologic studies of this
condition, a cause-and-effect relationship between neuroleptic use and
Tourette-like syndrome should be considered unproven.

# Clinical Assessment of a Patient
# With Movement Disorders

### History

1. If a patient has taken neuroleptics for fewer than 3 months, he or she
   does not meet research criteria for tardive dyskinesia. In clinical practice, however, tardive dyskinesia can develop with such a brief exposure to neuroleptics (Chouinard and Jones 1979). This is especially
   true in patients at increased risk for tardive dyskinesia, such as the elderly.
2. Recent use of other drugs that can produce dyskinesia (e.g., L-dopa
   and amphetamine) should be asked about. Most dyskinesias not induced by neuroleptics disappear when those medications are discontinued.
3. History of a neurologic illness—such as stroke, encephalitis, major
   head trauma, or symptoms suggestive of a tumor (e.g., headaches)—
   should lead to a search for a structural lesion affecting basal ganglia.
4. A positive family history for a movement disorder should suggest a possibility of hereditary disorders, such as Huntington's disease, Wilson's
   disease, or torsion dystonia. In such cases, details of the disorder in the
   affected family member should be sought. (There have been anecdotal reports of familial tardive dyskinesia—e.g., Weinhold et al. 1981.)

### Physical Examination

1. The specific types of abnormal involuntary movements present in a
   given patient (e.g., tremors, tics, and choreiform movements) should
   be identified.
2. Presence of signs of dementia may indicate a need to rule out such
   disorders as Huntington's disease, Wilson's disease, and brain tumor.
   (Some elderly patients may have both dementia and neuroleptic-
   induced tardive dyskinesia.)
3. Focal neurologic deficits—such as hemiparesis or gross asymmetry of
   reflexes—should lead to a search for structural brain lesions.
4. Patients should be examined for signs of metabolic (e.g., jaundice and
   hepatomegaly secondary to liver disease) and endocrine (e.g., tachy-

cardia, excessive sweating, and goiter due to hyperthyroidism) abnormalities.
5. Specific signs (e.g., Kayser-Fleischer rings in the cornea in Wilson's disease) should be looked for in appropriate cases.

### Laboratory Studies

It is unnecessary and impractical to subject all patients with possible tardive dyskinesia to a large battery of laboratory investigations. There are, however, some pointers in the history and physical examination that would suggest a need for further workup. These include severe or rapidly progressive dyskinesia, a history suggestive of brain lesion, a family history positive for a movement disorder, presence of dementia, and signs of other neurologic, metabolic, or endocrine abnormalities.

The laboratory workup includes the following:

1. Complete blood count—to rule out polycythemia vera and other disorders
2. Serum electrolytes—to exclude abnormalities of sodium and calcium metabolism that may cause movement disorders
3. Liver-function tests—to rule out Wilson's disease and other causes of liver dysfunction
4. Thyroid-function tests—to check for possible hyperthyroidism
5. Serum copper and ceruloplasmin, and urinary copper and amino acids in cases of suspected Wilson's disease
6. Connective tissue disease screen—to assess for SLE and other vasculitides
7. CT or MRI scan of head—may show atrophy of caudate in Huntington's disease, basal ganglia calcification in Fahr's syndrome, or a mass lesion in brain tumor.

The diagnosis of tardive dyskinesia is a clinical—not a laboratory—diagnosis. When the clinician is not certain of the diagnosis, it is advisable to follow the patient closely instead of bringing the diagnostic process to a premature close.

# References

Adams RD, Victor M: Principles of Neurology. New York, McGraw-Hill, 1977
Ayd FJ: A survey of drug-induced extrapyramidal reactions. JAMA 175:1054–1060, 1961
Baldessarini RJ, Cole JO, Davis J, et al: Tardive Dyskinesia: A Task Force Report of the American Psychiatric Association. Washington, DC, American Psychiatric Association, 1980

Barnes TRE: Movement disorder associated with antipsychotic drugs: the tardive syndromes. Int Rev J Psychiatry (in press)

Barnes TRE, Braude WM: Persistent akathisia associated with early tardive dyskinesia. Postgrad Med J 60:51–53, 1984

Barnes TRE, Braude WM: Akathisia variants and tardive dyskinesia. Arch Gen Psychiatry 42:874–878, 1985

Barnes TRE, Kidger T: The concept of tardive dyskinesia. Trends in Neurosciences 2:135–136, 1979

Barnes TRE, Kidger T, Gore SM: Tardive dyskinesia: a 3-year follow-up study. Psychol Med 13:71–81, 1983

Barnes TRE, Halstead SM, Little P: Akathisia variants: prevalence and iron status in an inpatient population with chronic schizophrenia. Schizophr Res 3:79, 1990

Bleuler EP: Dementia Praecox or the Group of Schizophrenias. (Monograph series on schizophrenia, No. 1). Translated by Zinkin J. New York, International Universities Press, 1950

Bobruff A, Gardos G, Tarsy D, et al: Clonazepam and phenobarbital in tardive dyskinesia. Am J Psychiatry 138:189–193, 1981

Braude WM, Barnes TRE, Gore SM: Clinical characteristics of akathisia: a systematic investigation of acute psychiatric inpatient admissions. Br J Psychiatry 143:139–150, 1983

Burke RE, Kang UJ: Tardive dystonia: clinical aspects and treatment, in Facial Dyskinesias. Edited by Jankovic J, Tolosa E. New York, Raven, 1988, pp 199–210

Burke RE, Fahn S, Jankovic J, et al: Tardive dystonia: late onset and persistent dystonia caused by antipsychotic drugs. Neurology 32:1335–1346, 1982

Burke RE, Kang UJ, Jankovic J, et al: Tardive akathisia: an analysis of clinical features and response to open therapeutic trials. Movement Disorders 4:157–175, 1989

Casey DE, Denney D: Pharmacological characterization of tardive dyskinesia. Psychopharmacology 54:1–8, 1977

Casey DE, Hammerstad JP: Sodium valproate in tardive dyskinesia. J Clin Psychiatry 40:483–485, 1979

Chouinard G, Jones BD: Early onset of tardive dyskinesia: case report. Am J Psychiatry 136:1323–1324, 1979

Cohen DJ, Riddle MA, Leckman JF, et al: Tourette's syndrome, in Neuropsychiatric Movement Disorders. Edited by Jeste DV, Wyatt RJ. Washington, DC, American Psychiatric Press, 1984, pp 19–52

Crane GE: Persistent dyskinesia. Br J Psychiatry 122:395–405, 1973

Crane GE, Naranjo EK, Chase C: Motor disorders induced by neuroleptics: a proposed new classification. Arch Gen Psychiatry 24:179–184, 1971

Cummings JL: Psychosomatic aspects of movement disorders. Adv Psychosom Med 13:111–132, 1985

Cummings JL, Benson DF: Dementia: A Clinical Approach. Boston, MA, Butterworth, 1983

Defendorf AR: Clinical Psychiatry (abstracted and adapted from the 6th German edition of Kraepelin's Lehrbuch Der Psychiatrie). London, Macmillan, 1902

Delwaide PJ, Desseilles M: Spontaneous buccolinguofacial dyskinesia in the elderly. Acta Neurol Scand 56:256–262, 1977

Drake RE, Erlich J: Suicide attempts associated with akathisia. Am J Psychiatry 142:499–501, 1985

Duvoisin RC: Meige syndrome: relief on high dose anticholinergic therapy. Clinical Neuropharmacology 6:63–66, 1983

Eldridge R, Gottlieb R: The primary hereditary dystonia: genetic classifications of 768 families and revised estimate of gene frequency, autosomal recessive form, and selected bibliography. Advanced Neurol 14:457–474, 1976

Engelhardt DM, Polizos P, Waizer J: CNS consequences of psychotropic drug withdrawal in autistic children: a follow-up report. Psychopharmacol Bull 11:6–7, 1975

Fahn S: Torscon dystonia: clinical spectrum and treatment. Semin Neurol 2:316–323, 1982

Fahn S: High dosage anticholinergic therapy in dystonia. Neurology 33:1255–1261, 1983

Fann WE, Lake CR, Gerber CJ, et al: Cholinergic suppression of tardive dyskinesia. Psychopharmacologia (Berlin) 37:101–107, 1974

Farran-Ridge C: Some syndromes referrable to the basal ganglia occurring in dementia praecox and epidemic encephalitis. J Mental Science 72:513–523, 1926

Feinglass EJ, Arnett FC, Dorsch LA, et al: Neuropsychiatric manifestations of systemic lupus erythematosus: diagnosis, clinical spectrum, and relationship to other features of the disease. Medicine 55:323–339, 1976

Gardos G, Cole JO, Sniffin C: An evaluation of papaverine in tardive dyskinesia. J Clin Pharmacol 16:304–310, 1976

Gauthier, Smith PC, Prankerd TA: Polycythemia vera and chorea. Acta Neurol Scand 43:357–364, 1966

Gilbert GJ: Familial spasmodic torticollis. Neurology 27:11–13, 1977

Glazer WM, Morgenstern H, Niedzwiecki D, et al: Heterogeneity of tardive dyskinesia: a multivariate analysis. Br J Psychiatry 152:253–259, 1988

Goldstein NP, Evert MA, Randall RV, et al: Psychiatric aspects of Wilson's disease (hepatolenticular degeneration): results of psychometric tests during long term therapy. Am J Psychiatry 124:1155–1161, 1968

Greil W, Haag H, Rossnagl G, et al: Effect of anticholinergics on tardive dyskinesia: a controlled study. Br J Psychiatry 145:304–310, 1985

Gureje O: The significance of subtyping tardive dyskinesia: a study of prevalence and associated factors. Psychol Med 19:121–128, 1989.

Gusella JF, Wexler NS, Conneally PM, et al: A polymorphic DNA marker genetically linked to Huntington's disease. Nature 306:234–238, 1983

Haskovec L: Nouvelles remarques sur l'akathisia. Nouv Iconogr Salpetriere Clin Maladies Systeme Nerv 16:287–293, 1903

Hayden MR: Huntington's Chorea. New York, Springer-Verlag, 1981

Hershon HI, Kennedy PF, McGuire RJ: Persistence of extrapyramidal disorders and psychiatric relapse after withdrawal of long-term phenothiazine therapy. Br J Psychiatry 120:41–50, 1972

Husby G, De Rign I, Zabriskie JB, et al: Antineuronal antibody in Sydenham's chorea. Lancet 2:1208, 1977

Jankovic J, Ford J: Blepharospasm and orofacial-cervical dystonia: clinical and pharmacological findings in 100 patients. Ann Neurol 13:402–411, 1983

Jayne D, Lees AJ, Stern GM: Remission of spasmodic torticollis. J Neurol Neurosurg Psychiatry 47:1236–1237, 1984

Jeste DV, Wyatt RJ: Understanding and Treating Tardive Dyskinesia. New York, Guilford, 1982

Jeste DV, Karson CN, Wyatt RJ: Movement disorders and psychopathology, in Neuropsychiatric Movement Disorders. Edited by Jeste DV, Wyatt RJ. Washington, DC, American Psychiatric Press, 1984, pp 119–150

Jeste DV, Wisniewski AA, Wyatt RJ: Neuroleptic-associated tardive syndromes. Psychiatr Clin North Am 9:183–192, 1986

Jones M, Hunter R: Abnormal movements in patients with chronic psychiatric illness, in Psychotropic Drugs and Dysfunctions of the Basal Ganglia (Publication No. 1938). Edited by Crane GE, Gardner R Jr. Washington, DC, U.S. Public Health Service, 1969, pp 53–65

Kang UJ, Burke RE, Fahn S: Natural history and treatment of tardive dystonia. Movement Disorders 1:193–208, 1986

Keegan DL, Rajput AH: Drug-induced dystonia tarda: treatment with L-dopa. Diseases of the Nervous System 38:167–169, 1973

Kennedy PF, Hershon HI, McGuire RJ: Extrapyramidal disorders after prolonged phenothiazine therapy. Br J Psychiatry 118:509–518, 1971

Kidger T, Barnes TRE, Trauer T, et al: Sub-syndromes of tardive dyskinesia. Psychol Med 10:513–520, 1980

Klawans HL: The pharmacology of tardive dyskinesias. Am J Psychiatry 130:82–86, 1973

Klawans HL, Shenker DM, Weiner WJ: Observations on the dopaminergic nature of hyperthyroid chorea, in Huntington's Chorea. Edited by Barbeau A, Chase TN, Paulson GW. New York, Raven, 1981, pp 543–549

Kraepelin EP: Dementia Praecox and Paraphrenia. Translated by Barclay RM. Edited by Robertson GM. Edinburgh, E & S Livingstone, 1919

Lidsky TI, Weinhold PM, Levine FM: Implications of basal ganglionic dysfunction for schizophrenia. Biol Psychiatry 14:3–12, 1979

MacKay AVP: Clinical controversies in tardive dyskinesia, in Neurology 2: Movement Disorders. Edited by Marsden CD, Fahn S. London, Butterworth Scientific, 1981, pp 249–262

Manschrek TC, Maher BA, Rucklos ME, et al: Disturbed voluntary motor activity in schizophrenic disorder. Psychol Med 12:73–84, 1982

Marsden CD: Blepharospasm-oromandibular dystonia syndrome (Breughel's syndrome). J Neurol Neurosurg Psychiatry 39:1204–1209, 1976

Marsden CD, Tarsy D, Baldessarini RJ: Spontaneous and drug-induced movement disorders in psychotic patients, in Psychiatric Aspects of Neurological Disease. Edited by Benson DF, Blumer D. New York, Grune & Stratton, 1975

McAndrew JB, Case Q, Treffert DA: Effects of prolonged phenothiazine intake on psychotic and other hospitalized children. J Autism Childhood Schizophrenia 2:75–91, 1972

Mettler FA, Crandell A: Neurologic disorders in psychiatric institutions. J Nerv Ment Dis 128:148–159, 1959

Mizrahi EM, Holtzman D, Tharp B: Haloperidol-induced tardive dyskinesia in a child with Gilles de la Tourette's disease. Arch Neurol 37:780–783, 1980

Nadeau SE, Watson RT: Neurologic manifestations of vasculitis and collagen vascular syndromes, in Clinical Neurology, Vol 4. Edited by Baker AB, Baker LH. New York, Harper & Row, 1983, pp 1–133

. National Institutes of Health: NIH Consensus Conference on the Clinical Use of Botulinin Toxin. Washington, DC, U.S. Government Printing Office, 1990

Nausieda PA, Crossman BJ, Koller WC, et al: Sydenham chorea: an update. Neurology 30:331–334, 1980

Ortiz A: Neuropharmacological profile of Meige's disease: overview and a case report. Clinical Neuropharmacology 6:297–304, 1983

Owens DGC: Involuntary disorders of movement in chronic schizophrenia—the role of the illness and its treatment, in Dyskinesia: Research and Treatment. Edited by Casey DE, Chase TN, Christensen AV, et al. Berlin, Springer-Verlag, 1985, pp 79–87

Owens DGC, Johnstone EC, Frith CD: Spontaneous involuntary disorders of movement: their prevalence, severity and distribution in chronic schizophrenics with and without treatment with neuroleptics. Arch Gen Psychiatry 39:452–461, 1982

Polizos P, Engelhardt DM, Hoffman SP, et al: Neurological consequences of psychotropic drug withdrawal in schizophrenic children. J Autism Childhood Schizophrenia 3:247–253, 1973

Rifkin A, Quitkin F, Kane J, et al: Are prophylactic antiparkinsonian drugs necessary: a controlled study of procyclidine withdrawal. Arch Gen Psychiatry 35:483–489, 1978

Robertson MM: The Gilles de la Tourette syndrome: the current status. Br J Psychiatry 154:147–169, 1989

Saltz BL, Woerner MG, Kane JM, et al: Prospective study of tardive dyskinesia incidence in the elderly. JAMA 266:2402–2406, 1991

Scheinberg IH, Sternlieb I: Wilson's Disease. Philadelphia, PA, WB Saunders, 1984

Schooler NR, Kane JM: Research diagnoses for tardive dyskinesia. Arch Gen Psychiatry 39:486–487, 1982

Schwartzman J: Chorea minor: review of 175 cases with reference to etiology, treatment and sequelae. Rheumatism 6:89–95, 1950

Segal DS, Janowsky DS: Psychostimulant-induced behavioral effect: possible models of schizophrenia, in Psychopharmacology: A Generation of Progress. Edited by Lipton MA, DiMascio A, Killam KF. New York, Raven, 1978, pp 1113–1123

Shapiro AK, Shapiro E, Bruun RD, et al: Gilles de la Tourette's Syndrome. New York, Raven, 1978

Simpson GM, Voitashevsky A, Young MA, et al: Deanol in the treatment of tardive dyskinesia. Psychopharmacology 52:257–261, 1977

Snyder SH: Amphetamine psychosis: a "model" schizophrenia mediated by catecholamines. Am J Psychiatry 130:61–67, 1973

Steck H: Le syndrome extrapyramidal et diencephalique au cours des traitments au largactil et au serpasil. Annales Medico Psychologigues 112:734–743, 1954

Thiebaut F: Sydenham's chorea, in Handbook of Clinical Neurology, Vol 6. Edited by Vinken PJ, Bruyn GW. Amsterdam, North-Holland, 1968, pp 409–434

Van Putten T: Why do schizophrenic patients refuse to take their drugs? Arch Gen Psychiatry 31:67–72, 1974

Waddington JL, Youssef HA, Dolphin C, et al: Cognitive dysfunction, negative symptoms and tardive dyskinesia in schizophrenia: their association in relation to topography of involuntary movements and criterion of their abnormality. Arch Gen Psychiatry 44:907–912, 1987

Weiner WJ, Luby ED: Persistent akathisia following neuroleptic withdrawal. Ann Neurol 13:466–467, 1983

Weiner WJ, Nausieda PA, Glantz RH: Meige syndrome (blepharospasm-oromandibular dystonia) after long term neuroleptic therapy. Neurology 31:1155–1156, 1981

Weinhold P, Wesner J, Kane JM: Familial occurrence of tardive dyskinesia: a case report. J Clin Psychiatry 42:165–166, 1981

Wexler N: Huntington's disease, in Neuropsychiatric Movement Disorders. Edited by Jeste DV, Wyatt RJ. Washington, DC, American Psychiatric Press, 1984, pp 53–65

Winsberg BG, Hurwic MJ, Perel J: Neurochemistry of withdrawal emergent symptoms in children. Psychopharmacol Bull 13:38–40, 1977

Yarden PE, Discipio WJ: Abnormal movements and prognosis in schizophrenia. Am J Psychiatry 128:317–323, 1971

Chapter 3

# Assessment of Tardive Dyskinesia

## Problems in Assessment

### The Tardive Dyskinesia Syndrome

There are several features peculiar to tardive dyskinesia that make accurate assessment a particular problem. One major problem is that the apparently mundane issue of what constitutes tardive dyskinesia remains unresolved. Without specific operational criteria for a diagnosis, prevalence figures have limited value and the results of studies on the course and prognosis of the syndrome are difficult to interpret. The lack of consistent criteria partly accounts for the wide variation in prevalence reported.

The core sign of tardive dyskinesia is orofacial dyskinesia, or the buccolinguomasticatory triad (Delwaide and Desseilles 1977; Faurbye et al. 1964; Sigwald et al. 1959), the most familiar and prevalent feature of the condition. It consists of involuntary movements of the tongue, face, or jaws; for example, protrusion or twisting of the tongue may be combined with lip smacking, cheek puffing, pursing and sucking actions of the lips, or chewing and lateral jaw motions. Involvement of the periorbital muscles, sometimes resembling blepharospasm, is also seen (Baldessarini et al. 1980; Barnes and Kidger 1979; Marsden et al. 1975). Clinical folklore suggests that fine vermicular (wormlike) movements of the tongue represent an early sign of tardive dyskinesia (Fann 1980; Jeste and Wyatt 1980), although no convincing evidence to support this notion has ever been presented. The particular combinations of movement seen vary considerably among patients but tend to be relatively consistent for an individual.

In addition to these orofacial phenomena, most descriptions of tardive dyskinesia include a variety of trunk and limb movements. The involuntary limb movements are purposeless and usually labeled as choreiform or choreoathetoid. Athetosis of the extremities and axial and limb dystonia are often listed as part of the syndrome, as are abnormalities of gait and trunk posture, such as lordosis, rocking and swaying, shoulder shrugging, and rotary movements of the pelvis (American College of Neuropsychopharmacology 1973; Marsden et al. 1975; Paulson 1975). Grunting and respiratory arrhythmias are also seen.

Although orofacial dyskinesia can be considered as a clinically discrete entity, this is not the case for abnormal involuntary trunk and limb movements. This may be partly explained by the difficulty in differentiating between the choreiform or choreoathetoid dyskinesia considered characteristic of tardive dyskinesia and the variety of other trunk and limb movements, due to other causes, seen in chronic psychiatric patients. For such movements, simple, quantitative measures of frequency, amplitude, or duration of movement may be inadequate, as they fail to discriminate between tardive dyskinesia of the trunk and limbs and other classes of abnormal movement that may be present.

### Additional Diagnostic Criteria

The evidence for a causal role of antipsychotic drugs in the genesis of tardive dyskinesia is overwhelming. Schooler and Kane (1982) suggested that the diagnosis of tardive dyskinesia should not be made in the absence of a minimum of three months of total cumulative administration of antipsychotic drugs. If the patient has been receiving drug treatment for less than this time, the diagnosis should be qualified as "less than three months' neuroleptic exposure." Nevertheless, accepting that many or all of the abnormal movements described as part of the condition can be drug-induced does not, in itself, establish the syndrome as a distinct nosological entity. Additional defining characteristics that have been suggested include the following. First, the movements are exacerbated or may be provoked by reduction or withdrawal of the antipsychotic drug. Also, increasing the drug dose will transiently suppress the movements (Baldessarini 1979). Second, the movements are unresponsive to anticholinergic drugs and may even be exacerbated by such medication (Gardos and Cole 1983). Third, the movements are sometimes aggravated with emotional stress. Lastly, the movements are reduced or disappear during sleep (Marsden et al. 1975). Such features have not been systematically validated for all of the types of movements described as part of the syndrome and are rarely employed as diagnostic criteria.

### Differential Diagnosis

In addition to the tardive dyskinesia syndrome, psychiatric patients receiving antipsychotic medication may manifest a range of abnormal, involuntary movements that can confound and confuse assessment. The potential causes of disordered movement in such patients that may lead to diagnostic confusion are discussed in Chapter 2.

If an attempt is made to classify the trunk and limb movements observed according to their nature, then a variety of movements—including choreiform movements, tardive dystonia, tardive akathisia, stereotypies, and mannerisms—can be identified (Barnes et al. 1983b). However, current rating methods do not allow for reliable discrimination between these phenomena. Indeed, although the basic conceptual distinctions between normal and abnormal, purposeful and purposeless, and drug-induced and schizophrenia-related movements are clear, clinically these categories of movement can be extremely difficult to distinguish.

### Intrapatient Variation

The spontaneous intrapatient variability in the site and severity of dyskinesia poses a problem for the interpretation of ratings based on observation of a patient for a short time (Barnes and Kidger 1979; Richardson et al. 1982). Such variability can influence the point prevalence figures in surveys of tardive dyskinesia in that false negative ratings may occur. Also, in a treatment study, spontaneous changes in the movements may be falsely attributed to a response to the therapy under test.

**Arousal.** Fluctuation in severity may be observed in association with change in the level of physiological arousal, posture, and mobility (Gardos and Cole 1980). Anxiety or volitional motor activity usually aggravates the dyskinesia, whereas attempts to voluntarily suppress the movements will commonly result in increased movement, particularly in those muscle groups that are not the focus of the patient's attention. The movements tend to improve with relaxation or sedation, and they disappear during sleep (Baldessarini and Tarsy 1978; Crane 1973).

**Temporal fluctuation.** Once tardive dyskinesia has developed, it does not seem to be a generally progressive condition. Rather than showing a steady increase in severity, the condition tends to follow a fluctuating course with spontaneous remissions (Barnes et al. 1983a; Casey 1985; Gardos and Cole 1980). Patients may show apparently spontaneous variation in the severity of movements from day to day or even within hours or minutes. Richardson et al. (1982) found these temporal variations to be of such magnitude that they could contribute to the likelihood of false negative assessments of tardive dyskinesia, particularly if short assessment periods of 1 minute or less were used.

### Change in Response to Medication

**Antipsychotic drugs.** A major source of variation in tardive dyskinesia is change in drug treatment. Change in the dosage or class of antipsychotic drug treatment can also influence the severity of the movements. An increase in plasma drug levels will tend to suppress the dyskinesia, whereas a reduction may exacerbate the problem. Even relatively subtle drug plasma level changes can affect the severity of movements, in patients on either oral (Gardos and Cole 1980) or depot (Barnes and Wiles 1983) preparations.

**Anticholinergics.** The administration, withdrawal, or change in dose of concomitant anticholinergic medication will influence tardive dyskinesia. It is a commonplace clinical observation that the administration of anticholinergic agents will aggravate the dyskinesia, whereas their discontinuation will invariably improve the condition; this observation is supported by experimental and clinical evidence (Greil et al. 1984; Kane and Smith 1982; Klawans and Rubovits 1974).

# Rating Methods

The various methods used to assess tardive dyskinesia can be loosely divided into those involving instrumentation (e.g., electromyography or ultrasound), frequency counts of movements, multi-item rating scales, and videotape.

## Instrumentation

One strategy adopted to overcome the problems involved in the quantitative assessment of tardive dyskinesia has been to develop objective, automated measurement techniques. The instrumental methods used for the quantitative assessment of neurological function in psychiatric patients have been reviewed by Gardos et al. (1977), Simpson (1982), May et al. (1983), and Simpson and Singh (1988).

**Vocal assessment.** Fann et al. (1977) assessed vocal function as a measure of dyskinesia, on the premise that articulation would be disturbed by the neuromuscular disorder. For example, they hypothesized that one consequence of orofacial dyskinesia would be an increase in the nasal component of speech. This was measured using a Tonar-II system, involving a sound separation microphone assembly, which could isolate the oral and nasal components of speech and present signal and frequency data for both. Nasality represented the ratio of the nasal signal to the sum of the nasal and oral signals.

**Electromyography.** Electromyographic procedures involve the recording of activity from electrodes placed over selected muscles. Studies have recorded movements from a variety of body sites, including the buccolingual region (Jus et al. 1973) and the fingers (Alpert et al. 1976; Gardos and Cole 1980; Young et al. 1975).

**Accelerometers.** Accelerometers have been employed for recording movements, particularly tremor of the limbs and face (Falek and Glanville 1962; Young et al. 1975). One of the main disadvantages of such a method is that only a limited number of body sites can be measured.

Fann et al. (1977) used triaxial vector accelerometry to provide a graphic display of the motion characteristics of a particular body site. The researchers standardized the system on normal subjects. To monitor drug-induced movement disorder, particularly parkinsonism and dyskinesia, miniature accelerometers are attached to such areas as the wrist, ankles, and chin. The system provided data on the total change of velocity and acceleration in the body parts over time.

Tryon and Pologe (1987) also used accelerometric recordings for detection of limb movement. They compared drug-treated schizophrenic patients with and without tardive dyskinesia, and obtained measures associated with resting the hand, posturing the arm, and moving the arm. Their findings included a greater amplitude of dyskinesia and a lower peak frequency in the various postures in the dyskinetic group.

**Ultrasound.** Systems using ultrasound to record movements have been employed in patients with affective disorder (Haines and Sainsbury 1972) and Huntington's disease (Leonard et al. 1974). A compact apparatus to record ocular movements, comprising a transducer attached to a pair of spectacles, was adapted to measure orofacial tardive dyskinesia (Resek et al. 1981). The transducer emits and detects ultrasound waves. Facial movements disturb the pattern of reflected waves, and their frequency is recorded on a digital counter. High test-retest reliability was demonstrated for the system, and concurrent validity was confirmed by comparing the ultrasound scores with time-sampled scores based on simultaneous videotape recordings.

Similarly, May et al. (1983) utilized an ultrasound system to provide activity counts for orofacial movement in patients with tardive dyskinesia. These investigators concluded that the orofacial counter was simple, easy to operate, and suitable for brief screening examinations and routine clinical monitoring. McClelland et al. (1987) also evaluated an ultrasound detector for the assessment of orofacial dyskinesia. The system was able to distinguish between normal volunteers and chronic psychotic inpatients with Abnormal Involuntary Movement Scale (AIMS) scores of at least 2 on an orofacial item. The concurrent validity of the system was demonstrated by the finding of significant correlations between the ultrasound scores and clinical AIMS ratings; however, these authors mentioned that some patients found the mechanical device difficult to tolerate, being unable to cooperate for more than 30 seconds.

Buruma et al. (1982) developed a method based on the principle of Doppler radar. Involuntary movements in patients with Huntington's disease and tardive dyskinesia were measured over the whole body. Patients were seated in a beam of electromagnetic waves. Reflected waves caused by body movements caused Doppler frequency shift, which a receiver and transducer converted into a parameter that the authors considered proportional to the number of movements, their amplitude, and the size of the involved body parts. In the patients with tardive dyskinesia, the Doppler radar scores showed good correlation with ratings of orofacial dyskinesia derived from videotape recordings of patients made simultaneously with the Doppler radar.

**Electromechanical instruments.** Denney and Casey (1975) developed a device for measuring oral movements that involved a piezoelectric transducer with a rubber bulb inserted in the mouth. Chien et al. (1977, 1980) used this system to provide a direct count of orofacial movements, which was compared with five clinical rating scales, including the AIMS. There was a problem with the acceptability of the apparatus, with only 9 of 15 patients holding the rubber bulb in the mouth long enough to complete the recording. For these 9 patients, for whom both piezoelectric data and clinical ratings were available, there were statistically significant correlations with four of the five scales.

Wirshing and Cummings (1988) referred to a battery of prototype electromechanical instruments that had been developed to measure and analyze the movements of tardive dyskinesia (May et al. 1983). Comparing 50 patients with no evidence of movement disorder other than tardive dyskinesia and 70 neurologically normal control subjects, the battery revealed differences between the two groups, such as a marked increase in orofacial movements during distracting tasks, and a greater variability in all movements in the dyskinetic group. One-third of the patients with tardive dyskinesia also showed an increase in the energy in the 3–5 Hz frequency band of measured hand movements, which the researchers interpreted as a manifestation of combined tardive dyskinesia and subclinical parkinsonian tremor.

This group of investigators (Bartzokis et al. 1989a, 1989b) also assessed a group of patients with tardive dyskinesia using ultrasound detectors to count facial and whole body movements, electromechanical frequency measures, and clinical ratings from videotaped AIMS examinations. Comparing these three measures, they found statistically significant correlations between orofacial ultrasound measures and the AIMS ratings; however, the clinical ratings did not show a significant correlation with the frequency measures. The investigators concluded that the electromechanical frequency measures revealed information not available from the clinical rating scale scores.

In summary, many of these automated techniques have shown acceptable levels of concordance with clinical assessments. Clinical utility has not been demonstrated for any of these techniques, however, and none has achieved widespread use. Nevertheless, the possibility remains that with further development such methods may be able to provide a more objective, quantitative assessment of tardive dyskinesia (Caligiuri et al. 1991; Wirsching and Cummings 1988; Wirsching et al. 1991).

### Frequency Counts

Frequency counts of abnormal movements might seem attractive as a method of rating, yielding an ostensibly precise and objective score—that is, the number of movements occurring within a certain observation time. To count the frequency of all body movements over a reasonable period, however, is likely to be immensely time consuming and is probably only possible from a videotape. In practice, investigators who have chosen this method have usually selected for assessment one specific movement that was prominent, clearly defined, and readily countable (Branchey et al. 1979; Richardson et al. 1982). Such a strategy limits the value of frequency counts for comparing the severity of the condition between patients. For example, comparison of a frequency count of tongue protrusion in one patient is not directly comparable with the count for choreiform, "piano-playing" movements of the fingers in another.

Further, the particular movements counted may bear little relationship to the overall severity of the condition in terms of the number of body sites affected and the magnitude and disabling nature of the abnormal movements present. Richardson et al. (1982) failed to find a significant correlation between the frequency count and total scores on the Simpson Abbreviated Dyskinesia Rating Scale (Simpson et al. 1979). The clinical relevance and validity of frequency counts for the assessment of tardive dyskinesia remain in doubt.

### Multi-Item Scales

**Advantages.**   Multi-item scales (see Table 3-1) have proved the most popular form of rating instrument in clinical research. Their main advantage is that a more comprehensive rating of the abnormal involuntary movements at the various body sites is generated than would be provided by frequency counts or simple global ratings. Many incorporate a standard procedure for examination of the patient, so the assessment is standardized to some degree. Thus data from different studies and centers can be considered relatively comparable. Gardos and Cole (1977) noted that the data generated by such scales are generally ordinal or interval in nature, suitable for manipulation by standard statistical techniques, including factor analysis.

**Table 3–1.**  Multi-item scales for tardive dyskinesia

| Scale | References |
|---|---|
| Crane Rating Scale | Crane et al. (1969) |
| | Heinrich et al. (1968) |
| | Hippius and Logemann (1970) |
| | Kennedy et al. (1971) |
| | Hershon et al. (1972) |
| Kazamatsuri Rating Scale | Kazamatsuri et al. (1972) |
| | Huang (1984) |
| St. Paul-Ramsey Hospital Scale | Reda et al. (1974) |
| | Escobar and Kemp (1975) |
| Withdrawal Emergent Symptom Checklist | Engelhardt (1974) |
| | Gualtieri et al. (1982) |
| Abnormal Involuntary Movements Scale (AIMS) | Guy (1976) |
| Smith Tardive Dyskinesia Scale | Smith et al. (1977) |
| | Tamminga et al. (1977) |
| Simpson Tardive Dyskinesia Rating Scale | Simpson et al. (1979) |
| Abbreviated (Simpson) Dyskinesia Rating Scale | Simpson and Singh (1988) |
| Gerlach/Sct. Hans Rating Scale for Extrapyramidal Syndromes | Gerlach (1979) |
| | Gerlach and Korsgaard (1983) |
| | Malt et al. (1990) |
| Tardive Dyskinesia Videotape Rating Technique | Barnes and Trauer (1982) |
| | Firth and Ardern (1985) |
| Dyskinesia Identification System— Coldwater (DIS-Co) | Sprague et al. (1984a, 1984b) |
| | Kalachnik et al. (1988) |
| Dyskinesia Identification System: Condensed User Scale | Sprague et al. (1989) |
| Scale for Abnormal Hyperkinetic Movements | Fleischhauer et al. (1985) |
| Sonoma Involuntary Movement | Stone et al. (1989) |

Early detection and systematic monitoring of tardive dyskinesia have been widely recommended, on the premise that reduction or discontinuation of antipsychotic medication early in the course of the condition may improve the prognosis (Baldessarini et al. 1980). Rating scales seem particularly suitable for screening populations for tardive dyskinesia (Ahrens et al. 1988; Munetz and Schulz 1986) in that they are relatively inexpensive and unobtrusive, take only a short time to administer, and may be applied to almost all patients.

**Disadvantages.** The multi-item, checklist scales already available, such as the AIMS, were originally research tools developed to quantify the severity of movements rather than to act as diagnostic instruments. Although they were not designed as diagnostic instruments, they usefully document the motor phenomena present and their level of severity, thereby contributing to the diagnostic process.

For these scales to function as diagnostic instruments, threshold scores must be employed. These are essentially arbitrary and refer to the severity rating and number of body sites displaying abnormal movements. The relevant questions are rarely addressed explicitly and include the following. First, how obvious or frequent must an orofacial movement be to be judged abnormal? Second, is the occurrence of dyskinesia limited to a single body site sufficient for a diagnosis of tardive dyskinesia? Most patients, and many normal, drug-free individuals, will manifest one or two ratable movements while under observation, but occasional tongue protrusion or puckering of the lips does not warrant a diagnosis of tardive dyskinesia.

The severity of an abnormal involuntary movement may be judged in terms of the quality, frequency, duration, and magnitude or amplitude of the movement or even the degree of disability associated (Barnes and Trauer 1982; Lane et al. 1985). Most of these rating scales, however, do not provide any criteria for severity. As Barnes and Trauer (1982) and Bergen et al. (1984) pointed out, the rater arrives at a global judgment of severity based on the character, amplitude, and frequency of the movement. Schooler and Kane (1982) suggested that to warrant a diagnosis of tardive dyskinesia, the abnormal, involuntary movements should be of at least "moderate" severity in one or more body areas, or of at least "mild" severity at two or more body sites. The question of what constituted mild or moderate severity was not answered other than by the recommendation that standardized rating scales, such as the AIMS, should be used to ascertain the presence of movements. These authors also asserted that "the diagnosis [of tardive dyskinesia] reported in the literature frequently represents little more than a score on a rating scale" (Schooler and Kane 1982, p. 486).

In treatment trials with patients ostensibly suffering from tardive dyskinesia of the trunk and limbs, the diagnostic criteria used are rarely declared except in terms of the rather ambiguous and limited definitions of the AIMS or similar scales. In research, the use of such scales as diagnostic instruments, with relatively arbitrary cutoff scores, can yield a sample of patients all qualifying for a diagnosis of tardive dyskinesia, but markedly heterogeneous with regard to type and distribution of movements. This is a critical issue if the research suggesting that there are regional subtypes of tardive dyskinesia is correct—that is, that orofacial and trunk and limb dyskinesias are subsyndromes that may be pathophysiologically distinct with different prognostic and etiologic determinants (Barnes et al. 1990; Glazer et al. 1988; Gureje 1989; Kidger et al. 1980). (See Chapter 2.)

The tongue-protrusion test is included in some of these scales. Marsden and Schacter (1981), in a review of assessment techniques for extrapyramidal disorders, considered that the duration of tongue extension was easily measured and widely applicable. On the basis of their own observations, however, Gardos and Cole (1980) expressed doubts about its correlation with orofacial movements and felt that the clinical value was limited. One major disadvantage of such a maneuver, as well as provocation tests with their necessary close inspection of the subject, is that the patient under scrutiny becomes aware of the specific interest in his or her movements and this may influence his or her presentation in repeat assessments.

Assessment using such scales involves some degree of social interaction between examiner and patient, which may be a confounding variable, influencing the signs and symptoms present. An unfamiliar examiner may provoke anxiety and apprehension in a patient, leading to an increase in dyskinesia, whereas a familiar examiner may invite conversation and thus complicate the assessment of mouth movements (Barnes and Trauer 1982).

**Reliability.** Gardos and Cole (1980) considered multi-item scales to be the most satisfactory of the rating methods. Reliability was summarized as variable, but satisfactory levels of interrater reliability have been demonstrated for several of the more widely used scales such as the AIMS (Chien et al. 1977; Lane et al. 1985; Smith et al. 1979a, 1979b; Whall et al. 1983), the Simpson Tardive Dyskinesia Rating Scale (Simpson et al. 1979), and the Sct. Hans scale (Gerlach and Korsgaard 1983; Malt et al. 1990). When Bergen et al. (1984) used the AIMS in an attempt to quantify the spontaneous fluctuations in tardive dyskinesia in a small group of patients, they found that within-rater variability dominated intrapatient variability. They pointed out that to assess the change in tardive dyskinesia genuinely attributable to a therapeutic intervention or the passage of time, there would need to be knowledge of the intrarater and intrapatient variability in the condition.

**Validity.** Gardos et al. (1977) defined validity as "the extent to which the instrument succeeds in measuring what it intends to measure" (p. 1210). They further defined face validity, concurrent validity, and construct validity with reference to rating scales for tardive dyskinesia. Examining first concurrent validity, this is the degree to which the assessment of tardive dyskinesia, using the scale, correlates with an established criterion measure. Gardos et al. (1977) pointed out that as no established criterion for the condition exists, concurrent validity is virtually impossible to demonstrate. The next best approach is to demonstrate that the rating method under scrutiny correlates with other measures of tardive dyskinesia, such as another, perhaps more established rating scale or the assessment of experienced clinicians, rating the same patients at the same time (Barnes and Trauer 1982). This consensual validity relies on rather circular reasoning, however.

Construct validity, in this context, refers to correlation between the measure of tardive dyskinesia and "the hypothetical constructs that have been generated to account for the nature and pathogenesis of the dyskinesias" (Gardos et al. 1977, p. 1210). Such theoretical constructs might include increased severity of tardive dyskinesia with reduction or withdrawal of antipsychotic drug dose, but stability of the condition over time if drug regimen is unchanged; an increase in severity with the addition of anticholinergic medication and a reduction if the anticholinergic drug is reduced or stopped; and an increase in severity and prevalence with age. In only a few cases has validation against such criteria been attempted.

More recent reviews of rating scales for tardive dyskinesia have not pursued the issue of validity much further (Simpson and Singh 1988; Sprague et al. 1984a, 1984b). Sprague et al. (1984a, 1984b) were critical of the lack of attention to the psychometric properties, such as interrater reliability, test-retest reliability, norms for a population, and the proportion of a population that can be assessed using the scale.

**Abnormal Involuntary Movements Scale.** The AIMS is discussed as a specific example of a widely used instrument, but it in no way implies superiority over other rating scales (see Appendix).

Smith et al. (1979a) wrote that none of the rating scales for tardive dyskinesia currently available had been "widely accepted as a reliable, valid and sensitive measure of this disorder" (p. 918). Since that time, the AIMS (Guy 1976), a 12-item scale, has become the most popular instrument for rating tardive dyskinesia, judging by the relative frequency of use in clinical research. In their early prevalence studies using this scale, Smith et al. (1979a, 1979b) found satisfactory interrater and test-retest reliability using the Pearson $r$ correlation coefficient. They concluded, however, that consistent bias may occur even with trained raters. Thus they cautioned against using AIMS raters interchangeably in longitudinal assessments. Lane et al. (1985) examined interrater reliability in 33 patients with tardive dyskinesia, using two experienced psychiatrists familiar with the AIMS and two residents with little previous exposure to patients with tardive dyskinesia. Interrater reliability was calculated using both the Pearson $r$ and the intraclass correlation coefficient recommended by Bartko and Carpenter (1976), on the suspicion that the former statistic provided an overestimate of the level of agreement. The correlations obtained by the two methods were very similar, and both showed high levels of agreement. The authors attributed these results, at least in part, to the conventions that had developed for scoring the AIMS. These put forward criteria for rating severity on the dimensions of quality, frequency, and amplitude and included guidelines for distinguishing between jaw and lip movement. The data revealed that the experienced raters obtained higher levels of agreement than the residents, and their scores were more consistent over time.

The AIMS scale ratings are based on a standard examination procedure (see Appendix) that the previous report on tardive dyskinesia by the American Psychiatric Association (Baldessarini et al. 1980) considered could be reliably employed in the routine clinical evaluation of the condition. Clinicians of various disciplines may be easily trained to conduct and score the AIMS examination, which in routine clinical practice can be completed within 5–10 minutes (Germer et al. 1984; Munetz and Schulz 1986).

In addition to the new scoring conventions and rating criteria proposed by Lane et al. (1985) and briefly mentioned above, Munetz and Benjamin (1988) also presented a revised and extended version of the guidelines for conducting the AIMS examination, based on their clinical experience with the scale. Some of the rating criteria proposed by Lane et al. (1985) were incorporated, but the two sets of scoring conventions differ in other respects. For example, Munetz and Benjamin (1988) suggested that all hyperkinetic movements are rated regardless of presumed etiology, so the dyskinesia of Huntington's disease and Tourette's syndrome would be rated, whereas Lane et al. (1985) stated that only movements of tardive dyskinesia should be rated and specified that movements due to Huntington's disease, tics, and tremors are excluded. Further, the original AIMS examination incorporated simple provocation tests, such as asking the patient to tap the tip of each finger in turn with the thumb. Any resultant "activated" movements that are observed are arbitrarily scored one point less than those occurring spontaneously. Scores for both types of movement are added together for each body-site rating. Potentially useful information is thus irretrievably buried within the total score (Barnes and Trauer 1982). Munetz and Benjamin (1988) proposed that a point is not subtracted from the score for movements seen only on activation. Their instruction is that the score should be determined "by considering the composite amplitude and frequency of movements that are qualitatively consistent with tardive dyskinesia" (p. 1176). Lane et al. (1985) also suggested that movements occurring on activation are scored the same as spontaneous movements, except in the upper limbs, where finger movements occurring "in the passive hand in parallel with elicitation are scored one [point] lower than finger movements not in parallel with elicitation" (p. 355). Addressing this same issue, the Sct. Hans scale distinguishes between hyperkinesia in the passive phase, when patients are sitting and relaxed, and movements observed in the active phase, when patients are speaking or performing motor tasks, such as writing or walking. The passive and active movement scores are added together for each of the body sites, and the mean score is calculated.

### Videotape Assessment

**Advantages.** Videotape recordings of patients would seem to have several practical advantages. First, videotapes can be stored for reassessment at any time. Second, if serial videotapes from a study are presented to a rater in random order, they allow blind ratings to be made. Third, close and prolonged observation is less intrusive than it would be with one or more clinical observers and less revealing of the true purpose of assessment. If patients are aware that their movements are the focus of attention, they might deliberately or involuntarily suppress or control their movements. Fourth, subtle abnormal movements may be more easily seen by an undistracted rater when viewing close-ups on a monitor screen than during clinical examination. Asnis et al. (1977) considered videotape recordings to be invaluable in increasing diagnostic sensitivity for tardive dyskinesia, particularly with regard to the detection of early signs of the condition. Fifth, all patients included in a study can be recorded in a standard fashion, engaged in the same activity (Barnes and Trauer 1982; Fann et al. 1977). For example, Fann et al. (1977) used a standard procedure for videotaping patients, following the order of the AIMS examination. Lastly, tapes may be used to train raters and establish interrater reliability for a rating instrument, at least with regard to observable phenomena (Gardos and Cole 1980; Marsden and Schacter 1981). For example, to help train the raters for their surveys of tardive dyskinesia in schizophrenic inpatients and outpatients, Smith et al. (1979a, 1979b) used standard tapes of AIMS examinations supplied by the Psychopharmacology Research Branch of the National Institute of Mental Health.

The Sct. Hans Rating Scale for Extrapyramidal Syndromes (see Table 3–1) was designed to be used for repeated evaluation, using videotape recordings. A standard video examination procedure is recommended, and the examination and recording take only 5–7 minutes (Gerlach and Korsgaard 1983). The scale covers parkinsonism, dystonia, and akathisia, as well as tardive dyskinesia. When rating from a videotape there is a problem rating parkinsonian features, such as rigidity and salivation, and the presence of these must be indicated by the examiner during the recording. This scale and the videotape recording procedure have been successfully employed in a clinical multicenter study (Nordic Dyskinesia Study Group 1986).

Similarly, the Tardive Dyskinesia Videotape Rating Scale (see Table 3-1) was designed for use with a standard videotape procedure (Barnes and Kidger 1979; Kidger et al. 1980). Interrater and test-retest reliability data for this scale are satisfactory (Barnes and Trauer 1982).

**Disadvantages.** First, patients may consciously limit their abnormal movements under the scrutiny of the camera. Second, the assessment is restricted by the quality of the recording and the length of the recording, with subtle, fine movements only ratable in body sites selected for close-up. Lastly, the necessary recording equipment can be relatively expensive.

### Comparison of Clinical and Videotape Assessment

Firth and Ardern (1985) compared the Tardive Dyskinesia Videotape Rating Scale (Barnes and Trauer 1982) with the Simpson Abbreviated Dyskinesia Rating Scale (ADRS; Simpson et al. 1979) in 10 chronic schizophrenic patients. The patients were rated on the ADRS and then videotaped according to the recommended procedure. Six months later, the videotapes were rated using the ADRS, by two raters, one of whom had originally made the clinical ratings.

Agreement was calculated between the clinical ratings and the videotape ratings using 10 of the 17 items of the ADRS. Seven items were excluded as being irrelevant to tardive dyskinesia (e.g., the restless movements of akathisia) are impossible to see on a videotape (e.g., intraoral tongue movements). The agreement coefficient was calculated using the method of Ciccheti (1976). Excluding items rated as "uncertain," the coefficients of agreement between the clinical rating and the two videotape ratings were .79 and .82, the latter figure referring to the clinical and videotape ratings by the same rater 6 months apart. The coefficient for the two videotape ratings was .77.

The mean total score for the clinical rating using the 10-item ADRS was slightly higher than either of the videotape scores, but not significantly so. Firth and Ardern (1985) concluded that there was "good, but not complete, agreement between clinical and videoraters for both specific and total scores," but the videorating tended to identify fewer movements (p. 725).

McCreadie et al. (1987) compared the same videotape rating assessment with the AIMS in 10 inpatients with chronic schizophrenia. As assessed by the AIMS, all patients had orofacial dyskinesia and 5 had distal dyskinesia, whereas the video ratings found only 6 patients with orofacial and 4 patients with distal dyskinesia. McCreadie et al. (1987) concluded that videotape assessment may be less sensitive in mild and moderate cases.

Fisk and York (1987) also employed the videotape assessment in a 6-week, double-blind trial of sodium valproate. In addition, each patient was rated "live" using the videotape assessment scale. The videotapes were used to provide two further blind ratings of tardive dyskinesia by "experienced independent raters." Concordance between the clinical and videotape ratings for tardive dyskinesia was significant (Kendall coefficient of concordance: $P < .005$). The authors considered that these results supported the reliability of the Tardive Dyskinesia Videotape Rating Scale.

## Assessment of Tardive Dyskinesia in Different Patient Populations

### Schizophrenia

Schizophrenia can be regarded as a psychomotor disorder, with a proportion of patients with the untreated illness manifesting neurologic features, such as cognitive impairment, structural brain pathology, and disorders of movement (Barnes 1988). The wide range of motor abnormalities, or catatonic phenomena, seen in such patients includes disturbances of voluntary motor activity, such as stereotypies, mannerisms, posturing (Marsden et al. 1975), and "spontaneous" dyskinesias, including choreiform and dystonic movements and orofacial dyskinesia (Casey and Hansen 1984). Spontaneous dyskinesia, as an expression of the schizophrenic illness, may appear identical to tardive dyskinesia, and the two conditions may share an association with similar clinical features. The designation of abnormal movements as either drug-related or intrinsically related to the schizophrenic illness on the basis of their characteristics is problematic (Barnes 1988; Owens 1985) (see Chapter 2). Thus a major methodological issue for investigators is the distinction between these various types of movement disorders.

Casey and Hansen (1984) suggested that the AIMS is an appropriate instrument for the assessment of spontaneous dyskinesia in schizophrenic patients, using the research diagnostic criteria of Schooler and Kane (1982) for tardive dyskinesia. Rogers (1985), however, developed a scale to assess movement disorders in schizophrenic patients, which avoided assumptions about a psychiatric or neurologic etiology. Items were grouped under such headings as disturbance of posture, tone, purposive movement, and speech. It was acknowledged that some of the movements rated would be regarded as drug-induced, whereas others were more typical of the classical catatonic features of schizophrenia. The scale also covered phenomena that did not readily fit into either category, such as abnormal eye movements, ticlike movements, and abruptness and rapidity of spontaneous movements.

The original scale has been modified (Lund et al. 1991). The revised version of the Rogers Motor Disorder Scale comprises 36 items, rating the severity of each abnormality on a three-point scale: absent (0), definitely present (1), and marked or pervasive (2). The abnormalities considered to represent drug-induced parkinsonian and dyskinetic phenomena are identified, and the authors of the scale claim that the exclusion of these after the scale has been completed allows for the isolation of presumptive catatonic features.

### Mental Handicap

Antipsychotic drugs are widely used in individuals with developmental disability (see Chapter 6). When assessing the occurrence and nature of tardive dyskinesia in this population, dyskinesia compatible with a diagnosis of tardive dyskinesia must be distinguished from abnormal movements—such as stereotypies, psychotic gestures and mannerisms, and imitating and adventitious movements—which are sometimes displayed (Campbell et al. 1983; Gualtieri et al. 1984).

The AIMS scale has been successfully employed in several surveys of tardive dyskinesia in mentally handicapped persons (Ganesh et al. 1989; Gualtieri and Hawk 1980; Rao et al. 1987). For example, Gualtieri et al. (1986) used the AIMS in a systematic survey of tardive dyskinesia in 38 mentally retarded children during withdrawal from antipsychotic medication. To tackle the problem of rating antipsychotic-induced dyskinesia in patients manifesting a variety of other abnormal movements, these investigators excluded all individuals with a known neurologic disorder and trained the raters to reliably identify and differentiate dyskinetic movements from stereotypies.

In this study (Gualtieri et al. 1986), videotape recordings were reviewed by assessors blind to each patient's diagnosis and drug status. These recordings were used to validate the diagnosis, in that, for a diagnosis of tardive dyskinesia to be conferred on a person, there had to be agreement between the videotape assessors and the clinicians originally examining the patient on the presence of tardive or withdrawal dyskinesia. Among the three clinical raters, mean interrater reliability for the assessment of dyskinetic movements using the AIMS was .83 (Cohen's kappa).

Rao et al. (1987) used the AIMS and the Simpson Tardive Dyskinesia Rating Scale to rate tardive dyskinesia on two occasions, 6 months apart, in 67 mentally handicapped subjects receiving antipsychotic medication. Interrater and test-retest reliabilities for both scales were high. The prevalence of tardive dyskinesia determined from the AIMS total score, with a threshold criterion score of more than 2, was 21%; the corresponding figure for the Simpson scale was 42%, using a criterion score of more than 43.

The development of the Dyskinesia Identification System—Coldwater (DIS-Co) focused on the assessment of mentally retarded individuals. This is a 34-item scale based on data from 519 "institutionalized mentally-retarded residents," 250 of whom had never received antipsychotic medication (Sprague et al. 1984a). Subsequently, Kalachnik et al. (1984) used the scale in a clinical study comparing three randomly assigned treatment groups: a group receiving gradual reduction of their antipsychotic medication, a group receiving antipsychotic drugs without reduction, and a group who had not received antipsychotic drugs for at least 5 years. Sprague et al. (1984b) then revised the DIS-Co, based on the data collected in these studies. They developed a method for selecting items for the rating scale based on six qualities, including interrater reliability, stability, and relationship with medication. The resulting 15-item scale, the Dyskinesia Identification System: Condensed User Scale (DISCUS), has been used in training clinicians to assess tardive dyskinesia (Kalachnik et al. 1988). The psychometric properties of the DISCUS—that is, the interrater reliability, test-retest reliability, and means and standard deviations for scale items—have been provided, based on 400 individuals with developmental disability (Sprague et al. 1989).

Stone et al. (1989) developed the Sonoma Involuntary Movement Assessment System to examine the prevalences and interrelationships of five movement disorders—dyskinesia, dystonia, akathisia, parkinsonism, and paroxysms—occurring within a large population of developmentally disabled individuals. The term *dyskinesia* is used rather than *tardive dyskinesia* because the former word does not presume the etiology or a delayed onset. The definition of *dyskinesia* is restricted to choreoathetoid movements.

Interrater and intrarater reliability were assessed using videotape recordings presenting discrete examples of the movement disorders under scrutiny. The raters involved varied in their amount of clinical experience and length of training with the scale. Interrater agreement for dyskinesia did not vary with length of previous experience but was higher in those raters who had longer periods of training with the scale. The validity of the hypothesis that the five movement disorders rated on the scale represented separate entities was tested by looking at the strength of the correlations among the five conditions, applying multivariate statistics on the data (a varimax principal components analysis), and examining the relationship between the emerging components and relevant clinical variables. Sprague et al. (1989) and Kalachnik et al. (1988) have emphasized the importance of training raters and have observed that initially inexperienced raters tend to rate higher than more experienced raters. The impact of inadequate training on epidemiological data, therefore, is a major concern.

### Children

Few systematic investigations of dyskinesias associated with antipsychotic drugs have been carried out in children (McAndrew et al. 1972; Polizos and Engelhardt 1980). These drugs are prescribed for a variety of childhood conditions, such as mental retardation (including autism), conduct disorders with aggression, hyperactivity failing to respond to stimulants, and Tourette's syndrome (Campbell et al. 1983).

Problems in assessment include the differentiation between drug-related dyskinesia and abnormal movements, such as stereotypies and grimacing, occurring as part of the clinical behavioral syndrome. Even a proportion of normal children without any antipsychotic drug treatment can exhibit orofacial movements like lip puckering and tongue movements (Campbell et al. 1983). Further, it may be difficult to obtain the cooperation of children with these conditions to allow adequate examination. In addition, the work of Polizos et al. (1973) and Engelhardt et al. (1975) suggests that dyskinesia in children most commonly occurs on drug withdrawal and tends to involve the trunk and limbs. This is in contrast to tardive dyskinesia in adults, for which development during long-term drug treatment and the presence of orofacial dyskinesia are sometimes taken as diagnostic features. Other investigators (Gualtieri et al. 1984; Paulson et al. 1975) contend, however, that orofacial movements are seen relatively commonly in children, even with withdrawal dyskinesia.

The AIMS scale has been used in children and adolescents with high interrater agreement (Campbell et al. 1983; Gualtieri et al. 1982, 1986), as has the ADRS (Campbell et al. 1983). Engelhardt (1974) developed the Withdrawal Emergent Symptom Check List for rating symptoms on drug withdrawal, and high interrater agreement has also been achieved with this instrument in samples of children with mental retardation (Gualtieri et al. 1982).

## Summary

Systematic and reliable assessment of tardive dyskinesia is essential in both research and clinical settings. The most popular rating method is the multi-item scale that provides a comprehensive rating of the abnormal involuntary movements at the various body sites. Some of these scales incorporate a standard procedure for the examination of patients, and reliability and validity data are available for the most widely used scales, such as the AIMS and the Simpson Tardive Dyskinesia Rating Scale. Other clinical methods of assessment are frequency counts of dyskinetic movements and ratings from standardized videotape recordings of patients. In addition, rating methods involving a range of electromechanical devices and other instrumentation have been developed. The advantages and disadvantages of these various methods are discussed.

Problems in the assessment of tardive dyskinesia include marked within-patient variation in severity over time and in response to change in medication or level of arousal. Difficulties also arise where the motor phenomena of tardive dyskinesia need to be distinguished from motor disturbance related to the condition for which antipsychotic drugs were originally prescribed. Although the standard multi-item scales have usually been considered appropriate for most patient populations, scales have also been specifically developed to address this issue. Thus, the Rogers Motor Disorder Scale was devised to assess movement disorder in schizophrenia, avoiding assumptions about etiology, and the DIS-Co was originally developed for individuals with mental handicaps.

It is critical to stress the fact that scores on a rating scale or the results of a particular assessment strategy cannot at present be used to make a diagnosis. Assessment techniques are important for identifying possible cases as well as for documenting severity and measuring treatment response or long-term outcome, but a process of clinical evaluation and differential diagnosis is necessary to establish the presence of tardive dyskinesia.

# References

Ahrens TN, Sramek JJ, Herrera JM, et al: Pharmacy-based screening program for tardive dyskinesia. Drug Intelligence and Clinical Pharmacy 22:205–208, 1988

Alpert M, Diamond F, Friedhoff AJ: Tremographic studies in tardive dyskinesia. Psychopharmacol Bull 12:5–7, 1976

American College of Neuropsychopharmacology, Food and Drug Administration Task Force: Neurological syndromes associated with antipsychotic drug use: a special report. ARch Gen Psychiatry 28:463–467, 1973

Asnis GM, Leopold MA, Buvoisin RC, et al: A survey of tardive dyskinesia in psychiatric outpatients. Am J Psychiatry 134:1367–1370, 1977

Baldessarini RJ: The "neuroleptic" antipsychotic drugs: neurologic side-effects. Postgrad Med J 65:123–128, 1979

Baldessarini RJ, Tarsy D: Tardive dyskinesia, in Psychopharmacology: A Generation of Progress. Edited by Lipton MA, DiMascio A, Killam KE. New York, Raven, 1978, pp 993–994

Baldessarini RJ, Cole JO, Davis JM, et al: Tardive dyskinesia: summary of Task Force Report of the American Psychiatric Association. Am J Psychiatry 137:1163–1172, 1980

Barnes TRE: Tardive dyskinesia: risk factors, pathophysiology and treatment, in Recent Advances in Clinical Psychiatry 6. Edited by Granville-Grossman K. London, Churchill Livingstone, 1988, pp 185–207

Barnes TRE: Movement disorder associated with antipsychotic drugs: the tardive syndromes. Int Rev Psychiatry 2:355–366, 1990

Barnes TRE, Kidger T: Tardive dyskinesia and problems of assessment, in Current Themes in Psychiatry, Vol 2. Edited by Gaind RN, Hudson BL. London, Macmillan, 1979, pp 145–162

Barnes TRE, Trauer T: Reliability and validity of a tardive dyskinesia videotape rating scale. Br J Psychiatry 140:508–515, 1982

Barnes TRE, Wiles DH: Variation in oro-facial tardive dyskinesia during depot antipsychotic drug treatment. Psychopharmacology 81:359–362, 1983

Barnes TRE, Kidger T, Gore SM: Tardive dyskinesia: a 3-year follow-up study. Psychol Med 13:71–81, 1983a

Barnes TRE, Rossor M, Trauer T: A comparison of purposeless movements in psychiatric patients treated with antipsychotic drugs, and normal individuals. J Neurol Neurosurg Psychiatry 46:540–546, 1983b

Bartko J, Carpenter W: On the methods and theory of reliability. J Nerv Ment Dis 163:307–317, 1976

Bartzokis G, Wirshing WC, Hill MA, et al: Comparison of electromechanical measures and observer ratings of tardive dyskinesia. Psychiatry Res 27:193–198, 1989a

Bartzokis G, Hill MA, Altshuler L, et al: Tardive dyskinesia in schizophrenic patients: correlation with negative symptoms. Psychiatry Res 28:145–151, 1989b

Bergen JA, Griffiths DA, Rey JM, et al: Tardive dyskinesia: fluctuating patient on fluctuating rater. Br J Psychiatry 144:498–502, 1984

Branchey MH, Branchey LB, Bark NM, et al: Lecithin in the treatment of tardive dyskinesia. Commun Psychopharmacol 3:303–307, 1979

Buruma OJS, Kemp B, Roos RAC, et al: Quantification of choreatic movements by Doppler radar. Acta Neurol Scand 66:363–368, 1982

Caligiuri MP, Lohr JB, Bracha HS, et al: Clinical and instrumental assessmen of neuroleptic-induced parkinsonism in patients with tardive dyskinesia. Biol Psychiatry 29:139–148, 1991

Campbell M, Grega DM, Green WH, et al: Neuroleptic-induced dyskinesias in children. Clinical Neuropharmacology 6:207–222, 1983

Casey DE: Tardive dyskinesia: reversible and irreversible, in Dyskinesia, Research and Treatment (Psychopharmacology Supplementum 2). Edited by Casey DE, Chase TN, Christensen AV, et al. Berlin, Springer-Verlag, 1985, pp 88–97

Casey DE, Hansen TE: Spontaneous dyskinesias, in Neuropsychiatric Movement Disorders. Edited by Jeste DV, Wyatt RJ. Washington, DC, American Psychiatric Press, 1984, pp 68–95

Chien C-P, Jung K, Ross-Townsend A, et al: The measurement of persistent dyskinesia by piezoelectric recording and clinical rating scales. Psychopharmacol Bull 13:34–36, 1977

Chien C-P, Ross-Townsend A, Donnelly M: Past history of drug and somatic treatments in tardive dyskinesia, in Tardive Dyskinesia, Research and Treatment. Edited by Fann WE, Smith RC, Davis JM, et al. New York, Spectrum, 1980, pp 233–241

Ciccheti DV: Assessing inter-rater reliability for rating scales: resolving some basic issues. Br J Psychiatry 129:452–456, 1976

Crane GE: Persistent dyskinesia. Br J Psychiatry 122:395–405, 1973

Crane GE, Ruiz P, Kernohan WJ: Effects of drug withdrawal on tardive dyskinesia. Act Nerv Super 11:30–35, 1969

Delwaide PJ, Desseilles M: Spontaneous buccolinguofacial dyskinesia in the elderly. Acta Neurol Scand 56:256–262, 1977

Denney D, Casey DE: An objective method for measuring dyskinetic movements in tardive dyskinesia. Electroencephalogr Clin Neurophysiol 38:645–646, 1975

Engelhardt DM: Withdrawal Emergent Symptom Checklist (WESC). Brooklyn, NY, Downstate Medical Center, State University of New York, 1974

Engelhardt DM, Polizos P, Waizer J: CNS consequences of psychotropic drug withdrawal in autistic children: a follow-up report. Psychopharmacol Bull 11:6–7, 1975

Escobar JI, Kemp KF: Dimethylaminoethanol for tardive dyskinesia. N Engl J Med 292:318, 1975

Fann WE: Tardive dyskinesia and other drug-induced movement disorders, in Tardive Dyskinesia, Research and Treatment. Edited by Fann WE, Smith RC, Davis JM, et al. New York, Spectrum, 1980, pp 215–231

Fann WE, Stafford JE, Malone RL, et al: Clinical research techniques in tardive dyskinesia. Am J Psychiatry 134:759–762, 1977

Faurbye A, Rasch PJ, Petersen PB, et al: Neurological symptoms in pharmacotherapy of psychoses. Acta Psychiatr Scand 40:10–27, 1964

Firth WR, Ardern MH: Measuring abnormal movements in tardive dyskinesia: a pilot study. Br J Psychiatry 147:723–726, 1985

Fisk GG, York SM: The effect of sodium valporate on tardive dyskinesia—revisited. Br J Psychiatry 150:542–546, 1987

Fleischhauer J, Kocher R, Hobi V, et al: Prevalence of tardive dyskinesia in a clinic population, in Dyskinesia—Research and Treatment (Psychopharmacology Supplementum 2). Edited by Casey DE, Chase TN, Christensen AV, et al. Berlin, Springer-Verlag, 1985, pp 162–172

Ganesh S, Rao JM, Cowie VA: Akathisia in neuroleptic medicated mentally handicapped subjects. J Ment Defic Res 33:323–329, 1989

Gardos G, Cole JO: Problems in the assessment of tardive dyskinesia, in Tardive Dyskinesia, Research and Treatment. Edited by Fann WE, Smith RC, Davis JM, et al. New York, Spectrum, 1980, pp 201–214

Gardos G, Cole JO: Tardive dyskinesia and anticholinergic drugs. Am J Psychiatry 140:200–202, 1983

Gardos G, Cole JO, La Brie R: The assessment of tardive dyskinesia. Arch Gen Psychiatry 34:1206–1212, 1977

Gerlach J: Tardive dyskinesia. Danish Med Bull 26:209–245, 1979

Gerlach J, Korsgaard S: Classification of abnormal involuntary movements in psychiatric patients. Neuropsychiatr Clin 2:201–208, 1983

Germer CK, Seraydarian L, McBrearty JF: Training hospital clinicians to diagnose tardive dyskinesia. Hosp Community Psychiatry 35:769–783, 1984

Glazer WM, Morgenstern H, Niedzwiecki D, et al: Heterogeneity of tardive dyskinesia: a multivariate analysis. Br J Psychiatry 152:253–259, 1988

Greil W, Haag H, Rossnagl G, et al: Effect of anticholinergics on tardive dyskinesia. Br J Psychiatry 145:304–310, 1984

Gualtieri CT, Hawk MS: Tardive dyskinesia and other drug-induced movement disorders among handicapped children and youth. Appl Res Ment Retard 1:55–69, 1980

Gualtieri CT, Breuning SE, Schroeder SR, et al: Tardive dyskinesia in mentally retarded children, adolescents and young adults: North Carolina and Michigan studies. Psychopharmacol Bull 18:62–65, 1982

Gualtieri CT, Quade D, Hicks RE, et al: Tardive dyskinesia and other clinical consequences of neuroleptic treatment in children and adolescents. Am J Psychiatry 141:20–23, 1984

Gualtieri CT, Schroeder SR, Hicks RE, et al: Tardive dyskinesia in young mentally retarded individuals. Arch Gen Psychiatry 43:335–340, 1986

Gureje O: The significance of subtyping tardive dyskinesia: a study of prevalence and associated factors. Psychol Med 19:121–128, 1989

Guy W: ECDEU Assessment Manual for Psychopharmacology, Revised Edition. Washington, DC, U.S. Department of Health, Education, and Welfare, 1976

Haines J, Sainsbury P: Ultrasound system for measuring patients' activity and movement disorder. Lancet 2:802–803, 1972

Heinrich K, Wegener I, Bender H-J: Spate extrapyramidale Hyperkinesen bei neuroleptischer Langzeittherapie. Pharmakopsychiatr Neuropsychopharmakol 1:169–195, 1968

Hershon HI, Kennedy PF, McGuire RJ: Persistence of extrapyramidal disorders and psychiatric relapse after withdrawal of long-term phenothiazine therapy. Br J Psychiatry 120:41–50, 1972

Hippius H, Logemann G: Zur Wirkung von Dioxyphenylalanin (L-Dopa) auf extrapyramidal-motorische Hyperkinesen nach langfristiger neuroleptischer Therapie. Arzneim Forsch 20:894–895, 1970

Huang CC: Follow-up studies of tardive dyskinesia. Wisconsin Medical Journal 83:27–29, 1984

Jeste DV, Wyatt RJ: Tardive dyskinesia: the syndrome. Psychiatric Annals 10:16/6–13/25, 1980

Jus K, Jus A, Villeneuve A: Polygraphic profile of oral tardive dyskinesia and of the rabbit syndrome. Diseases of the Nervous System 34:27–32, 1973

Kalachnik JE, Harder SR, Kidd-Nielsen P, et al: Persistent tardive dyskinesia in randomly assigned neuroleptic reduction, neuroleptic nonreduction, and non-neuroleptic history groups: preliminary results. Psychopharmacol Bull 20:27–32, 1984

Kalachnik JE, Sprague RL, Slaw KM: Training clinical personnel to assess for tardive dyskinesia. Neuropsychopharmacology and Biological Psychiatry 12:749–762, 1988

Kane JM, Smith JM: Tardive dyskinesia: prevalence and risk factors, 1959–1979. Arch Gen Psychiatry 39:473–481, 1982

Kazamatsuri H, Chien CP, Cole JO: Treatment of tardive dyskinesia, 1: clinical efficacy of a dopamine-depleting agent, tetrabenazine. Arch Gen Psychiatry 27:95–99, 1972

Kennedy PF, Hershon HI, McGuire RJ: Extrapyramidal disorders after prolonged phenothiazine therapy. Br J Psychiatry 118:509–518, 1971

Kidger T, Barnes TRE, Trauer T, et al: Subsyndromes of tardive dyskinesia. Psychol Med 10:513–520, 1980

Klawans HL, Rubovits R: Effect of cholinergic and anticholinergic agents on tardive dyskinesia. J Neurol Neurosurg Psychiatry 27:941–947, 1974

Lane RD, Glazer WM, Hansen TE, et al: Assessment of tardive dyskinesia using the Abnormal Involuntary Movement Scale. J Nerv Ment Dis 173:353–357, 1985

Leonard DP, Kidson MA, Shannon PJ, et al: Double-blind trial of lithium carbonate and haloperidol in Huntington's chorea. Lancet 2:1208–1209, 1974

Lund CE, Mortimer AM, Rogers D, et al: Motor, volitional and behavioural disorders in schizophrenia, 1: assessment using the Modified Rogers Scale. Br J Psychiatry 158:323–327, 1991

Malt UF, Bech P, Dencker SJ, et al: Sct. Hans Skala for vurdering av ekstrapyramidale symtomer (SHVES). Nordisk Psykiatrisk Tidsskrift 44:196–197, 1990

Marsden CD, Schacter M: Assessment of extrapyramidal disorders. Br J Clin Pharmacol 11:129–151, 1981

Marsden CD, Tarsy D, Baldessarini RJ: Spontaneous and drug-induced movement disorders in psychotic patients, in Psychiatric Aspects of Neurological Disease. Edited by Benson DF, Blumer D. New York, Grune & Stratton, 1975, pp 219–266

May PRA, Lee MA, Bacon RC: Quantitative assessment of neuroleptic-induced extrapyramidal symptoms: clinical and nonclinical approaches. Clinical Neuropharmacology 6 (suppl 1):35–51, 1983

McAndrew JB, Case Q, Treffert DA: Effects of prolonged phenothiazine intake on psychotic and other hospitalized children. J Autism Childhood Schizophrenia 2:75–91, 1972

McClelland HA, Fairbairn AF, McDonald M, et al: The evaluation of an ultrasound detector (UD) in the measurement of oro-facial dyskinesia. Int Clin Psychopharmacol 2:159–164, 1987

McCreadie RG, Razzak A, Mackay AVP: Difficulties in assessing tardive dyskinesia. Br J Psychiatry 150:410–411, 1987

Munetz MR, Benjamin S: How to examine patients using the Abnormal Involuntary Movement Scale. Hosp Community Psychiatry 39:1172–1177, 1988

Munetz MR, Schulz SC: Screening for tardive dyskinesia. J Clin Psychiatry 47:75–77, 1986

Nordic Dyskinesia Study Group: Effect of different neuroleptics in tardive dyskinesia and parkinsonism: a video-controlled multicenter study with chlorprothixene, perphenazine, haloperidol and haloperidol + biperiden. Psychopharmacology 90:423–429, 1986

Owens DGC: Involuntary disorders of movement in chronic schizophrenia in the role of the illness and its treatment, in Dyskinesia—Research and Treatment. Edited by Casey DE, Chase TN, Christensen AV, et al. Berlin, Springer-Verlag, 1985, pp 79–87

Paulson GW: Tardive dyskinesia. Ann Rev Med 26:75–81, 1975

Paulson GW, Rizvi CA, Crane GE: Tardive dyskinesia as a possible sequel of long-term therapy with phenothiazines. Clin Pediatr 14:953–955, 1975

Polizos P, Engelhardt DM: Dyskinetic and neurological complications in children treated with psychotropic medications, in Tardive Dyskinesia, Research and Treatment. Edited by Fann WE, Smith RC, Davis JM, et al. New York, Spectrum, 1980, pp 193–199

Polizos P, Engelhardt DM, Hoffman SP, et al: Neurological consequences of psychotropic drug withdrawal in schizophrenic children. J Autism Childhood Schizophrenia 3:247–253, 1973

Rao JM, Cowie VA, Mathew B: Tardive dyskinesia in neuroleptic medicated mentally handicapped subjects. Acta Psychiatr Scand 76:507–513, 1987

Reda FA, Scanlon JM, Kemp KF: Treatment of tardive dyskinesia with lithium carbonate. N Engl J Med 291:850, 1974

Resek G, Haines J, Sainsbury P: An ultrasound technique for the measurement of tardive dyskinesia. Br J Psychiatry 138:474–478, 1981

Richardson MA, Craig TJ, Branchey MH: Intra-patient variability in the measurement of tardive dyskinesia. Psychopharmacology 76:269–272, 1982

Rogers D: The motor disorders of severe psychiatric illness: a conflict of paradigms. Br J Psychiatry 147:221–232, 1985

Schooler NR, Kane JM: Research diagnosis for tardive dyskinesia. Arch Gen Psychiatry 39:486–487, 1982

Sigwald J, Bouthier D, Raymondeaud U, et al: Quatre cas de dyskinesie facio-bucco-linguo-masticatrice a evolution prolongee secondaire a traitment par les neuroleptiques. Revue Neurologique 100:751–755, 1959

Simpson GM: Neurological assessments, in Behavior of Psychiatric Patients: Quantitative Techniques for Evaluation. Edited by Burdock EI, Sudilovsky A, Gershon S. New York, Marcel Dekker, 1982, pp 103–114

Simpson GM, Singh H: Tardive dyskinesia rating scales. L'Encephale 14:175–182, 1988

Simpson GM, Lee JH, Zoubok B, et al: A rating scale for tardive dyskinesia. Psychopharmacology 64:171–179, 1979

Smith JM, Kucharski LT, Oswald WT, et al: A systematic investigation of tardive dyskinesia in inpatients. Am J Psychiatry 136:918–922, 1979a

Smith JM, Kucharski LT, Eblen C, et al: An assessment of tardive dyskinesia in schizophrenic outpatients. Psychopharmacology 64:99–104, 1979b

Smith RC, Tamminga CA, Haraszti J, et al: Cholinergic influences in tardive dyskinesia. Am J Psychiatry 134:763–768, 1977

Sprague RL, White DM, Ullmann R, et al: Methods for selecting items in a tardive dyskinesia rating scale. Psychopharmacol Bull 20:339–345, 1984a

Sprague RL, Kalachnik JE, Breuning SE, et al: The Dyskinesia Identification System—Coldwater (DIS-Co): a tardive dyskinesia rating scale for the developmentally disabled. Psychopharmacol Bull 20:328–338, 1984b

Sprague RL, Kalachnik JE, Shaw KM: Psychometric properties of the Dyskinesia Identification System: Condensed User Scale (DISCUS). Mental Retardation 27:141–148, 1989

Stone RK, May JE, Alvarez WF, et al: Prevalence of dyskinesia and related movement disorders in a developmentally disabled population. J Ment Defic Res
33:41–53, 1989

Tamminga CA, Smith RC, Ericksen SE, et al: Cholinergic influences in tardive dyskinesia. Am J Psychiatry 134:769–774, 1977

Tryon WW, Pologe B: Accelerometric assessment of tardive dyskinesia. Am J Psychiatry 144:1584–1587, 1987

Whall AL, Engle V, Edwards A, et al: Developmen of a screening programme for
tardive dyskinesia: feasibility issues. Nursing Research 32:151–156, 1983

Wirshing WC, Cummings JL: Electromechanical characteristics of tardive dyskinesia (abstract). Schizophr Res 1:234, 1988

Wirsching WC, Cummings JL, Dencker SJ, et al: Electromechanical characteristics
of tardive dyskinesia. Journal of Neuropsychiatry and Clinical Neurosciences
3:10–17, 1991

Young RR, Growdon JH, Shahani BT: Beta-adrenergic mechanisms in action
tremor. N Engl J Med 293:950–953, 1975

# Chapter 4

# Epidemiology, Risk Factors, and Outcome of Tardive Dyskinesia

$A$lthough there still remains some debate as to the extent to which antipsychotic drug treatment is either necessary or sufficient to produce abnormal involuntary movements in various psychiatric populations, in our view the consensus at the present time is that antipsychotic drugs do play a major role in producing, precipitating, or evoking abnormal involuntary movements. This conclusion recognizes the fact that abnormal involuntary movements occurring in schizophrenic patients were described in the preantipsychotic drug era by Kraepelin (1919), Bleuler (1950), and others and have been also been observed more recently among chronic schizophrenic patients never treated with antipsychotic drugs (Owens et al. 1982; Waddington and Youssef 1986). No doubt various other predisposing factors play a critical role in determining which individuals are most likely to develop the condition.

## Prevalence

Prevalence estimates indicate how many individuals in a given population are affected by a condition at any specified point in time. Numerous prevalence surveys of tardive dyskinesia have been conducted, and these have been extensively reviewed (Jeste and Wyatt 1982; Kane and Smith 1982). In general, prevalence surveys have helped to identify populations at particular risk, to suggest factors that may contribute to risk, and to establish the overall scope of the problem. The results from prevalence studies can be difficult to compare and contrast because of the diverse procedures used for data collection and analysis. Various assessment techniques with or without rating scales are used (see Chapter 3), with a lack of consistent criteria for defining a case of tardive dyskinesia. Further, the populations studied differ on patient characteristics, such as psychiatric diagnosis, inpatient or outpatient status, and age.

There are other factors that limit the usefulness of prevalence surveys, and some of these are consequences of the nature of the syndrome itself and its relationship to antipsychotic drugs. Although antipsychotic drugs are implicated in the development of tardive dyskinesia, they are also capable of masking the clinical manifestations of the disorder. Therefore, prevalence estimates may be inaccurate because most subjects are examined while receiving antipsychotic drugs and a proportion of non–tardive dyskinesia patients may be false negatives. The condition can wax and wane over days or even hours, and false negatives may occur if a patient is subjected to only brief assessment during a quiescent phase of the condition. Less commonly, false positives may occur in surveys, when psychiatric patients manifest abnormal involuntary movements that are unrelated to their drug treatment.

It is possible to estimate the rate of false negatives by withdrawing patients without evidence of tardive dyskinesia from antipsychotic drugs and determining the proportion who manifest covert or withdrawal dyskinesia. Our ability, however, to distinguish so-called spontaneous dyskinesias from antipsychotic drug-related dyskinesias is limited, making estimates of the proportion of false positives potentially less accurate. Although we are able to identify some neuromedical conditions that might be mistaken for tardive dyskinesia, we do not know what proportion of patients with a particular psychiatric diagnosis might develop movements in some way associated with their illness but not induced by antipsychotic drugs.

There are data to suggest that abnormal involuntary movements are seen infrequently at the onset of a schizophrenic or schizophreniform illness. The critical test would be the assessment of individuals with a long history of well-diagnosed schizophrenia who had never received antipsychotic drug treatment. The opportunity to examine such patients rarely presents itself, but Owens et al. (1982), while assessing movement disorder in a sample of 411 hospitalized schizophrenic patients, identified 47 who, as far as they could ascertain, had never been exposed to antipsychotic drugs. Comparison of the drug-treated and non-drug-treated groups failed to reveal many significant differences with regard to prevalence, severity, and distribution of abnormal, involuntary movements. Although movements were recorded using the Abnormal Involuntary Movement Scale (AIMS) and the Rockland/Simpson Tardive Dyskinesia Rating Scale, the authors refrained from applying diagnostic categories or classifying the movements in terms of their nature or characteristics.

Owens (1985) later analyzed the data further. When the age difference between the two patient samples was taken into account, there was a significant linear relationship between the prevalence of abnormal involuntary movements and exposure to antipsychotic medication. Further, grouping movements into clinically recognizable syndromes revealed a particular susceptibility to oro-facial dyskinesia in drug-treated patients. Owens pointed out, however, that such movements were seen in 30% of those cases never treated with drugs.

One inescapable conclusion from these findings is that spontaneous, involuntary, orofacial movements can be a feature of chronic schizophrenia that has not been modified by the administration of antipsychotic drugs. A proportion of such movements may merely represent "spontaneous" orofacial dyskinesia of the elderly, but Owens and Johnstone (1980) postulate that in some patients the syndrome reflects the pathological cerebral process underlying severe, chronic schizophrenia.

In an older study, Yarden and Discipio (1971) reported that in a cohort of young, first-episode schizophrenic patients, who had never been exposed to antipsychotic drugs, approximately 6% manifested choreiform and athetoid dyskinesia. In addition, when these patients were followed, it was the investigators' impression that those patients who exhibited abnormal involuntary movements tended to have an early onset, a steadily progressive course accompanied by marked deterioration and thought disorder, and a poor response to antipsychotic drug treatment.

The fact that abnormal involuntary movements are also seen following antipsychotic drug treatment in nonschizophrenic patients should also be considered in evaluating the role of antipsychotic drugs. In fact, some evidence suggests that patients with affective illness may be at greater risk for developing tardive dyskinesia, given the same length of antipsychotic drug exposure, than patients with schizophrenia.

Woerner et al. (1991) completed a large-scale prevalence survey designed to address some of the concerns alluded to above. In addition, an attempt was made to include as broad a spectrum of antipsychotic drug-treated patients as possible, drawn from different clinical facilities while utilizing the same assessment measures, case criteria, and rating team. In order to include a wide range of patients, three separate institutions providing inpatient and outpatient psychiatric care were included in the survey: a voluntary hospital in a middle-class neighborhood with a relatively young patient population, a U.S. Veterans Administration (VA) medical center serving a somewhat older and more chronic population, and a state facility located in New York City with greater numbers of elderly and very chronic patients. Among the antipsychotic drug-treated subjects at these institutions, the overall prevalence found was 23.4%. The prevalence figures at the three sites ranged from 13.3% for the sample of patients at the voluntary hospital to 36.1% for the patients at the state hospital. The proportion of apparent cases of tardive dyskinesia that could be attributed to other neuromedical conditions following clinical laboratory evaluation and examination by the neurologist experienced in the assessment of movement disorders was surprisingly low (0.1%). A somewhat larger subgroup (3.7%) had abnormal movements in the context of neuromedical illnesses that could possibly play some etiologic role; therefore, the most conservative estimate of prevalence was 19.6%.

In order to estimate the rate of false negative cases due to masking of the dyskinesia by antipsychotic drug at the time the patients were examined, antipsychotic medication was withdrawn from a subgroup of patients with no evidence of tardive dyskinesia. These cases were examined at weekly intervals for 3 weeks. For those cases exhibiting emergent tardive dyskinesia, follow-up was continued off antipsychotic drugs to assess persistence of movements. Seventy subjects were discontinued, and 24 (34%) of these showed emergent dyskinesia. Seven cases were designated persistent, 16 probable, and 1 transient, according to the research criteria for tardive dyskinesia. The rate of emergent tardive dyskinesia at the state facility was strikingly higher (67%) than at the voluntary hospital (18%) or the VA facility (17%).

Preliminary exploration of the variables related to withdrawal or covert tardive dyskinesia (Kane et al. 1988) indicated that patients discontinued from fluphenazine decanoate (a minimum of 5 weeks from the last injection) were less likely to show covert tardive dyskinesia than patients discontinued from oral medication, confirming the previous findings of Levine et al. (1980). The dose (in chlorpromazine equivalents a day) of antipsychotic drug prior to discontinuation was not related to the emergence of tardive dyskinesia. However, a history of treatment with very high doses of antipsychotic drugs (3,000 mg a day in chlorpromazine equivalents) was negatively correlated with covert tardive dyskinesia. Age and total months of antipsychotic drug treatment were found to be significantly positively correlated with emergent tardive dyskinesia.

## Tardive Dyskinesia in Children

Severe, persistent tardive dyskinesia does occur in children, sometimes after relatively short treatment periods (Campbell et al. 1983; Gualtieri and Hawk 1980). Most studies of tardive dyskinesia in children refer to three additional neuroleptic withdrawal syndromes or "withdrawal emergent symptoms": 1) transient withdrawal dyskinesia; 2) withdrawal symptoms like nausea, vomiting, anorexia, diaphoresis, and seizures; and 3) a behavioral analog of tardive dyskinesia (Davis and Rosenberg 1979), "tardive dysbehavior" (Gualtieri and Guimon 1981), or "supersensitivity psychosis" (Chouinard and Jones 1980; Gualtieri et al. 1984).

The first description of persistent choreoathetoid movement in children on long-term phenothiazine therapy was by McAndrew et al. (1972). In 125 hospitalized children age 4–16, 10 (8%) developed dyskinesia following neuroleptic withdrawal that persisted for 3–12 months. The dyskinetic group had been treated with phenothiazines at higher doses for longer periods of time (McAndrew et al. 1972).

Polizos and Engelhardt coined the term "withdrawal emergent symptoms" (Engelhardt et al. 1975; Polizos and Engelhardt 1978). Such symptoms occurred in 51% of a group of autistic and schizophrenic children within 2 weeks of neuroleptic withdrawal. Subsequent studies suggest that dyskinetic movements occurring in children are not topographically different from those seen in adults (Gualtieri et al. 1984; Paulson et al. 1975). Buccal-lingual-masticatory and facial movements predominate in children (Gualtieri et al. 1984) and in developmentally handicapped young adults (Gualtieri et al. 1986). Recent research indicates that withdrawal dyskinesia, defined in these studies as duration of 4 months or less, is the most common form of neuroleptic-induced dyskinesia in children (Gualtieri et al. 1984; Polizos and Engelhardt 1980). Cumulative neuroleptic dose does appear to be a relevant factor in the development of dyskinesias in this population (Gualtieri et al. 1984; Gualtieri et al. 1986).

The occurrence of transient periods of behavioral instability in children who are withdrawn from neuroleptic drugs has fed speculation concerning the existence of a "behavioral equivalent" of tardive or at least of withdrawal dyskinesia (Gualtieri and Guimond 1981). (See Chapter 9.)

At present we are lacking sufficient data with regard to prevalence, incidence, and course of tardive dyskinesia or related disorders in children and adolescents. The collection of such data should receive a high priority. It is clear, however, that movement disorders associated with long-term neuroleptic treatment can occur in children and adolescents, and this possibility should be considered in weighing the benefit-to-risk ratio of neuroleptic treatment as well as in the process of informed consent.

### Prevalence of Tardive Dyskinesia in Autistic Children

Polizos et al. (1973) developed a measuring device for detecting tardive dyskinesia in children, which they named withdrawal emergent symptoms (WES). In a study of five neuroleptic medications that had been given to 34 children diagnosed as having childhood schizophrenia with prominent autistic features, Polizos et al. (1973) reported an incidence of 41% for the withdrawal symptoms. Several of the medications had been given to the children for various periods of time. In another report with a somewhat larger sample ($N = 47$), Engelhardt et al. (1975) reported an incidence of 48% for withdrawal symptoms in these children.

M. Campbell's laboratory at New York University has followed up on these initial studies of autistic children. Using the AIMS and the Rockland Abbreviated Dyskinesia Rating Scale, Campbell et al. (1983) found that during a 2.5-year follow-up, 8 (22%) of 36 children developed abnormal movements. All of these subjects received the neuroleptic haloperidol.

In a study reported later with more subjects, Perry et al. (1985) examined 58 children. During a period of 3.5–42.5 months of observation, 13 (22%) of 58 "developed mild to moderate drug-related abnormal movements," which is a prevalence rate that exactly matched the rate found in their earlier study.

These four studies indicate that tardive dyskinesia may develop in very young and older autistic children if they are treated with neuroleptic medication; most information is available about haloperidol, since Campbell's laboratory has used this medication extensively.

### Prevalence of Tardive Dyskinesia in Mentally Retarded Populations

Kalachnik et al. (1984) presented a thorough summary of the studies that have attempted to assess the prevalence of tardive dyskinesia in a population of mentally retarded people. As could be expected, the methodologies used to assess tardive dyskinetic symptoms vary greatly from study to study and, again, as could be expected from these different methodological techniques, the percentages vary greatly.

Paulson et al. (1975), using clinical methods, found that 21 of 103 subjects had persistent tardive dyskinesia. In a more recent similar study, Gualtieri et al. (1986), using the AIMS, found that 13 (34.2%) of 38 had tardive dyskinesia. Using the research diagnosis for tardive dyskinesia (RD-TD) criterion of Schooler and Kane (1982), Kalachnik et al. (1984) followed 103 subjects in a medication-reduction study; they found that 9 months after the baseline, 17 (85%) of 20 of the medication-reduction group met the RD-TD criterion, 10 (33%) of 31 of the medication control group met the criterion, and 21 (40.4%) of 52 of the group with no neuroleptic medication and no recent history of medication administration met the criterion. The prevalence rates in this study were higher than those reported in the other studies, and the difference between the no-medication group or control group (40.4%) and the medication-reduction group (85%) was 45%, a figure considerably higher than the other studies reported.

### Limitations of Prevalence Surveys

Interpretation of the results of prevalence surveys, particularly with regard to evaluation of risk factors, is also complicated by the fact that prevalence estimates are influenced by the persistence of the disorder within a given population. Many cases of tardive dyskinesia will remit with antipsychotic drug discontinuation, dosage reduction, or even continued antipsychotic drug treatment; however, others may persist for months or years. Therefore, analysis of risk factors in prevalence surveys is complicated by those factors that influence outcome. It may be that risk factors for the development of tardive dyskinesia are also risk factors for the persistence of tardive dyskinesia, as appears to be the case for advancing age. This should not be assumed to be true without appropriate data, but if it were true, this would serve to exaggerate the influence of a particular risk factor. For example, if both the incidence and the likelihood of persistence increase with age, then the relationship between age and tardive dyskinesia in a prevalence survey will be even more striking.

The strategy of estimating prevalence in a specific population has limitations, and further advances in our understanding of tardive dyskinesia will require a different type of methodology. Nevertheless, there remain populations of considerable interest for which prevalence estimates would be useful, such as schizophrenic patients who have not received antipsychotic drug treatment, nonpsychotic patients receiving antipsychotic drugs, and individuals with Tourette's disorder. In addition, patients receiving compounds with dopamine antagonist effects (e.g., metoclopramide) for the treatment of gastrointestinal disorders may be at risk for the development of tardive dyskinesia; however, incidence or prevalence in that context has not been established.

# Incidence

Incidence refers to the number of new cases occurring in a given population over a specified interval. Some important progress has been made in the last several years involving prospective studies of tardive dyskinesia development. This strategy overcomes many, but not all, of the concerns discussed with regard to cross-sectional prevalence surveys and enables us to develop more accurate estimates of incidence and develop more reliable data bases relevant to the assessment of risk factors.

The limitations of this methodology include the need to maintain the cooperation of large numbers of patients and staff for the duration of a long-term study and the attraction of sufficient funding. In addition, populations with different diagnostic, demographic, and treatment history characteristics should be studied in order to generate results that are applicable and relevant to all types of patients who receive antipsychotic medication.

In follow-up studies, changes in the dose or class of antipsychotic drug in the intervening period between assessments might substantially influence the observed outcome of tardive dyskinesia. For example, an increase in the dose of an antipsychotic drug shortly before reexamination would probably suppress the movements. The condition might then be rated as improved or completely resolved, although the dyskinesia is likely to reappear eventually. In contrast, if antipsychotic drugs were reduced or withdrawn before assessment, this would tend to provoke or increase symptoms (Casey and Gerlach 1986).

Kane et al. (1984, 1986, 1988) reported interim results from a long-term prospective study of tardive dyskinesia. More than 850 patients have entered this study, which involves prospective assessment every 3 months. Patients entering the study are selected without regard to their psychiatric diagnosis or history of antipsychotic drug treatment. A subgroup of approximately 100 of the patients recruited into the study have never received antipsychotic drugs, and this helps to keep the raters blind to medication status.

The average age of the cohort was 29 years, and 43% were female. Of those patients with a history of antipsychotic drug therapy at entry to the study, the median length of lifetime exposure is 12 months, which indicates that patients are followed from a relatively early stage in their drug treatment. The findings thus far are that the cumulative incidence of tardive dyskinesia was 5% at 1 year, 10% at 2 years, 15% at 3 years, and 19% following 4 years of antipsychotic drug exposure. For the fifth and sixth years the figures have continued to increase, being 23% and 26%, respectively.

These results suggest that the cumulative incidence of tardive dyskinesia does increase with increasing duration of antipsychotic drug exposure and that at least for the first several years of such exposure the increase is linear. Whether at some point beyond that the risk decreases remains to be seen, but at the present time it is difficult to identify a period of maximum risk. These data strongly implicate antipsychotic drugs in the development of tardive dyskinesia.

Yassa et al. (1984a, 1984b) carried out a prospective study involving 108 patients (55 men and 53 women) who were assessed over a 2-year period. Almost two-thirds (65%) had a diagnosis of schizophrenia, 12% were suffering from manic depressive illness, 9% had a diagnosis of mental retardation, and 5% had an organic mental syndrome. In 8 patients the tardive dyskinesia persisted through at least two separate examinations at some time during the 2 years. The condition was considered to be of moderate severity in one case and mild in the remainder. An incidence of 7.4% for persistent tardive dyskinesia is given, but this figure is not based on a life-table analysis or a cumulative proportion remaining free of tardive dyskinesia, which would allow inclusion of the dropouts in the incidence calculation. The patients with tardive dyskinesia (mean age 57 years) were significantly older than the nondyskinetic patients (mean age 47 years). The former group had also received antipsychotic drugs for a significantly longer interval (mean 23 years) than the latter group (mean 17 years).

### Natural History

The point prevalence figures for tardive dyskinesia at the beginning and end of follow-up studies generally suggest that the proportion of patients with tardive dyskinesia is relatively stable for a few years. A closer examination of the findings of such studies reveals that underlying this apparent stability there is substantial change within individual patients, with spontaneous remissions being relatively common, particularly in younger patients. The results from two recent 10-year follow-up studies (Casey and Gardos 1990; Yagi and Itoh 1987) add to the weight of evidence for this view.

For example, Barron and McCreadie (1983) reported on 103 patients who were assessed on two occasions 1 year apart. The prevalence of tardive dyskinesia fell from 31% to 27% during the follow-up period. However, the authors suggested that if a move from "absent" to "mild" on the global scale of the AIMS could be taken as evidence for the development of tardive dyskinesia, this yielded a 1-year incidence rate of 3%. Fifty-five percent of the patients showed no evidence of tardive dyskinesia at either assessment, 18% had tardive dyskinesia on both occasions, 9% developed tardive dyskinesia, and 18% no longer had tardive dyskinesia.

Similarly, a 7-year follow-up in Hungarian patients (Gardos et al. 1988a) found a modest increase in prevalence from 27% to 38%, although within the patient cohort there were 12 resolved cases and 19 new cases. Even more strikingly, a further study by Richardson and Casey (1988) of 62 patients followed for 4 years reported the same prevalence of 69% at the beginning and end of the study period. This finding reflected that the 5 new cases of tardive dyskinesia were balanced by an equal number of patients in whom the condition resolved.

Chouinard et al. (1986) conducted a 5-year follow-up study of tardive dyskinesia. The initial sample included 256 schizophrenic patients receiving antipsychotic drug maintenance treatment, 31% of whom manifested tardive dyskinesia. One hundred thirty-two patients who did not initially manifest tardive dyskinesia were reexamined 5 years later. During this interval the policy of the clinic providing treatment had been to switch patients from oral medication to long-acting injectable antipsychotic drugs. Forty-six (35%) of the patients in this cohort manifested tardive dyskinesia at the follow-up examination. This provides an estimate of new cases but does not really allow an incidence calculation, since some patients may have developed tardive dyskinesia and remitted within the 5-year interval, and there is no way to determine when during the 5-year interval tardive dyskinesia developed among those experiencing it at follow-up. The authors also reported that of 38 patients having tardive dyskinesia at the first assessment, 9 had apparently remitted at the 5-year follow-up.

Barnes et al. (1983a) reported a 3-year follow-up of patients previously examined for tardive dyskinesia. Of an original cohort of 182 patients receiving maintenance antipsychotic drugs, 99 were available for reassessment. The point prevalence of dyskinesia increased from 39% to 47%

during the 3-year period. Tardive dyskinesia developed in 22 of the 60 patients who did not have the condition 3 years earlier, whereas remission occurred in 14 of the 39 patients who originally had tardive dyskinesia. The average ages of the patient cohorts studied by Chouinard et al. (1986) and Barnes et al. (1983a) were 42 years and 56 years, respectively, in contrast to 29 years in the Kane et al. (1984, 1986, 1988) study. The extent to which the differences in the mean ages of the populations studied might account for the differences in incidence of tardive dyskinesia between the studies is difficult to determine; however, the findings are generally consistent with other data suggesting a higher incidence of tardive dyskinesia in older populations. Toenniessen et al. (1985) retrospectively analyzed the relationship between duration of antipsychotic drug treatment and tardive dyskinesia in 57 elderly psychiatric inpatients and suggested that many of these patients developed tardive dyskinesia with less than 2 years of antipsychotic drug treatment. These results are also supported by a prevalence survey conducted in elderly populations by Lieberman et al. (1984a, 1984b).

Kane (1990) and Saltz et al. (1991) are engaged in a continuing prospective study of tardive dyskinesia development in a large cohort of elderly subjects, with a mean age of 77 years, none of whom had any evidence of abnormal involuntary movements prior to antipsychotic drug treatment. Fifty-eight percent of this sample had a diagnosis of organic mental syndrome, and 42% had a primary psychiatric diagnosis. The incidence of tardive dyskinesia after 43 weeks of cumulative antipsychotic drug exposure was 31%.

The data from follow-up studies suggest that tardive dyskinesia does not commonly progress but tends to follow a fluctuating course with spontaneous remissions (Gardos et al. 1988b), although there are occasional reports of tardive dyskinesia worsening during continued drug therapy (Casey and Gerlach 1986; Gardos and Cole 1983a; Jus et al. 1979; Levine et al. 1980; Mehta et al. 1977). Time may be the most important factor in outcome. Length of follow-up is positively correlated with increasing improvement or resolution of tardive dyskinesia. Thus studies evaluating outcome for more than 5 years provide results that are more favorable than the somewhat pessimistic reports from shorter follow-up periods. Symptom resolution from 5 to 10 years shows that approximately 50% of the patients will show at least a 50% improvement in dyskinesia whether or not antipsychotic drugs are continued throughout. If drug treatment is stopped, however, the tardive dyskinesia has a more favorable outcome (Casey 1985; Casey and Gerlach 1986). Glazer et al. (1990, 1991) reported the results of a retrospective follow-up study of 192 patients (mean age 46 years) with tardive dyskinesia, seen two or more times (average 7.7 visits) during a 3- to 55-month period while continuing to receive neuroleptics. One hundred twelve (58%) of the sample demonstrated a "chronic persistent" pattern in contrast to an intermittent pattern in the remainder of the patients. (The most important predictors of chronic persistent tardive dyskinesia using multiple logistic regression analysis included increased age and the presence of nonorofacial tardive dyskinesia at the baseline.)

Glazer et al. (1990, 1991) reported results on a separate cohort of tardive dyskinesia patients who underwent neuroleptic discontinuation and were reexamined monthly for a mean of 10 months. Complete and persistent reversibility of tardive dyskinesia was seen in only 2% of these patients, but many patients showed substantial improvement.

Most reports that have tracked tardive dyskinesia for long periods show that, with the exception of the rapidly reversing tardive dyskinesia, minimal changes in the condition occur within the first 6–12 months of follow-up. Rather, the course is one of gradual improvement or stabilization for many years. Just as it takes a long time for tardive dyskinesia to develop, so it may also take a long time to resolve or stabilize. This perspective supports the concept that tardive dyskinesia is best considered along a continuum of resolved or persisting. This is in contrast to the categorical concept of reversible or irreversible tardive dyskinesia.

Those abnormal involuntary movements that do appear to be irreversible, in that they persist for years after the withdrawal of antipsychotic drugs, may, in some cases, represent movements related to the relevant neuropsychiatric disorder or represent idiopathic dyskinesias seen in the elderly (Marsden 1985).

## Risk Factors

The identification of factors that contribute to individual susceptibility to tardive dyskinesia should be of help in predicting the condition and in the development of preventive strategies; however, there is a relative lack of long-term prospective studies testing the predictive value of potentially relevant patient and treatment variables. Therefore, reviews in this area must derive evidence from cross-sectional and retrospective studies, case reports, and short-term follow-up studies (Barnes 1988; Waddington 1989).

### Age

In numerous studies, age has been shown to be clearly associated with the prevalence of tardive dyskinesia. Extensive reviews of the topic (Kane and Smith 1982; Smith and Baldessarini 1980) have concluded that increasing age remains the most consistently implicated factor for the risk of development of tardive dyskinesia as well as developing more severe and persistent forms of the disorder. Although in many instances age and duration of antipsychotic drug exposure are confounded, clinical investigations have repeatedly shown that the effect of age is not attributable to longer duration of antipsychotic drug treatment (Kane and Smith 1982). Much of the variation in prevalence figures reported is likely to be due to age differences in the samples studied (Kane and Smith 1982). Jeste et al. (1983) calculated that in the sample of chronically ill schizophrenic inpatients they studied, the probability of having tardive dyskinesia was greater than .4 in those patients older than 65 years.

The elderly are also at risk for the development of spontaneous dyskinesias or abnormal involuntary movements related to a variety of neuromedical conditions independent of exposure to antipsychotic drugs (Blowers 1981; Blowers et al. 1982; Bourgeois et al. 1980a, 1980b; Brandon et al. 1971; Delwaide and Desseilles 1977; Molsa et al. 1982, 1984). Nevertheless, prevalence surveys of healthy elderly volunteers suggest that spontaneous dyskinesias are relatively uncommon in the absence of some form of brain disease or dysfunction, even later in life (Kane et al. 1982; Klawans and Barr 1982; Lieberman et al. 1984a, 1984b).

Examining pooled epidemiological data, Smith and Baldessarini (1980) found a strong linear correlation between age and both the prevalence and severity of tardive dyskinesia. Advancing age has been found to be associated with an increased occurrence of tardive dyskinesia, greater severity, and a reduced likelihood of spontaneous remission. Smith and Baldessarini (1980) found that tardive dyskinesia in those younger than 60 years of age was more than three times more likely to remit spontaneously. Certainly, the older a patient is when he or she first receives antipsychotic medication, the more likely he or she is to develop the condition early in treatment (Jus et al. 1976). The data from the prevalence and follow-up studies of Kidger et al. (1980) and Barnes et al. (1983a, 1983b) suggest that drug-treated patients in their sixth decade are at the highest risk of developing orofacial dyskinesia. It seems likely that the relationship between quantity of antipsychotic treatment and vulnerability to tardive dyskinesia systematically varies with age. Such a relationship has not been systematically tested, however. In the minority of studies where a relationship between specific drug variables and tardive dyskinesia has been found, it has been within the first few years of treatment.

Csernansky et al. (1983) suggested that in younger, less chronic patients, specific drug exposure may be more important. They considered that tardive dyskinesia developing in such cases may be more directly related to drugs than in cases where tardive dyskinesia develops after prolonged drug administration in patients who are likely to be older and in whom other nondrug variables are likely to be relevant and may obscure any positive relationship with drug variables. The distinction between early and late dyskinesia may be worthy of further study (Barnes 1987).

The prospective data of Kane (1990) and Saltz et al. (1991) suggest that the incidence of presumptive tardive dyskinesia in a sample of elderly patients (mean age 77 years) receiving neuroleptics for the first time is 31% after 1 year or almost 10-fold greater than the incidence seen in their younger cohort (Kane et al. 1984, 1986).

The potential mechanisms for the influence of age in tardive dyskinesia vulnerability remain speculative. Neuronal damage or degeneration, age-related changes in receptor number, sensitivity or plasticity, and the reduced efficiency of adaptive, homeostatic processes may be relevant to the susceptibility to certain drug-induced neurologic side effects in older patients. The development of supersensitive, postsynaptic, dopamine receptors in the basal ganglia was originally considered to be the pathophysiological basis of tardive dyskinesia. Such supersensitivity would seem to be an inevitable consequence of prolonged antipsychotic drug treatment, however, and is therefore insufficient to explain why only a proportion of patients on long-term medication develops dyskinesia (Jeste and Wyatt 1981). An interaction between drug-induced receptor changes in the striatum and age-related degenerative effects in the nigrostriatal system may be a factor contributing to the increased frequency of tardive dyskinesia in the elderly.

Pharmacokinetic mechanisms could also be relevant. Age-related changes in the absorption, metabolism, and excretion of drugs may lead to higher plasma drug levels and delayed clearance. Plasma levels of antipsychotic drugs have been found to be raised in the elderly, compared with younger patients (Jeste et al. 1979b; Yesavage et al. 1981).

## Sex

Looking at the influence of sex, a relatively stable finding has been that women show a greater prevalence of severe dyskinesia, although the available evidence suggests that this is limited to the geriatric age range (Kennedy et al. 1971; Siede and Muller 1967). Smith and Dunn (1979) identified 13 studies that reported statistically significant differences supporting female vulnerability but none indicating higher risk in males. The average unweighted female-to-male prevalence ratio in 13 patient samples was 1.69. Attempts to explain this difference have been generally unrewarding. It is possible that neuroendocrine factors play a role. For example, estrogen may influence striatal dopamine systems, although the nature of this influence is far from clearly established (Hruska 1985). Further, rather than a direct reflection of gender, it has been variously speculated that female sex is a proxy variable for longer duration of hospitalization, higher drug dose, and longer duration of treatment.

This sex difference has not been found so consistently in more recent studies, although Smith et al. (1979a, 1979b) suggested that it might only apply to the more severe cases. These investigators argued that the magnitude of sex differences in tardive dyskinesia is dependent on the severity of the criterion used to define the disorder as well as the age of the sample. Smith et al. (1979a, 1979b) pointed out that the ability to detect a significant sex effect is also influenced by the sample size and the base rate of tardive dyskinesia in the population under investigation.

The findings of Richardson et al. (1984) illustrate these points. These researchers reported that females showed an increase in prevalence of tardive dyskinesia in all age groups up to and older than 75 years, whereas males only demonstrated an increase up to 75 years, with a subsequent decline. The differences in prevalence between the sexes was minimal up to 64 years using mild severity to define a case, but female prevalence was substantially higher when a criterion of moderate-to-severe severity was applied.

### Psychiatric Diagnosis

**Schizophrenia.** Long before the advent of antipsychotic drugs in the early 1950s, various motor disorders were described in psychiatric patients, particularly those with catatonic schizophrenia (Bleuler 1950; Kahlbaum 1874; Kleist 1908), but also in other types of schizophrenia (Farran-Ridge 1926; Jones and Hunter 1969). As previously discussed (see Chapter 2), these movements would seem to be principally disturbances of voluntary motor activity and may be classified as stereotypies and mannerisms; perseverative movements; tics; grimaces; and general clumsiness, awkwardness, and lack of coordination, although Kraepelin (1919) and Farran-Ridge (1926) observed spasmodic movements, mainly involving the orofacial muscles, which they considered choreiform in nature. Kraepelin (1919) also reported "peculiar, sprawling irregular outspreading movements," which he termed "athetoid ataxia."

In a comprehensive review of this topic, Marsden et al. (1975) concluded that true chorea and athetosis were scarce in chronic psychiatric patients before drug treatment and that much of the motor disorder seen was attributable to organic neurologic disorder, such as encephalitis and syphilis. Kleist (1908) and Farran-Ridge (1926) commented that the similarity between the manifestations of dementia praecox and epidemic encephalitis was such that difficulties in differential diagnosis could arise.

There would seem to be three possible interpretations of these observations (Barnes and Liddle 1985). First, the type of motor disturbance described is not specifically associated with schizophrenia, but is the product of "organic" brain disease. The two conditions occur together when the brain disease is also responsible for schizophreniclike syndromes secondary to Axis III physical disorders, as, for example, when schizophrenia appears in patients with encephalitis, Wilson's disease, or Huntington's chorea, among other conditions (Davison and Bagley 1969). Second, the association of motor disturbance and schizophrenia may be more specific in that an underlying neuropathologic process is capable of producing both psychological and motor impairments. In other words, schizophrenia is a psychomotor disorder. Third, as Kraepelin (1919) and Bleuler (1950) tended to suggest, the movements may be secondary to the schizophrenic disturbance of will, thought, and emotion. The distinctions between the three explanations cannot be too sharply drawn, however, and more than one may be relevant.

Further evidence to support the notion of schizophrenia as a motor disorder is the occurrence of motor disturbance in amphetamine-induced psychosis. Chronic abuse of amphetamine can produce a paranoid state almost indistinguishable from paranoid schizophrenia (Snyder 1973). This may be accompanied by complex patterns of perseverative, stereotyped behavior and impulsive fidgety movements, as well as less complex phenomena, such as grimacing, chewing, and twisting of the trunk and limbs (Segal and Janowsky 1978).

Thus schizophrenia is associated with a tendency to develop abnormal involuntary movements, and Owens (1985) propounded the notion that antipsychotic drugs act, promote, or exacerbate a tendency to develop spontaneous movement disorders inherent in at least some forms of the illness. He suggested that tardive dyskinesia is part of the Type II syndrome of schizophrenia.

If this were true, one would expect tardive dyskinesia to be more common in patients with negative features of schizophrenia. Reviews of studies that have examined this issue seem to support this view (Barnes and Liddle 1985; Jeste et al. 1984; Waddington 1987). Tardive dyskinesia has been found to be consistently more common in patients with negative features. Most studies comparing dyskinetic and nondyskinetic schizophrenic patients have reported a significant association between tardive dyskinesia and such symptoms as emotional withdrawal, blunted affect, poverty of speech, motor retardation, and reduced social interest (Barnes et al. 1989a; Csernansky et al. 1983; Glazer et al. 1984; Guy et al. 1986; Itil et al. 1981; Jeste et al. 1984; McCreadie et al. 1982; Owens and Johnstone 1980; Waddington and Youssef 1986; Waddington et al. 1985). Four studies (Iager et al. 1986; Lindenmayer et al. 1984; Opler et al. 1984; Richardson et al. 1985), all involving younger patient samples, failed to find this relationship between dyskinesia and negative features.

There are various caveats that should be considered in drawing conclusions from these data. Most important, differentiating so-called negative symptoms from depression or drug-induced parkinsonism can frequently be difficult, particularly on a cross-sectional basis (Barnes et al. 1989a, 1989b; Craig et al. 1985; Lindenmayer and Kay 1989; McKenna et al. 1989; Prosser et al. 1987). Given the fact that affective disorders and vulnerability to drug-induced parkinsonian symptoms have both been implicated as risk factors, the potential for confounding variables becomes a particular concern.

Nevertheless, the main clinical implication of an association between tardive dyskinesia and negative symptoms is that schizophrenic patients developing dyskinesia may have a poorer prognosis than their nondyskinetic fellows. The predictive value of abnormal movements in this regard may be true for schizophrenic patients whether or not antipsychotic drugs have been administered (Yarden and Discipio 1971).

These findings within groups of schizophrenic patients should be seen in context. Commenting on the issue of psychiatric diagnosis as a risk factor, Casey and Keepers (1988) concluded that schizophrenic patients may be less vulnerable to tardive dyskinesia than either patients with other psychiatric disorders or individuals without psychiatric illness who are exposed to antipsychotics.

**Affective disorder.**   It has become increasingly clear that tardive dyskinesia is not seen exclusively in patients with schizophrenia; it is also seen in many other individuals receiving antipsychotic drugs for a variety of psychiatric and even nonpsychiatric conditions. This does not diminish the importance of considering the underlying central nervous system (CNS) dysfunction as playing a role in the evolution of involuntary movements, but it does necessitate integration of these cases into any generalizations regarding the etiology of tardive dyskinesia.

Davis et al. (1976) were struck by a relatively high prevalence of tardive dyskinesia among patients with primary affective disorder, especially depressed patients treated with antipsychotic drugs. From the preliminary data of the prospective study by Kane et al. (1985), psychiatric diagnosis does appear to be a relevant variable. A life-table analysis based on the length of drug administration, and comparing the cumulative incidence of tardive dyskinesia in patients with affective or schizoaffective disorder with that of patients with a diagnosis of schizophrenia, revealed that the former have a significantly greater incidence after 6 years of exposure to antipsychotic drugs. The incidence figures were 26% for affective and schizoaffective patients compared with 18% for those with schizophrenia.

Mukherjee et al. (1986) found persistent tardive dyskinesia in 35% of a sample of bipolar patients who had received maintenance antipsychotic drugs, whereas no patients without such a drug history had persistent dyskinesia. This work raises the possibility that bipolar patients treated with maintenance antipsychotic drugs may well be at a high risk for developing tardive dyskinesia, and this may tend to be the persistent type.

The accumulating evidence from these and other studies (Casey 1988a, 1988b; Rosenbaum et al. 1977; Rush et al. 1982) suggests that patients with affective disorder may be particularly at risk of tardive dyskinesia if administered long-term antipsychotic medication. Interpretation of this association is complicated, as the increased risk may not be directly related to the psychiatric diagnosis. A diagnosis of depression may be a proxy variable for intermittent antipsychotic drug administration, electroconvulsive therapy, the concurrent use of tricyclic antidepressants, or alcohol abuse, all factors that may be more common in depressed patients and underlie the vulnerability to tardive dyskinesia.

Given suggestions as to the differences in neurochemical or neurophysiological substrates of schizophrenic and affective illness, this is an area that deserves further exploration with creative strategies to address some of the potential confounds. In discussing affective disorders, it should also be noted that there is some suggestion that concurrent administration of lithium with antipsychotic drugs may help reduce the risk of tardive dyskinesia development (Kane et al. 1986).

Even within the schizophrenic patient population there have been some suggestions that the presence of a familial history of affective disorders may increase the risk of tardive dyskinesia. Wegner et al. (1985a, 1985b) reported that patients with tardive dyskinesia had a high prevalence of affective disorders among first-degree relatives compared with control subjects who did not have tardive dyskinesia. Similarly, in a small sample of young male schizophrenic patients, Richardson et al. (1985) found that a positive family history of affective disorder was associated with four times the likelihood of manifesting tardive dyskinesia. Interestingly, an earlier study by Galdi et al. (1981) found that a family history of affective illness in first-degree relatives was associated with an increased risk of developing drug-induced parkinsonian side effects.

There are various other psychiatric conditions, such as borderline personality disorder, anxiety disorders, and attention-deficit hyperactivity disorder, for which antipsychotic drugs are used in clinical practice with varying degrees of justification, but for which estimates of tardive dyskinesia prevalence or incidence are sorely lacking.

### Drug-Treatment Variables

**Drug type.** Considerable attention has been focused on drug type as to whether specific antipsychotic drugs or drug classes differ in their propensity to produce tardive dyskinesia. Unfortunately, most of this attention has focused on the implications of preclinical studies in animal models that may not be entirely analogous to the clinical condition.

We are not aware of any compelling data from prospective clinical studies that any currently available antipsychotic drug has a lower risk for tardive dyskinesia, with the possible exception of clozapine (Kane 1990). Retrospective studies are confounded by factors such as polypharmacy, uncertainties about compliance with medication, and the administration of other drugs. For example, some reports suggested that depot injectable forms of fluphenazine may carry an increased risk of tardive dyskinesia (Gardos et al. 1977; Smith et al. 1978); however, this could be an epiphenomenon of increased antipsychotic drug exposure due to guaranteed medication delivery. There are numerous other problems in drawing conclusions on the relative risk with specific drugs from studies with methodological shortcomings, such as a failure of random assignment of patients to treatment groups, a lack of systematic evaluation, and no control of such variables as length of drug exposure, dose equivalence, and age.

The long-term comparative drug studies that would be necessary to establish the relative risk of tardive dyskinesia for antipsychotic drugs would require groups of patients starting and remaining on a single antipsychotic drug for several years. Such studies have not been undertaken and would be difficult to conduct. Another, more realistic strategy would be the identification and inclusion of patients at particular risk for developing the disorder in smaller-scale studies that might produce meaningful results after relatively short intervals. Until some type of appropriately controlled methodology is applied to this question, however, it will be difficult to draw conclusions.

Clinical effects that might provide some indication of the relative risk for tardive dyskinesia with a particular drug could include the relative severity of dyskinesia provoked or exacerbated by withdrawal of the drug and the incidence figures for patients maintained on the drug alone. The ability to suppress tardive dyskinesia is common to virtually all antipsychotic drugs and is therefore unlikely to be of predictive value, although the relative rapidity with which the dyskinesia reappeared might be of interest.

Several pharmacological properties have been considered relevant. These include the relative affinities for $D_1$ and $D_2$ dopamine receptors, the ability to induce $D_2$ dopamine receptor supersensitivity, and a selective action on specific brain dopaminergic systems (Coward et al. 1989; Jenner et al. 1985). The extent to which these preclinical findings can predict the risk of tardive dyskinesia with a particular drug remains to be demonstrated.

The strongest claims for a reduced liability for tardive dyskinesia have been made for sulpiride and clozapine, and for both drugs various theories have been put forward to explain this potential advantage. Sulpiride is a substituted benzamide, a selective antagonist of $D_2$ dopamine receptors, and possibly a subgroup of these, with no significant effects on other types of receptor so far tested (Rupniak et al. 1984). Uncontrolled worldwide observations reveal only a relatively small number of patients receiving sulpiride who have developed tardive dyskinesia; however, claims for a lower risk of the condition remain to be substantiated. Clinically, the spectrum of side effects produced by the drug closely resembles other antipsychotics.

Even stronger claims for a low propensity for tardive dyskinesia have been made for clozapine. Recent data in the United States indicate that more than 15,000 patients have been treated with clozapine, and no cases of tardive dyskinesia clearly attributable to clozapine have been observed during its use (J. Schwimmer, September 1991, personal communication). In Europe there are several case reports of "dyskinesias" associated with clozapine; however, differentiation among acute, withdrawal, and tardive dyskinesias was not systematic (H. Krupp, September 1987, personal communication). Even if we were to assume that these cases represented true tardive dyskinesia, this would still represent an extremely low incidence, given the number of patients treated.

From his review of the available evidence, Casey (1988a, 1988b) also concluded that thus far the drug has a very low incidence of parkinsonism, and there are virtually no reports of akathisia or dystonia. Clozapine is associated with a relatively high rate of agranulocytosis. Experience in the United States to date reveals a cumulative incidence of 0.8% for this toxic effect after a year of treatment (Alvir and Lieberman 1991), and assiduous hematological monitoring is necessary. Considerable attention has been given to hypotheses that might explain clozapine's relative lack of extrapyramidal effects and low propensity to produce tardive dyskinesia. In the absence of clearly established pathophysiologic mechanisms, these hypotheses remain speculative. Clozapine has relatively strong affinity for $D_1$ receptors in contrast to most typical neuroleptics while also retaining some affinity for $D_2$ receptors. It is possible that this ratio is relevant to clozapine's atypical properties.

Whether the relative selectivity of drugs for $D_1$ and $D_2$ receptors is relevant to their ability to induce tardive dyskinesia remains unclear (Kistrup and Gerlach 1987). For example, from their own rodent studies, Jenner et al. (1985) considered that the low incidence of tardive dyskinesia claimed for both clozapine and sulpiride was related to the absence of change in $D_2$ function with chronic administration, coupled with an ability to enhance $D_1$ function. In the model employed by Chiodo and Bunney (1983), repeated treatment with clozapine resulted in depolarization, inactivation of $A_{10}$ neurons, but not $A_9$ neurons. Coward (1989) suggested that given the possible importance of "GABAergic" ($\gamma$-aminobutyric acid) functional involvement in the pathophysiology of tardive dyskinesia, clozapine's effects on this system may be particularly relevant. Others have suggested that clozapine's atypical properties may be due to its ratio of serotonin ($S_2$) and dopamine ($D_2$) receptor effects (Altar et al. 1983; Meltzer 1989). Any conclusions regarding these putative mechanisms must remain tentative, but the increasing availability of relatively specific receptor agonists and antagonists should help to clarify the roles of various CNS receptor systems in the clinical effects of antipsychotic medications.

**Drug dosage.** Although at some level there must be a relationship between dose, duration, and risk of tardive dyskinesia, this has been a very difficult relationship to establish. Perhaps this should not be surprising, since most patients do not develop tardive dyskinesia, so dose-response relationships would only be apparent in those individuals vulnerable to the disorder. It is likely that individual differences in the degree of vulnerability exist even within that subgroup, which may account for more than differences in dosage or duration.

The vast majority of cross-sectional studies (Jeste and Wyatt 1981) and follow-up studies (Gardos et al. 1988b) that have addressed this issue have failed to find a clear association between developing tardive dyskinesia and drug variables, such as the length of time a patient has been receiving medication, the total amount of drug administered, the type or class of drug, and current dosage (Barnes et al. 1983a, 1983b; Kane and Smith 1982; Morgenstern et al. 1987). Baldessarini et al. (1988) suggested that the absence of an apparent dose-response relationship in many studies may be due to excessive doses received by most patients. The use of high doses in most patients would tend to obscure any relationship between dose and risk of tardive dyskinesia. These authors considered that the risk of tardive dyskinesia may well turn out to be dependent on dose when low-effective doses are evaluated and excessive doses are avoided (Baldessarini et al. 1988).

Another factor relevant to the interpretation of these data is the tendency for older patients not only to be more likely to manifest tardive dyskinesia but also to be administered lower doses of antipsychotic medication. Thus, in a sample of schizophrenic inpatients, Barnes et al. (1983a, 1983b) found that those with orofacial tardive dyskinesia were apparently receiving significantly lower drug doses than those without such movements. Such a finding had been previously reported by Opler et al. (1984) and Waddington and Youssef (1986); however, this association between tardive dyskinesia and current dose of antipsychotic drug was no longer significant when a partial correlation, taking age into account, was calculated.

Kane and Smith (1982) pointed out that most studies that have reported a significant relationship between tardive dyskinesia and antipsychotic drug dosage or duration of treatment have involved samples of patients in the early years of drug treatment. It may be that the relationship between dose/duration and tardive dyskinesia is more of a factor or easier to document in the relatively early development of tardive dyskinesia as opposed to cases occurring after 5–10 years of antipsychotic drug treatment.

**Drug holidays.**  Recent emphasis on strategies to reduce cumulative antipsychotic drug exposure (see Chapter 7) has provided opportunities to explore these relationships in a more systematic, though somewhat truncated, fashion. For example, "drug holidays" for patients on long-term antipsychotic treatment was first advocated as a beneficial strategy by Ayd in 1966. He suggested that intermittent therapy might reduce the risk of developing tardive dyskinesia. The American College of Neuropsychopharmacology—Food and Drug Administration Task Force (1973) supported this notion. Originally, the concept of a drug holiday was that drugs were not taken on 1 or 2 days during each week. Given the relatively long elimination half-lives of antipsychotic drugs during chronic treatment, however, it is not clear that the intended effect would be accomplished. More important, no clinical trials have been conducted to assess the potential impact of this strategy on tardive dyskinesia. Many clinicians and investigators made intuitive assumptions that lengthier drug holidays—that is, greater than 2 months—might reduce the risk of tardive dyskinesia, but again, few data were available to address this issue. The findings of clinical studies that have investigated this treatment variable have suggested that rather than reduce the likelihood of tardive dyskinesia, interruptions of drug therapy may increase the risk of persistent dyskinesia as well as the risk of relapse (Goldman and Luchins 1984; Jeste et al. 1979a).

The recent findings of a follow-up study of a cohort of 100 patients with early tardive dyskinesia (Gardos et al. 1988a, 1988b) further complicate the picture. During an average follow-up period of 41 months, the investigators found that improvement in dyskinesia was associated with more continuous drug therapy before the onset of the condition and more drug interruptions after the tardive dyskinesia had developed. In general, the data are inadequate to allow the relative effects of interrupted and continuous drug therapy to be clearly evaluated.

**Low-dose and intermittent (targeted) treatment.**  Information on the dose-response relationship for tardive dyskinesia is also scant. Patients vulnerable to the development of the condition, perhaps on the basis of some of the risk factors already described, may develop dyskinesia on relatively modest doses of antipsychotic medication, whereas those without such a susceptibility may be at low risk of dyskinesia even when receiving doses above the normal range.

The data available from the controlled studies of low-dose drug treatment (Hogarty 1984; Hogarty et al. 1988; Kane et al. 1983; Marder et al.

1987) suggest that the potential benefits may include a reduced incidence of early signs of tardive dyskinesia as well as improved social functioning and sense of well-being. In a 1-year comparison of patients receiving standard doses of fluphenazine decanoate (12.5–50 mg every 2 weeks) or one-tenth of the usual doses, Kane et al. (1983) reported significantly fewer early signs of tardive dyskinesia on a rating scale among the patients receiving the lower dose. Marder et al. (1987) compared a basic treatment with standard dosage (25 mg fluphenazine decanoate every 2 weeks) with one-fifth of the standard dose. These investigators reported differences in parkinsonian side effects, but not tardive dyskinesia. The characteristics of schizophrenic patients who are likely to respond to low-dose drug therapy are not known. The principal risk is an increased tendency to relapse, which may not be apparent for several years if the reduction in dose is modest (Johnson et al. 1987).

Similar considerations apply to what has been called "brief intermittent" or "targeted" treatment, pioneered by Herz and Melville (1980). Maintenance medication is discontinued, but there is prompt but time-limited reinstitution of antipsychotic drug treatment when early signs of relapse appear. Patients and their relatives learn to recognize these early or "prodromal" signs. Close clinical surveillance of patients is required.

Recent studies employing an intermittent or targeted strategy have yet to be fully analyzed for the effects on tardive dyskinesia, and a large-scale study comparing intermittent, continuous low-dose, and standard-dose antipsychotic drug treatment is still under way. Carpenter et al. (1987) reported preliminary results involving 55 patients undergoing continuous antipsychotic drug treatment and 41 patients only receiving medication when early signs of relapse emerged. The probability of developing early signs of tardive dyskinesia was found to be almost three times higher in the continuously treated group. Similar studies by Herz and Glazer (1988) and Jolley et al. (1989) also found fewer signs of tardive dyskinesia in the patients receiving the intermittent treatment in the short term, but the results from follow-up for several years are required to evaluate the viability and clinical advantages and disadvantages of this treatment approach (Hirsch et al. 1990).

**Antipsychotic plasma levels.** Comparisons regarding dosage and duration are also complicated by enormous individual differences in the absorption and metabolism of antipsychotic drugs, so patients receiving similar oral doses of a particular drug may experience very different levels of active drug in relevant brain areas. This is not to suggest that blood levels are a critical factor in explaining differences in risk of tardive dyskinesia. Although some studies suggested that patients with tardive dyskinesia experienced higher blood levels following equivalent doses of antipsychotic drugs, other investigators have not found this to be the case (Dahl 1986). The point here is that comparisons between prescribed dosage regimens are a long way from accurately reflecting receptor exposure, further complicating our ability to identify dose-response curves for this disorder.

Several studies have examined the relationship between antipsychotic drug level and tardive dyskinesia, but the results are inconclusive. Most of the studies found no significant correlation (Fairbairn et al. 1983; Itoh et al. 1984; Jeste et al. 1981; Rowell et al. 1983). For example, in a small group of schizophrenic outpatients, Csernansky et al. (1983) failed to demonstrate a relationship between 1) serum neuroleptic levels and current daily dose of antipsychotic drug and 2) tardive dyskinesia. Other investigators, however, have reported that patients with tardive dyskinesia had higher drug serum levels (Jeste et al. 1982) and Smith and Leelavathi (1980) found an inverse relationship between antipsychotic plasma levels and the severity of tardive dyskinesia in a sample of 153 schizophrenic patients (possibly reflecting a masking phenomenon). Yesavage et al. (1987) found higher steady state neuroleptic levels in patients with tardive dyskinesia compared with control subjects after 5 days of fixed dose treatment.

## Concomitant Medications

**Anticholinergic drugs.** It is a common clinical observation that the addition of anticholinergic medication can exacerbate existing tardive dyskinesia and that stopping anticholinergics may improve the condition; this is supported by experimental and clinical evidence (Greil et al. 1985; Jus et al. 1977; Kane and Smith 1982; Klawans and Rubovits 1974). This observation has led to the hypothesis that these compounds might also contribute to the development of tardive dyskinesia; however, when Klawans et al. (1980) examined the evidence for the popular belief that long-term anticholinergic drug treatment predisposes a patient to develop tardive dyskinesia, they came to the conclusion that no increased prevalence of tardive dyskinesia in patients chronically treated with antiparkinsonian drugs has been definitely established. A more recent review by Gardos and Cole (1983b) also found little convincing evidence to support the notion of long-term anticholinergic medication as a risk factor for tardive dyskinesia, although this may partly reflect the lack of systematic study of this issue.

Another possible explanation for this suspected vulnerability to tardive dyskinesia associated with anticholinergic administration is that it is an epiphenomenon (Barnes 1990; Kane and Smith 1982). Anticholinergics are not administered on a random or universal basis. Patients who develop extrapyramidal side effects (EPS) are more likely to receive antiparkinsonian drugs and, as discussed elsewhere, there are data suggesting that the vulnerability to developing EPS may indicate an increased susceptibility to subsequently developing tardive dyskinesia.

It is difficult to make inferences regarding etiology based on effects on preexisting tardive dyskinesia (the ability of antipsychotic drugs to mask the condition is an example), but the chronic administration of cholinergic receptor antagonists has been shown in animal models to increase antagonist-induced supersensitivity of dopamine receptors. Evidence also suggests considerable differences among commonly used anticholinergic drugs in their relative affinities for different subtypes of muscarinic receptors—for example, the $M_1$ and $M_2$ receptors (Cortes and Palacios 1986; Gil and Wolff 1985; Schreiber et al. 1988). Further, antipsychotic drugs themselves possess varying degrees of intrinsic anticholinergic activity.

**Lithium.**    Some animal studies have explored the effect of concomitantly administered lithium on the development of dopamine receptor hypersensitivity (Pert et al. 1978). The results have been somewhat mixed with either no effect or some reduction in some measures of dopamine receptor hypersensitivity. Few clinical data are available, but in a prospective study, Kane et al. (1986) found an effect of concomitant lithium administration in reducing the incidence of tardive dyskinesia among a group of patients receiving neuroleptic treatment.

### Organic Brain Dysfunction

The extent to which preexisting evidence of CNS dysfunction may indicate increased vulnerability to tardive dyskinesia has been explored. This issue remains complicated, however, by our lack of knowledge about the presumed "organic" basis for schizophrenia itself and the various (nonbehavioral) ways in which this disease may manifest itself.

Various studies have also employed indirect or presumed measures of brain dysfunction or insult, such as epilepsy, alcoholism, relative abnormalities on brain imaging, neuropsychologic testing, and neuropathology. Some such studies have revealed an association between these indices of brain dysfunction and tardive dyskinesia (Chouinard et al. 1979; Edwards 1970; Perris et al. 1979). As a rule, one of three experimental designs has been employed: contrasting the frequency of the CNS dysfunction or abnormality measure in dyskinetic and nondyskinetic samples, contrasting the frequency of tardive dyskinesia in groups defined on the basis of a particular measure of brain dysfunction, and multiple regression analysis.

Hunter et al. (1964) and Crane and Paulson (1967) reported tardive dyskinesia to be more prevalent in patients with organic mental syndromes than in those with schizophrenia. In accord with this view, Wolf et al. (1982) reported an association between preexisting brain damage and tardive dyskinesia, specifically in patients with affective disorders. Providing further support, Yassa et al. (1984a, 1984b) examined more than 300 patients treated with antipsychotic drugs and reported a higher prevalence of tardive dyskinesia in those with organic mental syndromes, a category that included mental retardation, psychosis with alcoholism, and psychosis with epilepsy. Other investigators, however, have not found an association between diagnosed organic brain syndrome and tardive dyskinesia (Crane 1973, 1974; Fann et al. 1972; Greenblatt et al. 1968; Siede and Muller 1967).

### Structural Brain Pathology

Postmortem studies of patients with tardive dyskinesia have been infrequent, and the findings have been inconsistent (Waddington 1989). Hunter et al. (1978) reported abnormalities in one of three postmortem evaluations of patients with tardive dyskinesia, although no control subjects were employed. Christiansen et al. (1970) studied 28 patients with heterogeneous dyskinesias (21 were felt to have antipsychotic-drug-induced dyskinesias) and 28 control subjects matched by diagnoses. The patients showed a higher incidence of gliosis in the midbrain and brainstem and all degeneration in the substantia nigra as compared to control subjects. This study, however, has been criticized on a variety of methodologic grounds.

Campbell et al. (1985) reported increased evidence of iron deposition in the basal ganglia and substantia nigra in one patient with tardive dyskinesia. Arai et al. (1987) examined brains from drug-treated schizophrenic patients with orofacial dyskinesia and found markedly inflated neurons in the cerebellar dentate nucleus without accompanying neuronal loss or gliosis.

### Brain Imaging

Several investigators have reported the results of computed tomography studies in patients with tardive dyskinesia (Albus et al. 1985; Bartels and Themelis 1983; Brainin et al. 1983; Famuyiwa et al. 1979; Gelenberg 1976; Jeste et al. 1980; Kaufmann et al. 1986; Kolakowska et al. 1986; Owens et al. 1985; Sorokin et al. 1988). In general, the findings are mixed and a variety of methodologic problems also complicate the drawing of any conclusions. Waddington (1989) suggested that the positive associations found between indices of structural brain pathology—such as increased ventricular size— and measures of abnormal involuntary movement are more robust for orofacial dyskinesia than for trunk and limb dyskinesia.

More recently, the availability of magnetic resonance imaging (MRI) and positron-emission tomography (PET) has increased the potential for new knowledge in this area, but at present the techniques are sensitive to only relatively gross abnormalities and have yet to be widely applied to studies of tardive dyskinesia. An early MRI study (Besson et al. 1987) in schizophrenic patients has revealed an association between tardive dyskinesia and an increased spin lattice relaxation time ($T_1$ values) in the basal ganglia.

## Neuropsychologic Studies

The relationship between various measures of cognitive functioning and tardive dyskinesia has been addressed in several investigations. Given the fact that some degree of cognitive dysfunction is found in a substantial subgroup of patients with schizophrenia, it is not surprising that some patients with tardive dyskinesia exhibit cognitive impairment. The question remains as to whether such abnormalities are more common in schizophrenic patients who develop tardive dyskinesia than in those who do not; if so, is this a risk factor for developing tardive dyskinesia or a concomitant manifestation of neuroleptic toxicity?

Results from initial studies showing a higher rate of cognitive dysfunction in patients with tardive dyskinesia were interpreted as evidence of preexisting dementia or brain dysfunction that may place some patients at increased risk for developing tardive dyskinesia (Donnelly et al. 1981; Edwards 1970; Itil et al. 1981; Pryce and Edwards 1966). Data from a previously described prospective study (Kane et al. 1986) suggested that decreased scores on some cognitive tests were evident before the development of tardive dyskinesia and might be indicative of increased vulnerability (Struve and Willner 1983; Wegner et al. 1985a). Wegner et al. (1985b) also presented evidence that the cognitive impairment found in patients with tardive dyskinesia was associated with an increased prevalence of neurological soft signs, a history of premorbid asocial adjustment, and family loading for affective illness.

Waddington and Youssef (1986) and Waddington et al. (1987) suggested that cognitive impairment, blunted affect, and histories of muteness are seen more frequently in patients with tardive dyskinesia than in control subjects. The association between tardive dyskinesia, cognitive impairment, and other aspects of Crow's (1980) Type II subgroup have not been reported by all investigators (Gureje 1988). Waddington and Youssef (1986) and Waddington et al. (1987) did not find an association between cognitive impairment and neuroleptic treatment history variables; nor did Wade et al. (1989). Famuyiwa et al. (1979) and Thomas and McGuire (1986), however, did find a significant relationship between the degree of cognitive impairment and the duration of treatment. Thomas and McGuire (1986) reported such a relationship with a lifetime dosage of neuroleptics.

Waddington (1987) reviewed 11 studies in which schizophrenic patients with and without tardive dyskinesia underwent neuropsychological testing. Although these investigations involved a broad range of test measures and very heterogeneous patient populations, in 8 of these reports there was evidence supporting an association between cognitive dysfunction and prevalence of tardive dyskinesia. Waddington (1987) suggested that this association was more evident among patients with orofacial dyskinesia than in those with truncal and limb involvement. There have been various methodological issues that need to be addressed in this line of investigation. Many investigators failed to control for such potentially important variables as age and psychiatric diagnosis. A significant relationship between tardive dyskinesia and cognitive impairment has also been found in neuroleptic-treated bipolar patients (Waddington and Youssef 1988; Waddington et al. 1989).

A major methodologic concern in this literature has been the limitations of the cognitive test batteries themselves. Some of the major findings have come from studies with test batteries limited to one or two short cognitive screening instruments (Famuyiwa et al. 1979; Struve and Willner 1983; Waddington et al. 1987).

More extensive neuropsychological test batteries have been employed in some studies in an attempt to provide more reliable methods for detecting and characterizing cognitive deficits in patients with tardive dyskinesia. Most of those studies that assessed a wider range of cognitive functions have failed to detect significant differences between patients with and without tardive dyskinesia (Barr et al. 1987; Gold et al. 1989; Kolakowska et al. 1986; Myslobodsky 1990; Soni and Neill 1990). Some studies employing extensive neuropsychologic testing have only found significant associations when such variables as age, educational level, diagnosis, duration of illness, and duration of hospitalization have been factored out (Wade et al. 1987, 1989). Some studies have analyzed a large number of variables without sufficiently attending to the risk of a Type I error.

At present it is difficult to draw conclusions on the relationship between cognitive dysfunction and drug-induced movement disorders. Some investigators have hypothesized that the cognitive impairments seen in patients with tardive dyskinesia might be similar to those observed in movement disorders such as Huntington's disease or Parkinson's disease. We are aware of only one study that specifically attempted to test this hypothesis, and the results were negative (Wade et al. 1989). A more focused investigation of the attention, concentration, and memory deficits associated with the "subcorticol dementias" (Albert et al. 1974; Cummings and Benson 1984) would be of great interest in future studies of patients with tardive dyskinesia.

### Neurological Features

Numerous studies have reported an association between tardive dyskinesia and neurological abnormalities in terms of a B-mitten EEG pattern (Struve and Willner 1983) and EEG dysrhythmia (Wegner et al. 1979), abnormal evoked potentials (Zeithofer et al. 1984), the presence of "soft" neurological signs (Mukherjee et al. 1984; Wegner et al. 1985a, 1985b; Wilson et al. 1986), and the presence of developmental (or primitive) reflexes (Youssef and Waddington 1988).

Soft neurological signs, including such deficiencies as poor coordination, suggest neurological impairment, although they lack precise cerebral localization. Wegner et al. (1985a, 1985b) reported on a battery of tests to measure neurologic soft signs, which theoretically would not be confounded by the occurrence of dyskinetic movements, and found that schizophrenic patients with tardive dyskinesia had a significantly greater number of such signs.

Developmental reflexes—such as the grasp, palmomental, snout, corneomandibular, and glabellar reflexes—are normally present in infancy and may return with advancing age (Paulson and Gottlieb 1968). Their presence in adult life has usually been taken as evidence of cerebral immaturity or of cerebral dysfunction. These signs may be relatively common in patients with psychotic illness, and longitudinal studies of patients with psychotic illness suggest that primitive reflexes may emerge and then disappear in association with the onset and recovery of acute episodes of schizophrenic and affective psychosis (Burra et al. 1980; Keshavan and Yergani 1987; Lohr 1985).

Youssef and Waddington (1988) examined 66 patients with schizophrenia (mean age 67 years) and 18 patients with bipolar affective disorder and found that in both diagnostic groups, patients with orofacial tardive dyskinesia showed a significant excess of developmental reflexes compared with control subjects.

Chrichton et al. (1991) examined this relationship in 48 chronic schizophrenic patients (mean age 45 years), a somewhat younger sample than the schizophrenic patients studied by Youssef and Waddington (1988). Although the proportion of patients with two or more developmental reflexes was similar in the two studies (23% and 26%, respectively), Chrichton et al. (1991) found no significant association between orofacial dyskinesia and the presence or number of developmental reflexes.

### Early-Onset Movement Disorders

An intriguing hypothesis, first suggested by Crane (1972), is that those patients who evidence the greatest vulnerability to early antipsychotic drug-induced EPS are at greatest risk of subsequently developing tardive dyskinesia. The assumption that dopamine receptor blockade plays some role in each is also consistent with this possibility.

The literature contains few investigations that directly examine this issue. Jus et al. (1976) reported that in a sample of more than 300 patients the prevalence of a previous history of antipsychotic-drug-induced EPS was the same in patients with and without tardive dyskinesia. Nevertheless, Kane (1990), Kane et al. (1986), and Saltz et al. (1991) found, among both young adults and elderly subjects participating in two separate prospective studies, that early occurrence of these adverse effects appears to be associated with at least a threefold increase in the risk of tardive dyskinesia development.

Based on their clinical observations, Chouinard et al. (1979) concluded that patients with tremor or akathisia, which they described as "hyperkinetic" symptoms, of parkinsonism, were more likely to manifest tardive dyskinesia than patients with "hypokinetic" symptoms such as bradykinesia and rigidity. DeVeaugh-Geiss (1982) elaborated on this idea, suggesting that, in some cases, akathisia represented a stage in a progression from parkinsonism to the development of orofacial and trunk and limb dyskinesia. Consistent with this notion, Barnes and Braude (1985) found a significant association between choreoathetoid limb dyskinesia, orofacial dyskinesia, and the presence of chronic akathisia, in a sample of chronic schizophrenic outpatients. These investigators (Barnes and Braude 1984) also described two cases in which the appearance of akathisia at the beginning of drug therapy, which then persisted despite the reduction of drug dosage to maintenance levels, seemed to herald the early onset of tardive dyskinesia. A single case report from Goswami and Channabasavanna (1984) described a man with bipolar affective disorder who exhibited severe akathisia on therapeutic serum levels of lithium and then developed orofacial dyskinesia 2 weeks later, following additional treatment with an anticholinergic.

Similarly, from case-report material, Nasrallah et al. (1980) and Munetz (1980) raised the possibility that the appearance of acute dystonic reactions might predict a future predisposition to tardive dyskinesia. Thus various study findings and case reports suggest that those patients presenting with symptoms of parkinsonism, acute akathisia, and acute dystonic reactions early in treatment are more likely to manifest tardive dyskinesia with continued antipsychotic medication.

## Summary and Conclusions

Available epidemiologic data do suggest that neuroleptic drugs play an important role in producing or evoking abnormal involuntary movements in some patients. It is also clear that some individuals with schizophrenia and other psychotic disorders may have or develop abnormal involuntary movements unassociated with long-term treatment with antipsychotic drugs. This highlights the importance of carefully examining patients prior to initiating treatment with any dopamine antagonists in order to determine and document the presence of any existing abnormal involuntary movements.

Considerable progress has been made in recent years in developing prospective studies to provide better estimates of incidence and more meaningful data with regard to risk factors. The increasing cumulative incidence with increasing lengths of neuroleptic exposure again argues for the role of neuroleptics in the development of this condition. It is also clear that the incidence is significantly higher in elderly individuals. With regard to risk factors other than age, early occurrence of EPS has emerged in several studies as an important indicator of increased future risk of developing tardive dyskinesia.

Although the number of relevant studies is limited and there are various methodologic problems, it appears that patients with affective disorders may be at particular risk for the development of tardive dyskinesia. This is important clinically in assessing the benefit-to-risk ratio of neuroleptic treatment in such patients and also suggests that the occurrence of apparent drug-related movement disorders is not confined to schizophrenic patients.

The risk of tardive dyskinesia appears to be higher in older women, but the sex effect is not seen in every study and is not consistently found in every decade in late life.

With regard to drug-treatment variables, the results of dosage-reduction studies provide some encouragement but are also viewed by many as disappointing in their relative impact on the incidence of tardive dyskinesia. The problem here remains one of methodology, however, in that the impact of preventive strategies is difficult to document in a sample of patients, many of whom may not be at particular risk for the development of tardive dyskinesia during the course of the investigation. If studies were focused on individuals at increased risk, then the impact of preventive strategies might be easier to detect and more robust. At present there are limited data supporting significantly different degrees of risk associated with specific antipsychotic drugs or drug classes; however, sulpiride and clozapine appear to hold some promise in this regard. It is hoped that future studies will allow more definitive conclusions.

The last decade has provided considerable new data on the long-term outcome of tardive dyskinesia. Here, the results have provided some reassurance that this disorder, in most cases, is nonprogressive and that even with continued neuroleptic administration there may be improvement over time (particularly if the lowest effective dosage can be employed).

This does not diminish the potential importance of discontinuing neuroleptic drugs when feasible, but for those patients in whom benefit is sufficient to warrant continued administration, clinicians are unlikely to see a worsening of the condition. The problem remains, however, that a subgroup of patients do develop a severe and disabling form of the condition, and efforts to identify such patients remain critical.

# References

Albert ML, Feldman RG, Willis AL: The "subcortical dementia" of progressive supranuclear palsy. J Neurol Neurosurg Psychiatry 37:121–130, 1974

Albus M, Naber D, Muller-Spahn E, et al: Tardive dyskinesia: relation to computer tomographic, endocrine and psychopathological variables. Biol Psychiatry 20:1082–1089, 1985

Altar CA, Wasley DM, Neale RF, et al: Typical and atypical antipsychotic occupancy of D-2 and S-2 receptors: an auto-radiographic study in rat brain. Brain Res Bull 16:517–525, 1983

American College of Neuropsychopharmacology—Food and Drug Administration Task Force: Neurological syndromes associated with antipsychotic drug use. N Engl J Med 289:20–23, 1973

Arai N, Amano N, Iseki E, et al: Tardive dyskinesia with inflated neurons of the cerebellar dentate nucleus: case reports and morphometric study. Acta Neuropathol 73:38–42, 1987

Ayd FJ: Drug holidays: intermittent pharmacotherapy for psychiatric patients. Int Drug Ther Newsletter 8:1–3, 1966

Baldessarini RJ, Cohen BM, Teicher MH: Significance of neuroleptic dose and plasma level in the pharmacological treatment of psychosis. Arch Gen Psychiatry 45:79–91, 1988

Barnes TRE: The present status of tardive dyskinesia and akathisia in the treatment of schizophrenia. Psychiatric Developments 4:301–319, 1987

Barnes TRE: Tardive dyskinesia: risk factors, pathophysiology and treatment, in Recent Advances in Clinical Psychiatry 6. Edited by Granville-Grossman K. London, Churchill Livingstone, 1988, pp 185–207

Barnes TRE: Comment on the WHO Consensus Statement. Br J Psychiatry 156:413–414, 1990

Barnes TRE, Braude WM: Persistent akathisia associated with early tardive dyskinesia. Postgrad Med J 60:51–53, 1984

Barnes TRE, Braude WM: Akathisia variants and tardive dyskinesia. Arch Gen Psychiatry 42:874–878, 1985

Barnes TRE, Liddle PF: Tardive dyskinesia: implications for schizophrenia?, in Schizophrenia: New Pharmacological and Clinical Development. Edited by Schiff AA, Roth M, Freeman HL. London, Royal Society of Medicine Services, 1985, pp 81–87

Barnes TRE, Wiles DH: Variation in orofacial tardive dyskinesia during depot antipsychotic drug treatment. Psychopharmacology 81:359–362, 1983

Barnes TRE, Kidger T, Gore SM: Tardive dyskinesia: a 3-year follow-up study. Psychol Med 13:71–81, 1983a

Barnes TRE, Rossor M, Trauer T: A comparison of purposeless movements in psychiatric patients treated with antipsychotic drugs, and normal individuals. J Neurol Neurosurg Psychiatry 46:540–546, 1983b

Barnes TRE, Liddle PF, Curson DA, et al: Negative symptoms, tardive dyskinesia and depression in chronic schizophrenia. Br J Psychiatry 155 (suppl 7):99–103, 1989a

Barnes TRE, Curson DA, Liddle PF, et al: The nature and prevalence of depression in chronic schizophrenic inpatients. Br J Psychiatry 154:486–491, 1989b

Barr WB, Mukherjee M, Caracci G, et al: Neuropsychological studies in tardive dyskinesia: a possible relationship with anomalous dominance (abstract). Society of Biological Psychiatry 42nd Annual Convention and Scientific Program, 295, 1987

Barron ET, McCreadie RG: One-year follow-up of tardive dyskinesia. Br J Psychiatry 143:423–424, 1983

Bartels M, Themelis J: Computerized tomography in tardive dyskinesia. Evidence of structural abnormalities in the basal ganglia. Arch Psychiatr Nervenkr 233:371–379, 1983

Besson JAO, Corrigan FM, Cherryman GR, et al: Nuclear magnetic resonance brain imaging in chronic schizophrenia. Br J Psychiatry 150:161–163, 1987

Bleuler E: Dementia Praecox or the Group of Schizophrenias. 1911 Edition. Translated by Zinkin J. New York, International Universities Press, 1950

Blowers AJ: Epidemiology of tardive dyskinesia in the elderly. Neuropharmacology 20:1339–1340, 1981

Blowers AJ, Borison RL, Blowers CM, et al: Abnormal involuntary movements in the elderly. Br J Psychiatry 139:363–364, 1982

Bourgeois M, Bouilh P, Tignol J, et al: Spontaneous dyskinesia versus neuroleptic-induced dyskinesia in 270 elderly subjects. J Nerv Ment Dis 168:177–178, 1980a

Bourgeois M, Boueilh P, Tignol J: Dyskinesies spontanees senile idiopathiques et dyskinesies tardive des neuroleptiques. L'Encephale 6:37–39, 1980b

Brainin M, Reisner IT, Zeithofer J: Tardive dyskinesia: clinic correlation with computed tomography in patients aged less than 60 years. J Neurol Neurosurg Psychiatry 46:1037–1040, 1983

Brandon S, McClelland MA, Protheroe C: A study of facial dyskinesia in a mental hospital population. Br J Psychiatry 118:171–184, 1971

Burra P, Powles WE, Riopelle RJ, et al: Atypical psychoses with reversible primitive reflexes. Am J Psychiatry 25:74–77, 1980

Campbell M, Grega DM, Green WH, et al: Review: neuroleptic-induced dyskinesias in children. Clinical Neuropharmacology 6:207–222, 1983

Campbell WG, Raskin MA, Gordan T, et al: Iron pigment in the brain of a man with tardive dyskinesia. Am J Psychiatry 142:364–365, 1985

Carpenter WT, Heinrichs DW, Hanlan TE: A comparative trial of pharmacologic strategies in schizophrenia. Am J Psychiatry 144:1466–1470, 1987

Casey DE: Tardive dyskinesia: reversible and irreversible, in Dyskinesia—Research and Treatment. Edited by Casey DE, Chase TN, Christensen AV, et al. Berlin, Springer-Verlag, 1985, pp 88–97

Casey DE: Neuroleptic-induced EPS and TD. Paper presented at Clozapine (Leponex/Clozaril) Scientific Update meeting. Montreux, Switzerland, October 31–November 1, 1988a

Casey DE: Affective disorders and tardive dyskinesia. L'Encephale 14:221–226, 1988b

Casey DE, Gardos G: Tardive dyskinesia: outcome at 10 years. Schizophr Res 3:11, 1990

Casey DE, Gerlach J: Tardive dyskinesia: what is the long-term outcome, in Tardive Dyskinesia and Neuroleptics: From Dogma to Reason. Edited by Casey DE, Gardos G. Washington, DC, American Psychiatric Press, 1986, pp 75–97

Casey DE, Keepers GA: Neuroleptic side effects: acute extrapyramidal syndromes and tardive dyskinesia, in Psychopharmacology: Current Trends. Edited by Casey DE, Christensen AV. Berlin, Springer-Verlag, 1988, pp 74–93

Chiodo LA, Bunney BS: Typical and atypical neuroleptics: differential effects of chronic administration on the activity of A9 and A10 midbrain dopaminergic neurons. J Neurosci 3:1607–1619, 1983

Chouinard G, Jones BD: Neuroleptic-induced supersensitivity psychosis: clinical and pharmacologic characteristics. Am J Psychiatry 137:16–21, 1980

Chouinard G, Annable L, Ross-Chouinard A, et al: Factors related to tardive dyskinesia. Am J Psychiatry 136:79–83, 1979

Chouinard G, Annable L, Mercier P, et al: A five-year follow-up study of tardive dyskinesia. Psychopharmacol Bull 22:259–263, 1986

Chrichton P, Barnes TRE, Nelson HE, et al: Primitive reflexes, tardive dyskinesia, and intellectual impairment in schizophrenia. Paper presented at the annual meeting of the Royal College of Psychiatrists, Brighton, England, July 1991

Christiansen E, Moller J, Faurbye A: Neuropathological investigation of 28 brains from patients with dyskinesia. Acta Psychiatr Scand 46:14–23, 1970

Collerton D, Fairbairn A, Britton P: Cognitive performance of medicated schizophrenics with tardive dyskinesia. Psychol Med 15:311–315, 1985

Cortes R, Palacios JM: Muscarinic cholinergic receptor subtypes in the rat brain: quantitative autoradiographic studies. Brain Res 362:227–238, 1986

Coward DM, Imperato A, Urwyler S, et al: Biochemical and behavioural properties of clozapine. Psychopharmacology 99:S6–S12, 1989

Craig TJ, Richardson MA, Pass R, et al: Measurement of mood and affect in schizophrenic patients. Am J Psychiatry 142:1272–1277, 1985

Crane GE: Pseudoparkinsonism and tardive dyskinesia. Arch Neurol 27:426–430, 1972

Crane GE: Persistent dyskinesia. Br J Psychiatry 122:395–405, 1973

Crane GE: Factors predisposing to drug-induced neurological effects, in The Phenothiazines and Structurally Related Drugs. Edited by Forrest IS, Carr CV, Usdin E. New York, Raven, 1974, pp 269–279

Crane GE, Paulson G: Involuntary movements in a sample of chronic mental patients and their relation to the treatment with neuroleptics. Int J Neurol 3:286–291, 1967

Crow TJ: Molecular pathology of schizophrenia: more than one disease process? Br Med J 280:66–68, 1980

Csernansky JG, Kaplan J, Holman CA, et al: Serum neuroleptic activity, prolactin and tardive dyskinesia in schizophrenic outpatients. Psychopharmacology 81:115–118, 1983

Cummings JL, Benson DF: Subcortical dementia: review of an emerging concept. Arch Neurol 41:874–879, 1984

Dahl SG: Plasma level monitoring of antipsychotic drugs: clinical utility. Clin Pharmacokinetics 11:36–61, 1986

Davis KL, Rosenberg GS: Is there a limbic system equivalent of tardive dyskinesia? Biol Psychiatry 14:699–703, 1979

Davis K, Berger P, Hollister L: Tardive dyskinesia and depressive illness. Psychopharmacol Communications 2:125–130, 1976

Davison K, Bagley C: Schizophrenia-like psychoses associated with organic disorders of the CNS: a review of the literature, in Current Problems in Neuropsychiatry. Edited by Herrington RN. (Br J Psychiatry Special Publ No 4). Ashford, Kent, UK, Headley Brothers, 1969, pp 113–184

Delwaide PJ, Desseilles M: Spontaneous buccolinguofacial dyskinesia in the elderly. Acta Neurol Scand 56:256–262, 1977

DeVeaugh-Geiss J: Prediction and prevention of tardive dyskinesia, in Tardive Dyskinesia and Related Involuntary Movement Disorders. Edited by DeVeaugh-Geiss J. Bristol, UK, John Wright, 1982, pp 161–178

Donnelly EF, Jeste DV, Wyatt RJ: Tardive dyskinesia and perceptual dysfunction. Percept Mot Skills 53:689–690, 1981

Edwards H: The significance of brain damage in oral dyskinesia. Br J Psychiatry 116:271–275, 1970

Engelhardt DM, Polizos P, Waizer J: CNS consequences of psychotropic drug withdrawal in autistic children: a follow-up report. Psychopharmacol Bull 11:6–7, 1975

Fairbairn AF, Rowell FJ, Hui SM, et al: Serum concentration of depot neuroleptics in tardive dyskinesia. Br J Psychiatry 142:579–583, 1983

Famuyiwa OO, Eccleston D, Donaldson AA, et al: Tardive dyskinesia and dementia. Br J Psychiatry 135:500–504, 1979

Fann WE, Davis JM, Janowsky DS: The prevalence of tardive dyskinesia in mental hospital patients. Diseases of the Nervous System 33:182–186, 1972

Farran-Ridge C: Some symptoms referrable to the basal ganglia occurring in dementia praecox and epidemic encephalitis. J Mental Science 72:513–523, 1926

Galdi J, Rieder RO, Silber D, et al: Genetic factors in response to neuroleptics: a psychopharmacogenetic study. Psychol Med 11:713–728, 1981

Gardos G, Cole JO: The prognosis of tardive dyskinesia. J Clin Psychiatry 44:177–179, 1983a

Gardos G, Cole JO: Tardive dyskinesia and anticholinergic drugs. Am J Psychiatry 140:200–202, 1983b

Gardos G, Cole JO, La Brie RA: Drug variables in the etiology of tardive dyskinesia: application of discriminant function analysis. Prog Neuro-psychopharmacol 1:147–154, 1977

Gardos G, Perenyi A, Cole JO, et al: Seven-year follow-up of tardive dyskinesia in Hungarian outpatients. Neuropsychopharmacology 1:169–172, 1988a

Gardos G, Cole JO, Haskell D, et al: The natural history of tardive dyskinesia. J Clin Psychopharmacol 8 (suppl 4):31–33, 1988b

Gelenberg AJ: Computerized tomography in patients with tardive dyskinesia. Am J Psychiatry 133:578–579, 1976

Gil DW, Wolff BB: Pirenzepine distinguishes between muscarinic receptor-mediated phosphoinositide breakdown and inhibition of adenylate cyclase. J Pharmacol Exp Ther 232:608–616, 1985

Glazer WM, Moore DC, Schooler NR, et al: Tardive dyskinesia, a discontinuation study. Arch Gen Psychiatry 41:623–627, 1984

Glazer WM, Morgenstern H, Schooler N, et al: Predictors of improvement in tardive dyskinesia following discontinuation of neuroleptic medication. Br J Psychiatry 157:585–592, 1990

Glazer WM, Morgenstern H, Doucette JT: The prediction of chronic persistent versus intermittent tardive dyskinesia: a retrospective follow-up study. Br J Psychiatry 158:822–828, 1991

Gold J, Egan M, Goldberg T, et al: Cognitive impairment and tardive dyskinesia (abstract). Schizophr Res 2:236, 1989

Goldman MB, Luchins DJ: Intermittent neuroleptic therapy and tardive dyskinesia: a literature review. Hosp Community Psychiatry 35:1215–1219, 1984

Goswami U, Channabasavanna SM: Is akathisia a forerunner of tardive dyskinesia? Clin Neurol Neurosurg 86:107–110, 1984

Greenblatt DL, Dominick RN, Stotsky BA, et al: Phenothiazine-induced dyskinesia in nursing-home patients. J Am Geriatr Soc 16:27–34, 1968

Greil W, Haag H, Rossnagl G, et al: Effect of anticholinergics on tardive dyskinesia: a controlled study. Br J Psychiatry 145:304–310, 1985

Gualtieri CT, Guimond M: Tardive dyskinesia and behavioral consequences of chronic neuroleptic treatment. Developmental Medicine and Child Neurology 23:225–259, 1981

Gualtieri CT, Hawk B: Tardive dyskinesia and other drug-induced movement disorders among handicapped children and youth. J App Res Ment Ret 1:55–69, 1980

Gualtieri CT, Quade D, Hicks RE, et al: Tardive dyskinesia and the clinical consequences of neuroleptic treatment in children and adolescents. Am J Psychiatry 141:21–23, 1984

Gualtieri CT, Schroeder SR, Hicks RE, et al: Tardive dyskinesia in young mentally retarded individuals. Arch Gen Psychiatry 43:335–340, 1986

Gureje O: Topographic subtypes of tardive dyskinesia in schizophrenic patients aged less than 60 years: relationship to demographic, clinical, treatment and neuropsychological variables. J Neurol Neurosurg Psychiatry 51:1525–1530, 1988

Guy W, Ban TA, Wilson WH: The prevalence of abnormal involuntary movements among chronic schizophrenics. Int Clin Psychopharmacol 1:134–144, 1986

Herz MI, Melville C: Relapse in schizophrenia. Am J Psychiatry 137:801–805, 1980

Herz MI, Glazer W: Intermittent medication in schizophrenia—preliminary results. Schizophr Res 1:224–225, 1988

Hirsch SR, Jolley AG, Morrison E, et al: Trial of brief intermittent neuroleptic prophylaxis for selected outpatients: clinical and social outcome at 2 years. Schizophr Res 3:40, 1990

Hogarty GE: Depot neuroleptics: the relevance of psychosocial factors—a United States prospective. J Clin Psychiatry 45(5):36–42, 1984

Hogarty GE, Macave JP, Munetz M, et al: Dose of fluphenazine, familial expressed emotion, and outcome in schizophrenia. Arch Gen Psychiatry 45:797–805, 1988

Hruska RE: Sex hormone exposure and non-reproductive behavior. Int J Mental Health 14:112–134, 1985

Hunter R, Earl CJ, Thornicroft S: An apparently irreversible syndrome of abnormal movements following phenothiazine medication. Proc R Soc Med 57:758–762, 1964

Hunter R, Blackwood W, Smith MC, et al: Neuropathological findings in three cases of persistent dyskinesia following phenothiazine medication. J Neurol Sci 7:268–273, 1978

Iager AC, Kirsch DG, Jeste DV, et al: Defect symptoms and abnormal involuntary movements in schizophrenia. Biol Psychiatry 21:751–755, 1986

Itil TM, Reisberg B, Huque M, et al: Clinical profiles of tardive dyskinesia. Compr Psychiatry 22:282–290, 1981

Itoh H, Yagi G, Tateyama M, et al: Monitoring of haloperidol serum levels and its clinical significance. Prog Neuropsychopharmacol Biol Psychiatry 8:51–62, 1984

Jenner P, Rupniak NMJ, Marsden CD: Differential alteration of striatal D-1 and D-2 receptors induced by the long-term administration of haloperidol, sulpiride or clozapine to rats, in Dyskinesia—Research and Treatment. Edited by Casey DE, Chase TN, Christensen AV, et al. Berlin, Springer-Verlag, 1985, pp 174–181

Jeste DV, Wyatt RJ: Changing epidemiology of tardive dyskinesia: an overview. Am J Psychiatry 138:297–309, 1981

Jeste DV, Wyatt RJ: Therapeutic strategies against tardive dyskinesia. Arch Gen Psychiatry 39:803–816, 1982

Jeste DV, Potkin SG, Sinha S, et al: Tardive dyskinesia, reversible and persistent. Arch Gen Psychiatry 36:585–590, 1979a

Jeste DV, Rosenblatt JE, Wagner RL, et al: High serum neuroleptic levels in tardive dyskinesia (letter). N Engl J Med 301:1184, 1979b

Jeste DV, Weinberger DR, Zaclam S, et al: Computed tomography in tardive dyskinesia. Br J Psychiatry 136:606–608, 1980

Jeste DV, Linnoila M, Wagner RL, et al: Serum neuroleptic concentrations and tardive dyskinesia. Psychopharmacology 76:377–386, 1982

Jeste DV, De Lisi LE, Zaleman S, et al: A biochemical study of tardive dyskinesia in young male patients. Psychiatry Res 4:327–331, 1981

Jeste DV, Jeste SD, Wyatt RJ: Reversible tardive dyskinesia: implications for therapeutic strategy and prevention of tardive dyskinesia, in New Directions in Tardive Dyskinesia Research. Edited by Bannet J, Belmaker RH. Basel, Switzerland, Karger, 1983, pp 34–48

Jeste DV, Karson CM, Iager AC, et al: Association of abnormal involuntary movements and negative symptoms. Psychopharmacol Bull 20:380–381, 1984

Johnson DAW, Ludlow JM, Street K, et al: Double-blind comparison of half-dose and standard-dose flupenthixol decanoate in the maintenance treatment of stabilized outpatients with schizophrenia. Br J Psychiatry 151:634–663, 1987

Jolley AG, Hirsch SR, McRink A, et al: Trial of brief intermittent neuroleptic prophylaxis for selected schizophrenic outpatients: clinical outcome at one year follow-up. Br Med J 298:985–990, 1989

Jones M, Hunter R: Abnormal movements in patients with chronic psychiatric illness, in Psychotropic Drugs and Dysfunction of the Basal Ganglia (U.S. Public Health Service Publication No. 1938). Edited by Crane GE, Gardner RE. Washington, DC, U.S. Public Health Service, 1969, pp 53–65

Jus A, Pineau R, Lachance R, et al: Epidemiology of tardive dyskinesia, part I. Diseases of the Nervous System 37:210–214, 1976

Jus A, Gautier J, Villeneuve A, et al: Chronology of combined neuroleptics and antiparkinsonian administration. Am J Psychiatry 134:1157, 1977

Jus A, Jus K, Fontaine P: Long-term treatment of tardive dyskinesia. J Clin Psychiatry 40:72–77, 1979

Kahlbaum KL: Die Katatonie Oder das Spannungsirresein. Berlin, Hirschwald, 1974

Kalachnik JE, Harder SR, Kidd-Nielson P, et al: Persistent TD in randomly assigned neuroleptic reduction, neuroleptic no-reduction and no-neuroleptic history groups: preliminary results. Psychopharmacol Bull 20:27–32, 1984

Kane J: Tardive dyskinesia. Paper presented at the annual meeting of the New Clinical Drug Evaluation Unit, Key Biscayne, FL, June 1990

Kane JM, Smith JM: Tardive dyskinesia: prevalence and risk factors, 1959–1979. Arch Gen Psychiatry 39:473–481, 1982

Kane JM, Weinhold P, Kinon B, et al: Prevalence of abnormal involuntary movements ("spontaneous dyskinesia") in the normal elderly. Psychopharmacology 77:105–108, 1982

Kane JM, Rifkin A, Woerner M, et al: Low-dose neuroleptic treatment of outpatient schizophrenics. Arch Gen Psychiatry 40:893–896, 1983

Kane J, Woerner M, Weinhold P, et al: Incidence of tardive dyskinesia: five year data from a prospective study. Psychopharmacol Bull 20:387–389, 1984

Kane JM, Woerner M, Leiberman J: Tardive dyskinesia: prevalence, incidence and risk factors, in Dyskinesia—Research and Treatment. Edited by Casey DE, Chase TN, Christensen AV, et al. Berlin, Springer-Verlag, 1985, pp 72–78

Kane J, Woerner M, Borenstein M: Integrating incidence and prevalence of tardive dyskinesia. Psychopharmacol Bull 22:254–258, 1986

Kane JM, Honigfeld G, Singer J, et al: Clozapine for the treatment-resistant schizophrenic. Arch Gen Psychiatry 45:789–796, 1988

Kaufmann CA, Jeste DV, Shelton RC, et al: Noradrenergic and neuroradiologic abnormalities in tardive dyskinesia. Biol Psychiatry 21:799–812, 1986

Kennedy PF, Hershon HI, McGuire RJ: Extrapyramidal disorders after prolonged phenothiazine therapy. Br J Psychiatry 118:509–518, 1971

Keshavan MS, Yergani VK: Primitive reflexes in psychiatry. Lancet 1:1264, 1987

Kidger T, Barnes TRE, Trauer T, et al: Subsyndromes of tardive dyskinesia. Psychol Med 10:513–520, 1980

Kistrup K, Gerlach J: Selective $D_1$ and $D_2$ receptor manipulation in cebus monkeys: relevance for dystonia and dyskinesia in humans. Pharmacol Toxicol 61:157–161, 1987

Klawans HL, Barr A: Prevalence of spontaneous lingual-facial-buccal dyskinesia in the elderly. Neurology 32:558–559, 1982

Klawans HL, Rubovits R: Effect of cholinergic and anticholinergic agents on tardive dyskinesia. J Neurol Neurosurg Psychiatry 27:741–747, 1974

Klawans HL, Goetz CG, Perlik S: Tardive dyskinesia, review and update. Am J Psychiatry 137:900–908, 1980

Kleist K: Studies of Psychomotor Symptoms in Mental Patients. Leipzig, Germany, Klinkhardt, 1908

Kolakowska T, Williams AO, Ardern M, et al: Tardive dyskinesia in schizophrenics under 60 years of age. Biol Psychiatry 21:161–169, 1986

Kraepelin EP: Dementia Praecox and Paraphrenia. Translated by Barclay RM. Edited by Robertson GM. Edinburgh, E & S Livingstone, 1919

Levine J, Schooler N, Severe J, et al: Discontinuation of oral and depot fluphenazine in schizophrenic patients after one year of continuous medication: a controlled study. Psychopharmacology 24:483–493, 1980

Lieberman J, Kane J, Woerner M, et al: Prevalence of tardive dyskinesia in elderly patients. Psychopharmacol Bull 20:22–26, 1984a

Lieberman J, Kane J, Woerner M, et al: Prevalence of tardive dyskinesia in elderly samples. Psychopharmacol Bull 20:382–386, 1984b

Lindenmayer JP, Kay SR: Depression, affect and negative symptoms in schizophrenia. Br J Psychiatry 155 (suppl 7):108–114, 1989

Lindenmayer JP, Kay SR, Opler L: Positive and negative subtypes in acute schizophrenia. Compr Psychiatry 25:455–464, 1984

Lohr JB: Transient grasp reflexes in schizophrenia. Biol Psychiatry 20:172–175, 1985

Marder SR, Van Putten T, Mintz J: Low- and conventional-dose maintenance therapy with fluphenazine decanoate: two-year outcome. Arch Gen Psychiatry 44:518–521, 1987

Marsden CD: Is tardive dyskinesia a unique disorder?, in Dyskinesia—Research and Treatment. Edited by Casey DE, Chase TN, Christensen AV, et al. Berlin, Springer-Verlag, 1985, pp 64–71

Marsden CD, Tarsy D, Baldessarini RJ: Spontaneous and drug-induced movement disorders in psychotic patients, in Psychiatric Aspects of Neurological Disease. Edited by Benson DF, Blumer D. New York, Grune & Stratton, 1975, pp 219–266

McAndrew JB, Case Q, Treffert DA: Effects of prolonged phenothiazine intake on psychotic and other hospitalized children. J Autism Childhood Schizophrenia 2:75–91, 1972

McCreadie RG, Barron ET, Winslow GS: The Nithsdale schizophrenia survey, II: abnormal movements. Br J Psychiatry 140:587–590, 1982

McKenna PJ, Lund CE, Mortimer AM: Negative symptoms: relationships to other schizophrenic symptom classes. Br J Psychiatry 155 (suppl 7):104–107, 1989

Mehta D, Mehta S, Mathew P: Tardive dyskinesia in psychogeriatric patients: a five-year follow-up. J Am Geriatr Soc 25:545–547, 1977

Meltzer HY: Clinical studies on the mechanism of action of clozapine: the dopamine serotonin hypothesis of schizophrenia. Psychopharmacology 99:S18–S27, 1989

Molsa PK, Martilla RJ, Rinne UK: Extrapyramidal symptoms in dementia. Acta Neurol Scand 65 (suppl 90):298–299, 1982

Molsa PK, Martilla RJ, Rinne UK: Extrapyramidal signs in Alzheimer's disease. Neurology 34:1114–1116, 1984

Morgenstern H, Glazer WM, Gibowski LD, et al: Predictors of tardive dyskinesia: results of a cross-sectional study in an outpatient population. J Chronic Dis 40:319–327, 1987

Mukherjee S, Shukla S, Rosen A: Neurological abnormalities in patients with bipolar disorder. Biol Psychiatry 19:337–345, 1984

Mukherjee S, Rosen AM, Caracci G, et al: Persistent tardive dyskinesia in bipolar patients. Arch Gen Psychiatry 43:342–346, 1986 .

Munetz MR: Oculogyric crisis and tardive dyskinesia. Am J Psychiatry 137:1628, 1980

Myslobodsky MS: Anosognosia in tardive dyskinesia: "tardive dysmentia" or "tardive dementia." Schizophr Bull 12:1–6, 1986

Nasrallah HA, Pappas NJ, Crowe BR: Oculogyric dystonia in tardive dyskinesia. Am J Psychiatry 137:850–851, 1980

Opler LA, Kay SR, Rosado V, et al: Positive and negative syndromes in chronic schizophrenic patients. J Nerv Ment Dis 172:317–325, 1984

Owens DGC: Involuntary disorders of movement in chronic schizophrenia: the role of the illness and its treatment, in Dyskinesia: Research and Treatment. Edited by Casey DE, Chase TN, Christensen AV, et al. Berlin, Springer-Verlag, 1985, pp 79–87

Owens DGC, Johnstone EC: The disabilities of chronic schizophrenics: their nature and the factors contributing to their development. Br J Psychiatry 136:384–395, 1980

Owens DG, Johnstone EC, Frith CD: Spontaneous involuntary disorders of movement. Arch Gen Psychiatry 39:452–461, 1982

Owens DGC, Johnstone EC, Crow TJ, et al: Lateral ventricular size in schizophrenia: relationship to the disease process and its clinical manifestations. Psychol Med 15:27–41, 1985

Paulson G, Gottlieb G: Developmental reflexes: the reappearance of foetal and neonatal reflexes in aged patients. Brain 91:37–52, 1968

Paulson GW, Rizvi CA, Crane GE: Tardive dyskinesia as a possible sequel of long-term therapy with phenothiazines. Clin Pediatr 14:953–955, 1975

Perris C, Dimitrijevic P, Jacobsson L, et al: Tardive dyskinesia in psychiatric patients treated with neuroleptics. Br J Psychiatry 135:509–514, 1979

Perry R, Campbell M, Green WH, et al: Neuroleptic-related dyskinesia in autistic children: a prospective study. Psychopharmacol Bull 21:140–143, 1985

Pert A, Rosenblatt JE, Sivit C, et al: Long-term treatment with lithium prevents the development of dopamine receptor supersensitivity. Science 201:171–173, 1978

Polizos P, Engelhardt D: Dyskinetic phenomena in children treated with psychotropic medications. Psychopharmacol Bull 14(4):65–68, 1978

Polizos P, Engelhardt DM: Dyskinetic and neuroleptic complications in children treated with psychotropic medication, in Tardive Dyskinesia: Research and Treatment. Edited by Fann WE, Smith RC, Davis JM, et al. New York, Spectrum, 1980, pp 193–199

Polizos P, Engelhardt DM, Hoffman SP, et al: Neurological consequences of psychotropic drug withdrawal in schizophrenic children. J Autism Childhood Schizophrenia 3:247–253, 1973

Prosser ES, Csernansky JG, Kaplan J, et al: Depression, parkinsonian symptoms and negative symptoms in schizophrenics treated with neuroleptics. J Nerv Ment Dis 175:100–105, 1987

Pryce IG, Edwards H: Persistent oral dyskinesia in female mental hospital patients. Br J Psychiatry 112:48–54, 1966

Richardson MA, Casey DE: Tardive dyskinesia status: stability or change. Psychopharmacol Bull 24:471–475, 1988

Richardson MA, Pass R, Craig TJ, et al: Factors influencing the prevalence and severity of tardive dyskinesia. Psychopharmacol Bull 20:33–38, 1984

Richardson MA, Pass R, Bregman Z, et al: Tardive dyskinesia and depressive symptoms in schizophrenics. Psychopharmacol Bull 21:130–135, 1985

Rosenbaum AH, Niven RG, Hanson HP, et al: Tardive dyskinesia: relationship with primary affective disorder. Diseases of the Nervous System 38:423–426, 1977

Rowell FJ, Rich CG, Hall G, et al: Serum chlorpromazine levels in tardive dyskinesia. Br J Clin Pharmacol 15:141–142, 1983

Rupniak NMJ, Mann S, Hall MD, et al: Differential effects of continuous administration for 1 year of haloperidol or sulpiride on striatal dopamine function in the rat. Psychopharmacology 84:503–511, 1984

Rush M, Diamond F, Alpert M: Depression as a risk factor in tardive dyskinesia. Biol Psychiatry 17:387–392, 1982

Saltz B, Woerner M, Kane J, et al: Prospective study of tardive dyskinesia in the elderly. JAMA 266:2402–2406, 1991

Schooler NR, Kane JM: Research diagnosis for tardive dyskinesia (RD-TD). Arch Gen Psychiatry 39:486–487, 1982

Schreiber C, Avissar S, Umansky R, et al: Implications of muscarinic receptor heterogeneity for research on tardive dyskinesia, in Tardive Dyskinesia: Biological Mechanisms and Clinical Aspects. Edited by Wolf ME, Mosnaim AD. Washington, DC, American Psychiatric Press, 1988, pp 25–28

Segal DS, Janowsky DS: Psychostimulant-induced behavioural effects: possible models of schizophrenia, in Psychopharmacology: A Generation of Progress. Edited by Lipton MA, DiMascio AD, Killam KF. New York, Raven, 1978, pp 1113–1123

Siede H, Muller HR: Choreiform movements as side effects of phenothiazine medication in geriatric patients. J Am Geriatr Soc 15:517–522, 1967

Smith JM, Baldessarini RJ: Changes in prevalence, severity and recovery in tardive dyskinesia with age. Arch Gen Psychiatry 37:1368–1373, 1980

Smith JM, Dunn DD: Sex differences in the prevalence of severe tardive dyskinesia. Am J Psychiatry 136:1080–1082, 1979

Smith RC, Strizich M, Klass D: Drug history and tardive dyskinesia. Am J Psychiatry 135:1402–1403, 1978

Smith JM, Kucharski LT, Oswald WT, et al: A systematic investigation of tardive dyskinesia in inpatients. Am J Psychiatry 136:918–922, 1979a

Smith JM, Kucharski LT, Eblen C, et al: An assessment of tardive dyskinesia in schizophrenic outpatients. Psychopharmacology 64:99–104, 1979b.

Smith RC, Leelavathi DE: Behavioural and biochemical effects of chronic neuroleptic drugs: interaction with age, in Tardive Dyskinesia: Research and Treatment. Edited by Fann WE, Smith RC, Davis JM. New York, Spectrum Publications, 1980, pp 65–88

Snyder SH: Amphetamine psychosis: a "model" schizophrenia mediated by cate-cholamines. Am J Psychiatry 130:61–67, 1973

Soni SD, Neill D: Tardive dyskinesia and cognitive functions in schizophrenia (abstract). Schizophr Res 3:78, 1990

Sorokin JE, Giordani B, Mohs RC, et al: Memory impairment in schizophrenic patients with tardive dyskinesia. Biol Psychiatry 23:129–135, 1988

Struve FA, Willner AE: Cognitive dysfunction and tardive dyskinesia. Br J Psychiatry 143:597–600, 1983

Thomas P, McGuire R: Orofacial dyskinesia, cognitive dysfunction and medication. Br J Psychiatry 149:216–220, 1986

Toenniessen LM, Casey DE, McFarland BH: Tardive dyskinesia in the aged. Arch Gen Psychiatry 42:278–284, 1985

Waddington JL: Tardive dyskinesia in schizophrenia and other disorders: association with aging, cognitive dysfunction and structural brain pathology in relation to neuroleptic exposure. Human Psychopharmacol 2:11–22, 1987

Waddington JL: Schizophrenia, affective psychoses, and other disorders treated with neuroleptic drugs: the enigma of tardive dyskinesia, its neurobiological determinants, and the conflict of paradigms. Int Rev Neurobiol 31:297–353, 1989

Waddington JL, Youssef HA: Late onset involuntary movements in chronic schizophrenia: relationship of "tardive" dyskinesia to intellectual impairment and negative symptoms. Br J Psychiatry 149:616–620, 1986

Waddington JL, Youssef HA: Tardive dyskinesia in bipolar affective disorder: aging, cognitive dysfunction, course of illness and exposure to neuroleptics and lithium. Am J Psychiatry 145:613–616, 1988

Waddington JL, Youssef HA, Molloy AG, et al: Association of intellectual impairment, negative symptoms and aging with tardive dyskinesia. J Clin Psychiatry 46:29–33, 1985

Waddington JL, Youssef HA, Dolphin C, et al: Cognitive dysfunction, negative symptoms and tardive dyskinesia in schizophrenia: their association in relation to topography of involuntary movements and criterion of their abnormality. Arch Gen Psychiatry 44:907–912, 1987

Waddington JL, Brown K, O'Neill J: Cognitive impairment, clinical course and treatment history in outpatients with bipolar affective disorder: relationship to tardive dyskinesia. Psychol Med 19:897–902, 1989

Wade JB, Taylor MA, Kasprisin A, et al: Tardive dyskinesia and cognitive impairment. Biol Psychiatry 22:393–395, 1987

Wade JB, Lehmann L, Hart R, et al: Cognitive changes associated with tardive dyskinesia. Neuropsychiatry Neuropsychology Behav Neurol 1:217–227, 1989

Wegner J, Struve F, Kane JM, et al: The relationship between the B-mitten EEG pattern and tardive dyskinesia: a pilot control study. Arch Gen Psychiatry 36:599–603, 1979

Wegner JT, Catalano F, Gibralter J, et al: Schizophrenics with tardive dyskinesia: neuropsychological deficit and family psychopathology. Arch Gen Psychiatry 42:860–865, 1985a

Wegner JT, Kane JM, Weinhold P, et al: Cognitive impairment in tardive dyskinesia. Psychiatry Res 16:331–337, 1985b

Wilson A, King DJ, Cooper SJ, et al: Proceedings of the Irish Neuroscience Group, Galway, 1986

Woerner M, Kane JM, Lieberman J, et al: The prevalence of tardive dyskinesia. J Clin Psychopharmacol 11:34–42, 1991

Wolf ME, Ryan JJ, Mosnaim AD: Organicity and tardive dyskinesia. Psychosomatics 23:475–480, 1982

Wolf ME, Ryan JJ, Mosnaim AD: Cognitive functions in tardive dyskinesia. Psychol Med 13:671–674, 1983

Yagi G, Itoh H: Follow-up study of 11 patients with potentially reversible tardive dyskinesia. Am J Psychiatry 144:1496–1498, 1987

Yarden PE, Discipio WJ: Abnormal movements and prognosis in schizophrenia. Am J Psychiatry 128:317–323, 1971

Yassa R, Nair V, Schwartz G: Tardive dyskinesia: a two-year follow-up study. Psychosomatics 25:852–855, 1984a

Yassa R, Nair V, Schwartz G: Tardive dyskinesia and the primary psychiatric diagnosis. Psychosomatics 25:135–138, 1984b

Yesavage JA, Holman CA, Becker JMT, et al: Correlation of age and acute thiothixine serum levels. Psychopharmacology 74:170–172, 1981

Yesavage JA, Tauke ED, Sheikh: Tardive dyskinesia and steady-state serum levels of thiothixene. Arch Gen Psychiatry 44:913–915, 1987

Youssef HA, Waddington JL: Primitive (developmental) reflexes and diffuse cerebral dysfunction in schizophrenia and bipolar affective disorder: overrepresentation in patients with tardive dyskinesia. Biol Psychiatry 23:791–796, 1988

Zeithofer J, Brainin M, Reisner T: BAEP abnormalities in tardive dyskinesia. J Neurol 231:266–268, 1984

# Chapter 5

# Treatment of Tardive Dyskinesia

N umerous studies of the treatment of tardive dyskinesia have been published since the previous report of the American Psychiatric Association Task Force (1980), yet the overall conclusion that there is no consistently effective treatment still remains valid.

Table 5–1 lists selected studies published from 1979 through 1987. A detailed analysis of the results may be found in a review by Jeste et al. (1988).

The studies published during the 1980s were generally superior to earlier investigations in that a much larger proportion used double-blind design and employed such rating scales as the Abnormal Involuntary Movement Scale (National Institute of Mental Health 1976) or the Rockland/Simpson Tardive Dyskinesia Rating Scale (Simpson et al. 1979). Nonetheless, several methodologic deficiencies have continued to plague the published investigations, most notably small sample sizes and relatively short duration of trials.

## Individual Treatments

### Neuroleptic Withdrawal

Since neuroleptics induce tardive dyskinesia, discontinuation of these drugs would obviously be the ideal treatment. Unfortunately, this often poses a problem because of a risk of worsening or relapse of psychotic symptoms. Nonetheless, it is usually prudent to attempt a progressive dose reduction and, if feasible, a discontinuation of neuroleptics in patients with tardive dyskinesia. Neuroleptic withdrawal is likely to be followed in the shorter run by a temporary aggravation of tardive dyskinesia, after which the severity of dyskinesia will usually stabilize. Subsequently, in a proportion of cases, there will be a reduction in intensity of tardive dyskinesia. In an open trial, Jeste et al. (1979) showed that discontinuation of neuroleptics in a sample of mostly schizophrenic patients for 3 months or longer resulted in improvement in approximately 40% of the patients.

**Table 5–1.** Treatment studies in tardive dyskinesia, 1979–1987

| Treatment | Number of studies | Drugs | References | Total number of patients | Number of patients improved |
|---|---|---|---|---|---|
| Neuroleptic withdrawal | 5 | | Jeste, et al. (1979) | 18 | 10 |
| | | | Itoh and Yagi (1979) | 17 | 11 |
| | | | Jeste and Wyatt (1982a) | 14 | 4 |
| | | | Klawans et al. (1984) | 6 | 6 |
| | | | Fahn (1985) | 22 | 13 |
| Anticholinergic withdrawal | 2 | | Reunanen et al. (1982) | 12 | 6 |
| | | | Yassa (1985) | 3 | 3 |
| Neuroleptics | 11 | Haloperidol | Jus et al. (1979) | 28 | 24 |
| | | Thiopropazate | Smith and Kiloh (1979) | 10 | 7 |
| | | Reserpine | Jus et al. (1979) | 36 | 28 |
| | | Reserpine | Huang et al. (1980) | 10 | NS |
| | | Reserpine | Huang et al. (1981) | 20 | 12 |
| | | Clozapine | Caine et al. (1979) | 2 | 0 |
| | | Clozapine | Cole et al. (1980) | 27 | 9 |
| | | Clozapine | Gerbino et al. (1980) | 23 | 23 |
| | | Fluphenazine decanoate | Barnes and Wiles (1983) | 6 | 4 |
| | | Fluperlapine | Korsgaard et al. (1984) | 11 | 0 |
| | | Molindone | Glazer et al. (1985a, 1985b, 1985c) | 6 | NS |
| | | Dogmatil | Haggstrom (1985) | 6 | 3 |
| | | Dogmatil | Quinn and Marsden (1985) | 9 | 7 |
| Norepinephrine antagonists | 5 | Propranolol | Schrodt et al. (1982) | 4 | 2 |
| | | Clonidine | Freedman et al. (1982) | 8 | NS |
| | | Clonidine | Nishikawa et al. (1980, 1983, 1984) | 23 | 18 |

| Category | N | Drug | Reference | | |
|---|---|---|---|---|---|
| Other catecholamine antagonists | 23 | Metoclopramide (iv) | Bateman et al. (1979) | 8 | 3 |
| | | Metoclopramide (iv) | Doongaji et al. (1982) | 81 | 35 |
| | | Sulpiride | Casey et al. (1979) | 11 | 10 |
| | | Oxyperomide | Casey and Gerlach (1980) | 10 | 6 |
| | | CF 25-397 | Frattola et al. (1980) | 4 | 0 |
| | | CF 25-397 | Tamminga and Chase (1980) | 8 | 2 |
| | | Oxypertine | Freedman and Sony (1980) | 10 | NS |
| | | Oxypertine | Kazamatsuri (1980) and 4 other studies (cited by Freedman and Sony 1980) | 50 | 29 |
| | | Alpha-methyldopa | Huang et al. (1980) | 10 | NS |
| | | Papaverine | Cole et al. (1980) | 41 | 6 |
| | | Apomorphine (sc) | Cole et al. (1980) | 7 | 1 |
| | | Bromocriptine | Tamminga and Chase (1980) | 7 | 0 |
| | | Apomorphine (sc) | Jeste et al. (1981) | 3 | 0 |
| | | Alpha-methylparatyrosine | Nasrallah et al. (1982, 1986) | 10 | 5 |
| | | Alpha-methylparatyrosine | Lang and Marsden (1982) | 3 | 0 |
| | | Tiapride | Pollak et al. (1985) | 10 | 3 |
| | | Tiapride | Perenyi et al. (1985) | 10 | NS |
| GABAergic drugs | 18 | Sodium valproate | Casey and Hammerstad (1979) | 1 | 1 |
| | | Sodium valproate | Nagao et al. (1979) | 7 | 3 |
| | | Diazepam | Singh et al. (1980) | 14 | 9 |
| | | Gamma-acetylenic GABA | Casey et al. (1980) | 10 | 4 |
| | | Clonazepam | Cole et al. (1980) | 6 | NS |
| | | Sodium valproate | Singh et al. (1980) | 1 | 0 |
| | | Sodium valproate | Pandurangi et al. (1980) | 2 | 0 |
| | | Diazepam | Singh et al. (1982, 1983) | 20 | 11 |
| | | Sodium valproate | Friis et al. (1983) | 6 | 3 |
| | | Sodium valproate | Nasrallah et al. (1986) | 10 | 0 |
| | | Gamma-vinyl GABA | Lambert et al. (1982) | 10 | 5 |

**Table 5–1.** Treatment studies in tardive dyskinesia, 1979–1987 (continued)

| Treatment | Number of studies | Drugs | References | Total number of patients | Number of patients improved |
|---|---|---|---|---|---|
| GABAergic drugs (continued) | 18 | Gamma-vinyl GABA | Stahl et al. (1985) | 5 | 1 |
| | | amma-vinyl GABA | Thaker et al. (1987) | 7 | 2 |
| | | THIP | Korsgaard et al. (1982a, 1982b) | 14 | NS |
| | | Baclofen | Stewart et al. (1982) | 13 | 6 |
| | | Baclofen | Glazer et al. (1985a, 1985b, 1985c) | 16 | 3 |
| | | Piracetam | Kabes et al. (1982) | 19 | NS |
| Cholinergic drugs | 26 | Deanol | Jeste et al. (1979) | 7 | 0 |
| | | Deanol | Casey (1979) | 31 | 14 |
| | | Deanol | Amsterdam and Mendels (1979) | 1 | 0 |
| | | Deanol | Paulson (1975) | 4 | 1 |
| | | Deanol | Betts et al. (1979) | 1 | 0 |
| | | Deanol | De Montigny et al. (1979) | 10 | NS |
| | | Deanol | Lonowski et al. (1979) | 4 | 1 |
| | | Choline | Gelenberg et al. (1979) | 5 | 1 |
| | | Lecithin | Gelenberg et al. (1979) | 4 | 1 |
| | | Lecithin | Jackson et al. (1979) | 6 | 6 (probably) |
| | | Lecithin | Branchey et al. (1979) | 8 | 0 |
| | | Lecithin | Singh et al. (1980) | 1 | 0 |
| | | Choline | Rosenbaum et al. (1980) | 1 | 0 |
| | | Deanol | Tamminga et al. (1980) | 6 | 0 |
| | | Deanol | Amsterdam and Mendels (1980) | 1 | 0 |
| | | Deanol | Weiss et al. (1980) | 1 | 0 |
| | | Deanol | Moore and Bowers (1980) | 10 | 3 |
| | | Deanol | Singh et al. (1980) | 3 | 0 |

| | Drug | Reference | n | Improved |
|---|---|---|---|---|
| | Physostigmine (iv) | Weiss et al. (1980) | 2 | 0 |
| | Physostigmine (iv) | Nasrallah (1980) | 1 | 0 |
| | Physostigmine (iv) | Moore and Bowers (1980) | 10 | 1 |
| | Deanol | George et al. (1981) | 11 | 1 |
| | Lecithin | Anderson et al. (1982) | 9 | 0 |
| | Choline | Nasrallah et al. (1984) | 11 | 0 |
| | RS 86 (specific muscarinic) | Noring et al. (1984) | 10 | 0 |
| | Meclofenoxate | Izumi et al. (1986) | 11 | 5 |
| Anticholinergic drugs | 6 | | | |
| | Procyclidine | Chouinard et al. (1979) | 20 | NS |
| | Benztropine (iv) | Moore and Bowers (1980) | 10 | 0 |
| | Trihexyphenidyl | Burnett et al. (1980) | 7 | 0 |
| | Various anticholinergic drugs | Burnett et al. (1980) | 10 | NS |
| | Biperiden | Friis et al. (1983) | 7 | 0 |
| | Trihexyphenidyl | Wolf and Koller (1985) | 3 | 2 |
| Catecholaminergic drugs | 14 | | | |
| | L-dopa | Betts et al. (1979) | 1 | 0 |
| | Amantadine | Weiss et al. (1980) | 1 | 0 |
| | L-dopa | Alpert and Friedhoff (1980) | 3 | 3 |
| | L-dopa | Pandurangi et al. (1980) | 1 | 0 |
| | L-dopa | Cole et al. (1980) | 3 | 0 |
| | d-amphetamine | Smith et al. (1980) | 8 | 0 |
| | Apomorphine | Jeste et al. (1981) | 5 | 1 |
| | Amantadine and neuroleptics | Allen (1982) | 6 | 6 |
| | Bromocriptine | Jeste et al. (1983) | 5 | 3 |
| | Bromocriptine | Lenox et al. (1985) | 12 | NS |
| | Levodopa | Alpert et al. (1982) | 15 | NS |
| | Levodopa | Casey et al. (1982) | 13 | 1 |
| | Levodopa | Fahn (1985) | 4 | 1 |
| | Levodopa | Nasrallah et al. (1986) | 10 | 0 |

**Table 5–1.** Treatment studies in tardive dyskinesia, 1979–1987 (continued)

| Treatment | Number of Studies | Drugs | References | Total number of patients | Number of patients improved |
|---|---|---|---|---|---|
| Miscellaneous drugs | 26 | Lithium | Ereshefsky et al. (1979) | 1 | 1 |
| | | Cyproheptadine | Nagao et al. (1979) | 5 | 1 |
| | | Baclofen | Amsterdam and Mendels (1979) | 1 | 1 |
| | | Baclofen | Amsterdam and Mendels (1979) | 1 | 0 |
| | | Propranolol | Moreira and Karnio (1979) | 1 | 1 |
| | | Propranolol | Bacher and Lewis (1980) | 10 | 7 |
| | | Propranolol | Kulik and Wilbur (1980) | 3 | 3 |
| | | Amitriptyline | Rosenbaum et al. (1980) | 20 | 9 |
| | | Conjugated estrogens | Villeneuve et al. (1980) | 20 | 10 |
| | | Enkephalin—FK33-824 | Bjorndal et al. (1980) | 8 | 2 |
| | | Morphine | Bjorndal et al. (1980) | 8 | NS |
| | | Naloxone | Bjorndal et al. (1980) | 8 | 1 |
| | | Clonidine | Freedman et al. (1980) | 2 | 1 |
| | | Baclofen | Feder and Moore (1980) | 1 | 1 |
| | | Lithium | Rosenbaum et al. (1980) | 20 | 9 |
| | | 5-hydroxy-tryptophan | Nasrallah et al. (1982, 1986) | 10 | 0 |
| | | Hydergine | Rastogi et al. (1982) | 40 | NS |
| | | Lithium | Yassa et al. (1984) | 6 | 0 |
| | | Estrogen | Koller et al. (1982) | 10 | 2 |
| | | Estrogen | Glazer et al. (1985a, 1985b, 1985c) | 5 | 1 |
| | | Destyrosine-gamma-endorphin | Korsgaard et al. (1982a, 1985b) | 4 | 0 |
| | | Alpha-tocopherol (vitamin E) | Lohr et al. (1987) | 15 | 7 |
| | | Ceruletide | Nishikawa et al. (1987) | 2 | 1 |

*Note.* iv, intravenous; sc, subcutaneous; GABA, γ-aminobutyric acid; THIP, tetrahydroisoxazolopyridinol; NS, not significant.
*Source.* Adapted in part from Jeste and Wyatt 1982b and Jeste et al. 1988.

Generally, the longer the period off neuroleptics, the greater the likelihood of eventual remission of tardive dyskinesia, as reported by Klawans et al. (1984). When there is neuroleptic-withdrawal-induced worsening of tardive dyskinesia, palliative treatments, such as benzodiazepines, may be tried to help tide patients over the crisis.

A decision to discontinue neuroleptics in a patient with tardive dyskinesia must take into account the likely deleterious effects of this strategy on the patient's psychotic symptoms. In a tardive dyskinesia patient without a history of psychotic symptoms, a far greater justification is needed to continue neuroleptics.

### Anticholinergic Withdrawal

Although there is no evidence to show that anticholinergic agents produce tardive dyskinesia, these drugs do sometimes worsen it and are not effective in alleviating tardive dyskinesia. Such drugs as procyclidine, benztropine, trihexyphenidyl, and biperiden have not produced improvement in tardive dyskinesia, although they may be helpful in some cases of tardive dystonia, as will be discussed subsequently. (See *anticholinergic drugs* in Table 5–1.) Improvement was defined as a 50% reduction in movement disorder. In a double-blind trial of 4 weeks duration, Friis et al. (1983) found that biperiden doses of 6–18 mg per day worsened tardive dyskinesia in 7 of 7 patients. Hence, discontinuation of anticholinergics would be advisable in a large proportion of tardive dyskinesia patients. Reunanen et al. (1982) and Yassa (1985) reported that tardive dyskinesia improved in 9 of 15 patients who were withdrawn from anticholinergic drugs.

### Neuroleptics

Neuroleptics tend to be potent suppressors of tardive dyskinesia, at least in the short term. As mentioned in Chapter 4, in some cases the signs of dyskinesia continue to be suppressed by neuroleptics for months or even years. The suggestion that neuroleptics mask rather than cure tardive dyskinesia is based on the fact that, in most such cases, neuroleptic withdrawal results in a relatively acute worsening of tardive dyskinesia. Use of neuroleptics specifically to treat tardive dyskinesia is not indicated unless the dyskinesia is severe or disabling.

In the studies listed in Table 5–1, approximately 66% of the patients treated with neuroleptics had 50% or greater improvement in tardive dyskinesia. The individual investigations differed in terms of length of trial, dose used (in milligrams equivalent of chlorpromazine), sample size, and so forth, making a valid comparison of the results difficult. Overall, the improvement in tardive dyskinesia with neuroleptics was greater than that produced by either a placebo or most other sedative drugs, suggesting that neuroleptics appear to have a specific dyskinesia-suppressant effect (Jeste and Wyatt 1982a).

The available evidence does not demonstrate any significant difference among the commonly used neuroleptics in terms of masking tardive dyskinesia. Although it has been claimed by some investigators that neuroleptics that are less potent in masking tardive dyskinesia are also less likely to induce tardive dyskinesia, so far there is no satisfactory evidence to support this hypothesis. Further experience will clarify whether an atypical neuroleptic, such as clozapine, may be an effective treatment for tardive dyskinesia, rather than being just a suppressant. At present there are insufficient data to draw conclusions in this regard. Given clozapine's apparent reduced propensity to produce tardive dyskinesia (see Chapter 4), its use in the management of patients who require ongoing neuroleptic treatment but have developed moderate or severe tardive dyskinesia seems reasonable. The extent to which this indication is consistent with present U.S. Food and Drug Administration–approved indications is open to interpretation; therefore, the use of clozapine requires particularly careful assessment of relative risk and benefit and alternative treatments with appropriate informed consent. There are studies under way that should help to clarify clozapine's role in this context.

### Noradrenergic Antagonists

There are data suggesting noradrenergic hyperactivity in a subset of patients with tardive dyskinesia (Kaufmann et al. 1986). For example, Jeste et al. (1984) reported higher cerebrospinal fluid concentrations of norepinephrine in patients with tardive dyskinesia compared to patients without tardive dyskinesia. Norepinephrine is synthesized from dopamine in noradrenergic neurons, and there is evidence of a synergy between central dopaminergic and noradrenergic activities in terms of locomotor function. Many drugs, including neuroleptics and stimulants, have effects on both dopaminergic and noradrenergic systems. Several studies have shown that alpha-1-adrenergic agonists (such as clonidine) and beta-adrenergic blockers (such as propranolol) are useful in the treatment of tardive dyskinesia in some patients. In a double-blind study investigating the effect of 0.2–0.9 mg of clonidine on tardive dyskinesia, Freedman et al. (1982) found a mean 63 reduction in tardive dyskinesia score. Nishikawa et al. (1980, 1983, 1984) reported improvement in tardive dyskinesia in 18 of 23 patients. Such agents as clonidine appear to be promising, and additional studies are warranted. These drugs do have side effects, however—such as hypotension—and, therefore, need careful monitoring.

### Other Catecholamine Antagonists

Tardive dyskinesia is usually thought to be associated with catecholaminergic hyperactivity. It is, therefore, not surprising that various catechol-amine antagonists have been tried in the treatment of tardive dyskinesia. These include a number of putative dopamine antagonists, such as alpha-methylparatyrosine and tiapride. The latter treatments were based on the previously popular hypothesis associating tardive dyskinesia with dopa-mine receptor supersensitivity. The overall success rate with dopamine an-tagonists (other than neuroleptics) has been rather low (less than 40% in the studies listed in Table 5–1), confirming the weaknesses of the dopaminergic supersensitivity hypothesis of tardive dyskinesia. The length of treatment in these studies was 6 weeks or less. There is, to date, no satisfactory evidence that continued long-term use of nonneuroleptic do-pamine antagonists is beneficial in the general treatment of tardive dyski-nesia. Also, several of the agents tried have been experimental drugs that are not yet available for clinical use, and they all have their own adverse effects.

**Catecholamine depleters.** One class of catecholamine antagonists that needs separate mention is catecholamine depleting agents. Such drugs as reserpine, tetrabenazine, and oxypertine, which work by depleting cate-cholamines (and even serotonin) from nerve terminals, are used relatively commonly as antidyskinetic agents. Reserpine depletes presynaptic stores of the monoamines, whereas tetrabenazine both depletes presynaptic stores and blocks postsynaptic dopamine receptors. Oxypertine is a rela-tively potent depleter of noradrenaline, its dopamine-depleting activity being less than that of reserpine or tetrabenazine. These agents have been claimed to produce tardive dyskinesia less often than "typical" neuroleptics (Lang and Marsden 1982), although this claim remains to be substanti-ated.

There are only a few early trials assessing the value of reserpine in tard-ive dyskinesia (Duvoisin 1972; Fahn 1985; Sato et al. 1971). Tetrabenazine has been investigated more extensively, and numerous case reports and treatment studies have found tetrabenazine to be a useful therapeutic agent, not only in tardive dyskinesia but also in a range of hyperkinetic movement disorders, such as Huntington's disease and dystonic phenom-ena (Fahn 1985; Lang and Marsdan 1982). Double-blind controlled stud-ies of tardive dyskinesia found that in a dose range of 50–200 mg/day, the drug suppressed the movements of tardive dyskinesia, although there were hints that the beneficial effect might diminish over time.

Such side effects as drowsiness, akathisia, and depression are relatively common with both reserpine and tetrabenazine, and they are probably best avoided in depressed patients. Compared with reserpine, tetrabena-zine has fewer peripheral effects, such as postural hypotension. Neverthe-less, when starting treatment with either drug, the dosage should be gradually increased to minimize adverse effects.

An antidyskinetic action for oxypertine was first described by Eckmann (1968); subsequently, the drug has been subjected to a number of therapeutic trials in tardive dyskinesia (Kazamatsuri 1980; Soni et al. 1984). In doses of 60–120 mg/day, the drug seems to be effective in a proportion of patients with tardive dyskinesia, but double-blind, placebo-controlled studies in larger samples are required to establish its value as a treatment for this condition.

### GABAergic Drugs

GABA (γ-aminobutyric acid) is an inhibitory neurotransmitter and is linked with nigrostriatal dopamine functions. Some investigators have suggested a reduction in nigrostriatal GABAergic activity in tardive dyskinesia. The evidence in favor of this hypothesis is mostly indirect. GABAergic agents, such as benzodiazepines, sodium valproate, and gamma-vinyl GABA, might be useful for treating tardive dyskinesia through their inhibition of the catecholaminergic hyperactivity in the nigrostriatum. The results with these agents have remained somewhat equivocal. In the studies listed in Table 5–1, 47% of the patients had improvement in tardive dyskinesia with these drugs. Problems with the development of tolerance and side effects (including sedation and occasional exacerbation of psychosis) are among the limiting factors. Nonetheless, commonly used agents with relatively low toxicity (e.g., benzodiazepines) are often of clinical value in the temporary management of moderate or severe tardive dyskinesia.

### Cholinergic Drugs

During the 1970s there was considerable interest in the hypothesis of cholinergic hypofunction in tardive dyskinesia, along with the use of cholinergic agents—such as deanol, choline, and lecithin—in the treatment of tardive dyskinesia. Basic and clinical research clearly points to an interaction between catecholaminergic (especially dopaminergic) and cholinergic interaction in the basal ganglia. The role of such interaction in the pathophysiology of tardive dyskinesia is, however, unclear. Studies using cholinergic agents, including specific muscarinic agonists (Izumi et al. 1986; Nasrallah et al. 1984; Noring et al. 1984), have yielded rather disappointing results. Only 21% of the patients treated with cholinergic drugs listed in Table 5–1 had improvement. It is conceivable that a specific subset of tardive dyskinesia patients improves with these agents. The side effects include depression, diarrhea, and bronchoconstriction.

### Anticholinergic Drugs

Several studies have shown the efficacy of anticholinergic drugs (often in relatively high doses) in tardive dystonia (Burke et al. 1982; Fahn 1985). In nondystonic tardive dyskinesia, the efficacy of anticholinergic drugs is limited; in a number of cases, the drugs may even worsen the dyskinesia.

As discussed before, withdrawal of anticholinergic drugs leads to improvement in tardive dyskinesia in some patients. Four studies using benztropine, trihexyphenidyl, or biperiden reported that only 2 of 27 patients had 50% or greater improvement in tardive dyskinesia (Burnett et al. 1980; Friis et al. 1983; Moore and Bowers 1980; Wolf and Koller 1985). Furthermore, these drugs have adverse effects, such as dryness of mouth, constipation, blurring of vision, and confusion. Hence, their use should generally be restricted to cases of tardive dystonia.

## Catecholaminergic Drugs

In view of the evidence for catecholamine overactivity in tardive dyskinesia, drugs with catecholaminergic action would be expected to aggravate tardive dyskinesia, and in a number of cases they do. Occasionally, however, agents such as bromocriptine, when used in a specific fashion, may help tardive dyskinesia. In a double-blind study investigating the effect of bromocriptine on tardive dyskinesia (Jeste et al. 1983), 3 of 5 patients improved. A possible explanation for the improvement in tardive dyskinesia is that bromocriptine has a biphasic effect; in lower doses it stimulates dopamine autoreceptors, thereby reducing the synaptic release of dopamine. The overall rate of improvement with catecholaminergic agents listed in Table 5–1 was only 25%. These agents also carry a risk of hypertension and an aggravation of psychotic symptoms as well as of dyskinesia.

One agent of some interest is amantadine, a dopaminergic drug useful in the treatment of Parkinson's disease as well as neuroleptic-induced parkinsonism. Allen (1982) reported improvement in tardive dyskinesia with a combination of amantadine and neuroleptics in all of the six patients so treated. This finding has not yet been replicated in a larger sample. Given the propensity of amantadine (especially in higher doses) to exacerbate psychosis as well as dyskinesia, the clinical value of this agent as a general treatment of tardive dyskinesia is limited.

## Miscellaneous Drugs

Various compounds, such as lithium and Hydergine, have been used in treating tardive dyskinesia. Rastogi et al. (1982) showed that at 4.5 mg/day of Hydergine, mean tardive dyskinesia score decreased 37% versus 29% for placebo. The results with lithium have been variable and often disappointing. The number of studies with most of the other agents has been too small to make any definitive conclusions.

Recently, there have been claims for the efficacy of calcium channel blockers and alpha-tocopherol or vitamin E in the treatment of tardive dyskinesia. Barrow and Childs (1986) and Ross et al. (1987) reported improvement in tardive dyskinesia with verapamil and diltiazem, respectively, which are both calcium channel blockers. Similarly, Lohr et al. (1987) and Elkashef et al. (1990) found vitamin E to be efficacious in reducing tardive dyskinesia in some patients. The use of vitamin E, a relatively nontoxic antioxidant and a scavenger of free radicals, has been based on a hypothesis that some cases of tardive dyskinesia are associated with a neuronal dysfunction or damage resulting from excessive free radical activity. In daily doses of 400–1200 mg/day, vitamin E was reported to improve tardive dyskinesia of relatively shorter duration and had no noticeable adverse effects apart from diarrhea. Although potentially promising, the general clinical value of the calcium channel blockers and vitamin E in tardive dyskinesia needs to be established with larger-scale and longer-term treatment studies.

### Other Treatments

There have been anecdotal case reports of improvement in tardive dyskinesia in depressed patients treated with electroconvulsive therapy (ECT) (Chacko and Root 1983; D. Hay, personal communication, February 1991; Rosenbaum et al. 1980). There are no sufficient data yet to assess the value of ECT as a treatment for tardive dyskinesia. Nonetheless, it seems that in some depressed patients with tardive dyskinesia, ECT may produce improvement in both depression and tardive dyskinesia.

# Discussion

The most logical treatment for neuroleptic-induced tardive dyskinesia is neuroleptic withdrawal. This may not, however, be practical when there is a risk of worsening or relapse of psychotic symptoms. In patients without a history of psychotic symptoms, neuroleptic dose reduction and then discontinuation would be especially advisable, unless the patient and his or her physician believe that the risk of neuroleptic withdrawal outweighs the likely benefits. It is necessary to stress that, in a majority of tardive dyskinesia patients, the dyskinesia is mild and may not require any specific treatment (apart from neuroleptic dose reduction or withdrawal, if feasible).

When continuation of neuroleptic treatment is necessary (for treatment of the underlying condition, such as chronic schizophrenia), an attempt at dose reduction should be considered seriously. A switch to a different class of neuroleptics (e.g., from a phenothiazine to a butyrophenone) may be useful, but controlled trials are lacking. Noradrenergic antagonists (e.g., propranolol and clonidine) and GABAergic agents (e.g., benzodiazepines) may be helpful in subsets of patients, at least on a temporary basis. Anticholinergic drugs deserve a trial in patients with tardive dystonia. Use of neuroleptics specifically for treating tardive dyskinesia is usually not justified, except in severe tardive dyskinesia, physically or socially disabling tardive dyskinesia, or treatment-resistant cases. Other types of drugs (possibly including such potentially promising agents as vitamin E or calcium channel blockers) may be tried in individual patients with moderate to severe tardive dyskinesia. It is important to bear in mind that any pharmacologic agents used have their own side effects, and should be employed only after consideration of their own risk-to-benefit ratios. Long-term value of most of the drug treatments for tardive dyskinesia has not been established.

It is likely that there are biochemical-pharmacological subtypes of tardive dyskinesia, and specific types of agents may benefit specific types of patients (e.g., cholinergic drugs in patients with cholinergic deficiency). At present, however, there are no established ways of identifying a possible biochemical-pharmacological subset to which a given patient belongs. Hence, a cautious trial-and-error approach is indicated.

# References

Allen RM: Palliative treatment of tardive dyskinesia with combination of Adineneuroleptic administration. Biol Psychiatry 17:719–727, 1982

Alpert M, Friedhoff AJ: Clinical application of receptor modification, in Tardive Dyskinesia: Research and Treatment. Edited by Fann WE, Smith RC, Davis JM, et al. New York, SP Medical & Scientific Books, 1980

Alpert M, Diamond F, Friedhoff AJ: Receptor sensitivity modification in the treatment of tardive dyskinesia. Psychopharmacol Bull 90–92, 1982

American Psychiatric Association: Tardive Dyskinesia: A Task Force Report of the American Psychiatric Association. Washington, DC, American Psychiatric Association, 1980

Anderson BG, Recker D, Ristich M, et al.: Lecithin treatment of tardive dyskinesia—a progress report. Psychopharmacol Bull 18:87–88, 1982

Bacher NM, Lewis HA: Low-dose propranolol in tardive dyskinesia. Am J Psychiatry 137:495–497, 1980

Barnes TRE, Wiles DH: Variation in oro-facial tardive dyskinesia during depot antipsychotic drug treatment. Psychopharmacology 81:359–362, 1983

Barrow N, Childs A: An anti-tardive dyskinesia effect of verapamil. Am J Psychiatry 143:1485, 1986

Bateman DN, Dutta DK, McClelland HA, et al: Metoclopromide and haloperidol in tardive dyskinesia. Br J Psychiatry 135:505–508, 1979

Betts WC, Johnston FS, Pratt MJ: An effective palliative treatment for phenothiazine-induced tardive dyskinesia. N Carolina Med J 40:286, 1979

Bjorndal N, Casey DE, Gerlach J: Enkephalin, morphine, and naloxone in tardive dyskinesia. Psychopharmacology 69:133–136, 1980

Branchey MH, Branchey LB, Bark NM, et al: Lecithin in the treatment of tardive dyskinesia. Communications in Psychopharmacology 3:303–307, 1979

Burke RE, Fahn S, Jankovic J, et al: Tardive dyskinesia: Late-onset and persistent dystonia caused by antipsychotic drugs. Neurology 32:1335–1346, 1982

Burnett GB, Prange AJ, Wilson IC, et al: Adverse effects of anticholinergic antiparkinsonian drugs in tardive dyskinesia. Neuropsychobiology 6:109–120, 1980

Caine ED, Polinsky RJ, Kartzinel R, et al: Trial use of clozapine for abnormal involuntary movement disorders. Am J Psychiatry 136:317–320, 1979

Casey DE: Mood alterations during deanol therapy. Psychopharmacology 62:187–191, 1979

Casey DE, Gerlach J: Oxiperomide in tardive dyskinesia. Journal of Neurology, Neurosurgery, and Psychiatry 43:264–267, 1980

Casey DE, Hammerstad JP: Sodium valproate in tardive dyskinesia. J Clin Psychiatry 40:483–485, 1979

Casey DE, Gerlach J, Magelund G, et al: γ-Acetylenic GABA in tardive dyskinesia. Arch Gen Psychiatry 37:1376–1379, 1980

Casey DE, Gerlach J, Bjorndal N: Levodopa and receptor sensitivity modification in tardive dyskinesia. Psychopharmacology 78:89–92, 1982

Chacko RC, Root L: ECT and tardive dyskinesia: two cases and a review. J Clin Psychiatry 44:265–266, 1983

Chouinard G, DeMontigny C, Annable L: Tardive dyskinesia and parkinsonian medication. Am J Psychiatry 136:228–229, 1979

Cole JO, Gardos G, Tarsy D, et al: Drug trials in persistent dyskinesia, in Tardive Dyskinesia: Research and Treatment. Edited by Fann WE, Smith RC, Davis JM, et al. New York, SP Medical & Scientific, 1980

DeMontigny C, Chouinard G, Annable L: Ineffectiveness of deanol in tardive dyskinesia: a placebo-controlled study. Psychopharmacology 65:219–222, 1979

Doongaji DR, Jeste DV, Jape NM, et al: Study of acute metoclopramide in 81 patients with tardive dyskinesia. J Clin Psychopharmacol 2:376–379, 1982

Duvoisin RC: Reserpine for tardive dyskinesia. N Engl J Med 286:611, 1972

Eckman F: Problematic von Dauerschaden nach neuroleptischer Langzeitbehandelung. Therapie der Gegenwart (Berlin) 197:316–323, 1968

Elkashef AM, Ruskin PE, Bacher N, et al: Vitamin E in the treatment of tardive dyskinesia. Am J Psychiatry 147:505–506, 1990

Ereshefsky L, Rubin TN, Friedman S: Treatment of tardive dyskinesia with RBC lithium determinations. Am J Psychiatry 136:570–573, 1979

Fahn S: A therapeutic approach to tardive dyskinesia. J Clin Psychiatry 464 (suppl):19–24, 1985

Frattola L, Albizzati MG, Bassi S, et al: Treatment of dyskinetic and dystonic with CF 25-397: clinical and pharmacological aspects, in Ergot Compounds and Brain Function. Edited by Goldstein M, Caine DB, Lieberman A, et al. New York, Raven, 1980

Freedman H, Sony SD: Oxypertine for tardive dyskinesia. Br J Psychiatry 137:522–523, 1980

Freedman R, Kirch D, Bell J, et al: Clonidine treatment of schizophrenia: double-blind comparison to placebo and neuroleptic drugs. Acta Psychiatr Scand 65:35–45, 1982

Friis T, Christensen TR, Gerlach J: Sodium valproate and biperiden in neuroleptic-induced akathisia, parkinsonism and hyperkinesia. Acta Psychiatr Scand 67:178–187, 1983

Gelenberg AJ, Doller-Wojcik JC, Growdon JH: Choline and lecithin in the treatment of tardive dyskinesia: preliminary results from a pilot study. Am J Psychiatry 136:772–776, 1979

George J, Pridmore S, Aldous D: Double blind controlled trial of deanol in tardive dyskinesia. Aust N Z J Psychiatry 15:68–71, 1981

Gerbino L, Shopsin B, Collora M: Clozapine in the treatment of tardive dyskinesia: an interim report, in Tardive Dyskinesia: Research and Treatment. Edited by Fann WE, Smith RC, Davis, JM, et al. New York, SP Medical & Scientific, 1980

Glazer WM, Hafez HM, Benarroche CL: Molindone and haloperidol in tardive dyskinesia. J Clin Psychiatry 46 (suppl):4–7, 1985a

Glazer WM, Moore DC, Bowers MB, et al: The treatment of tardive dyskinesia with baclofen. Psychopharmacology 87:480–483, 1985b

Glazer WM, Naftolin F, Morgenstern H, et al: Estrogen replacement and tardive dyskinesia. Psychoendocrinology 10:345–350, 1985c

Haggstrom JE: Efficacite possible du dogmatil dans le controle des dyskinesia tardives: etudes cliniques et experimentations animales. Sem Hop Paris 61:1365–1368, 1985

Huang CC, Wang RIH, Hasegawa A, et al: Evaluation of reserpine and alphamethyldopa in the treatment of tardive dyskinesia. Psychopharmacol Bull 16(3):41–43, 1980

Huang CC, Wang RIH, Hasegawa A, et al: Reserpine and alpha-methyldopa in the treatment of tardive dyskinesia. Psychopharmacology 73:359–362, 1981

Itoh H, Yagi G: Reversibility of tardive dyskinesia. Folia Psychiatric et Neurologica Japonica 33:43–54, 1979

Izumi K, Tominaga H, Koja T, et al: Meclofenate therapy in tardive dyskinesia: a preliminary report. Biol Psychiatry 21:151–160, 1986

Jeste DV, Wyatt RJ: Therapeutic strategies against tardive dyskinesia: two decades of experience. Arch Gen Psychiatry 39:803–816, 1982a

Jeste DV, Wyatt RJ: Understanding and Treatment of Tardive Dyskinesia. New York, Guilford, 1982b

Jeste DV, Potkin SG, Sinha S, et al: Tardive dyskinesia: reversible and persistent. Arch Gen Psychiatry 36:585–590, 1979

Jeste DV, De Lisi LE, Zalcman S, et al: A biochemical study of tardive dyskinesia in young male patients. Psychiatric Research 4:327–331, 1981

Jeste DV, Cutler NR, Kaufmann CA, et al: Low-dose apomorphine and bromocriptine in neuroleptic-induced movement disorders. Biol Psychiatry 18:1085–1091, 1983

Jeste DV, Doongaji DR, Linnoila M: Elevated cerebrospinal fluid noradrenaline in tardive dyskinesia. Br J Psychiatry 144:177–180, 1984

Jeste DV, Lohr JB, Clark C, et al: Pharmacological treatment of tardive dyskinesia in the 1980's. J Clin Psychopharmacol 8 (suppl):38S–48S, 1988

Kabes J, Sikora J, Pisvejc J, et al: Effect of piracetam on extrapyramidal side effects induced on neuroleptic drugs. Int Pharmacopsychiat 17:185–192, 1982

Kaufmann CA, Jeste DV, Shelton RC, et al: Noradrenergic and neurological abnormalities in tardive dyskinesia. Biol Psychiatry 21:799–812, 1986

Kazamatsuri H: Treatment of tardive dyskinesia with oxypertine: preliminary clinical experience and a brief review of the literature. Compr Psychiatry 21:352–357, 1980

Klawans HL, Tanner CM, Barr A: The reversibility of "permanent" tardive dyskinesia. Clin Neuropharmacol 7:153–159, 1984

Koller WC, Barr A, Biary N: Estrogen treatment of dyskinetic disorders. Neurology 32:547–549, 1982

Korsgaard S, Casey D, Gerlach J: High-dose destyrosine-γ-endorphin in tardive dyskinesia. Psychopharmacology 78:285–286, 1982a

Korsgaard S, Casey DE, Gerlach J, et al: The effect of tetrahydroisoxazolopyridinol (THIP) in tardive dyskinesia. A new aminotyric acid agonist. Arch Gen Psychiatry 39:1017–1021, 1982b

Korsgaard S, Noring U, Gerlach J: Fluperlapine in tardive dyskinesia and parkinsonism. Psychopharmacology 84:76–79, 1984

Kulik FA, Wilbur R: Propranolol for tardive dyskinesia and extrapyramidal side effects (pseudoparkinsonism) from neuroleptics. Psychopharmacol Bull 16(3):18–19, 1980

Lambert PA, Cantiniaux P, Chabannes J-P, et al: Essai therapeutique du vinyl GABA un inhibiteur de la GABA-transaminase, dans les skinesies tardives induites par les neuroleptiques. L'Encephale 8:371–376, 1982

Lang AE, Marsden CD: Alphamethylparatyrosine and tetrabenzine in movement disorders. Clinical Neuropharmacology 5:375–387, 1982

Lenox RH, Weaver LA, Saran BM: Tardive dyskinesia: clinical and neuroendocrine response to low dose bromocriptine. J Clin Psychopharmacol 5:286–292, 1985

Lohr JB, Cadet JL, Lohr MA, et al: Alpha-tocopherol in tardive dyskinesia. Lancet 1:913–914, 1987

Moore DC, Bowers MB Jr: Identification of subgroup of tardive dyskinesia patients by pharmacologic probes. Am J Psychiatry 137:1202–1205, 1980

Moreira MJC, Karnio IG: Improvement of tardive dyskinesia with high doses of propranolol: a case report. Revista Paulista de Medicina 93:76–78, 1979

Nagao T, Ohshimo T, Mitsunobu K, et al: Cerebrospinal fluid monoamine metabolites and cyclic nucleotides in chronic schizophrenic patients with tardive dyskinesia or drug-induced tremor. Biol Psychiatry 14:509–523, 1979

Nasrallah HA, Pappas NJ, Crowe RR: Oculogyric dystonia in tardive dyskinesia. Am J Psychiatry 137:850–851, 1980

Nasrallah HA, Smith RE, Dunner FJ, et al: Serotonin precursor effects in tardive dyskinesia. Psychopharmacology 77:234–235, 1982

Nasrallah HA, Dunner FJ, Smith RE, et al: Variable clinical response to choline in tardive dyskinesia. Psychol Med 14:697–700, 1984

Nasrallah HA, Dunner FJ, McCalley-Whitters M, et al: Pharmacologic probes of neurotransmitter systems in tardive dyskinesia: implications for clinical management. J Clin Psychiatry 47:56–59, 1986

National Institute of Mental Health; Alcohol, Drug Abuse, and Mental Health Administration; Public Health Service; U.S. Department of Health, Education, and Welfare: Abnormal Involuntary Movement Scale. Early Clinical Drug Evaluation Unit Intercom 4:3–6, 1975

Nishikawa T, Tanaka M, Koga I, et al: Tardive dyskinesia treated with clonidine. Kurume Med J 27:209–210, 1980

Nishikawa T, Tanaka M, Koga I, et al: Combined treatment of tardive dyskinesia with clodine and neuroleptics: a follow-up study of three cases for three years. Psychopharmacology 80:374–375, 1983

Nishikawa T, Tanaka M, Tsuda A, et al: Clonidine therapy for tardive dyskinesia and related syndromes. Clinical Neuropharmacology 7:239–245, 1984

Nishikawa T, Tanaka M, Tsuda A, et al: Ceruletide for tardive dyskinesia (letter). Biol Psychiatry 22:797–798, 1987

Noring U, Povlsen UJ, Casey DE, et al: Effect of a cholinomimetic drug (RS 86) in tardive dyskinesia and drug-related parkinsonism. Psychopharmacology 84:569–571, 1984

Pandurangi AK, Devi V, Channabasavanna SM: Caudate atrophy in tardive dyskinesia: a pneumoencephalographic study. J Clin Psychiatry 41:229–231, 1980

Paulson GW: Tardive dyskinesia. Ann Rev Med 26:75–81, 1975

Pollak P, Gaio J-M, Hommel M, et al: Effects of tiapride in tardive dyskinesia. Psychopharmacology 85:236–239, 1985

Quinn N, Marsden CD: Essai en double insu du dogmatil dans la choree de Huntington et al dyskinesie tardive. Sem Hop Paris 61:1376–1380, 1985

Rastogi SC, Blowers AJ, Gibson AC: Co-dergocne (hydergine) in the treatment of tardive dyskinesia. Psychol Med 12:427–429, 1982

Reunanen M, Kaarnen P, Vaisanen E: The influence of anticholinergic treatment on tardive dyskinesia caused by neuroleptic drugs. Acta Neurol Scand 65 (suppl 90):278–279, 1982

Rosenbaum AH, O'Connor MK, Duane DD, et al: Treatment of tardive dyskinesia in an agitated, depressed patient. Psychosomatics 21:765–766, 1980

Ross JL, Mackenzie TB, Hanson DR, et al: Diltiazem for tardive dyskinesia. Lancet 1:268, 1987

Sato S, Daly R, Peters H: Reserpine therapy of phenothiazine induced dyskinesia. Diseases of the Nervous System 32:680–685, 1971

Schrodt GR, Wright JH, Simpson R, et al: Treatment of tardive dyskinesia with propranolol. J Clin Psychiatry 43:328–331, 1982

Simpson GM, Lee JH, Zoubok B, et al: A rating scale for tardive dyskinesia. Psychopharmacology 64:171–179, 1979

Singh MM, Nasrallah HA, Lal H, et al: Treatment of tardive dyskinesia with diazepam: indirect evidence for the involvement of limib, possibly GABAergic mechanisms. Brain Res Bull 5 (Suppl 2):673–680, 1980

Singh MM, Becker R, Pitman RK, et al: Diazepam-induced changes in tardive dyskinesia: suggestions for a new conceptual model. Biol Psychiatry 17:729–742, 1982

Soni SD, Freeman HL, Hussein EM: Oxypertine in tardive dyskinesia: an 8-week controlled study. Br J Psychiatry 144:48–52, 1984

Stahl SM, Thornton JE, Simpson ML, et al: Gamma-vinyl-GABA treatment of tardive dyskinesia and other movement disorders. Biol Psychiatry 20:888–893, 1985

Stewart RM, Rollins J, Beckham B, et al: Baclofen in tardive dyskinesia patients maintained on neuroleptics. Clin Neuropharmacol 5:365–373, 1982

Tamminga CA, Chase TN: Bromocriptine and CF 25-397 in the treatment of tardive dyskinesia. Arch Neurol 37:204–205, 1980

Thaker GK, Tamminga CA, Alphs LD, et al: Brain gamma-aminobutyric acid abnormality in tardive dyskinesia. Arch Gen Psychiatry 44:522–529, 1987

Villeneuve A, Cazejust T, Cote M: Estrogens in tardive dyskinesias in male psychiatric patients. Neuropsychobiology 6:145–151, 1980

Weiss KJ, Ciraulo DA, Shader RI: Physostigmine test in rabbit syndrome and tardive dyskinesia. Am J Psychiatry 137:627–628, 1980

Wolf ME, Koller WC: Tardive dystonia: treatment with trihexyphenidyl. J Clin Psychopharmacol 5:247–248, 1985

Yassa R: Antiparkinsonian medication withdrawal in the treatment of tardive dyskinesia: a report of three cases. Can J Psychiatry 30:440–442, 1985

Yassa R, Archer J, Cordozo S: The long-term effect of lithium carbonate on tardive dyskinesia. Can J Psychiatry 29:36–37, 1984

Chapter 6

# Neuroleptic Drugs: Indications, Efficacy, and Therapeutic Dosages

Although the focus of this report is tardive dyskinesia, the task force felt it would be useful to provide a summary of the indications for and efficacy of neuroleptic drugs in the treatment of a variety of conditions. This review is intended to provide a framework for developing appropriate benefit and risk assessments of neuroleptic treatment. This chapter is in no way intended to substitute for textbooks in clinical diagnosis and psychopharmacology, but it can help to place the risk of tardive dyskinesia in an appropriate context.

The use of antipsychotic or neuroleptic drugs remains a matter of clinical judgment that must be made on an individual basis, but clinicians must weigh the relative indications for these drugs or alternative pharmacologic agents when neuroleptics are not the only available treatment.

The overall indications for both short-term and long-term utilization of neuroleptics have not changed appreciably in the past decade. The primary indications for short-term use include 1) the treatment of an acute episode or exacerbation of a schizophrenic illness, 2) delusional disorder and other psychotic disorders, 3) the manic phase of bipolar disorder when very rapid control is necessary in a highly agitated patient or when lithium treatment is inadequate, 4) the treatment of agitation or psychosis in some organic mental disorders, 5) major depressive episodes with psychotic features, and 6) neurologic or psychiatric manifestations of certain neuropsychiatric conditions, such as Huntington's disease and Tourette's disorder. In addition, a brief therapeutic trial of neuroleptics may be indicated in some severe personality disorders. In children or adolescents, neuroleptics may be indicated in schizophrenia, autism, pervasive developmental disorder, Tourette's disorder, attention deficit disorder with hyperactivity, conduct disorder, and in some cases of aggressive and nonspecific behavioral symptoms associated with mental retardation. In general, the

121

use of antipsychotic or neuroleptic drugs remains a matter of clinical judgment that must be made on an individual basis.

Indications for neuroleptics may be influenced by the relative efficacy of other treatments in a given individual. For example, the use of neuroleptics in the treatment of mania will be influenced by the severity of agitation or excitement and the previous response to lithium or electroconvulsive therapy (ECT) (and possibly carbamazepine). The use of neuroleptics in psychotic depression may be influenced by the previous response to tricyclics or the willingness of the patient to undergo ECT. As a result, it is impossible to make sweeping generalizations that will apply to all patients. It is critical, however, that clinicians weigh the relative indications for alternative treatments when neuroleptics are not the only available treatment and document the process of clinical judgment in the medical record (see Chapter 10).

The efficacy of neuroleptic medication is by far best studied and best confirmed in the acute and long-term treatment of schizophrenia. The therapeutic benefits of these drugs in this context have been established in numerous random-assignment, placebo-controlled, double-blind trials (Davis et al. 1980; Kane and Lieberman 1987; Klein and Davis 1969).

The long-term efficacy of neuroleptics in the treatment of delusional disorders, bipolar disorder, major depression with psychotic features, organic mental disorders, and chronic characterologic disorders has not been addressed in controlled clinical trials; however, clinical experience would suggest that prolonged neuroleptic therapy may be of benefit in some such individuals. The critical factor in such utilization is the appropriate consideration of alternative therapeutic (pharmacologic or nonpharmacologic) approaches and objective documentation of significant benefit from neuroleptic treatment.

# Antipsychotic Drugs in the Treatment of Schizophrenia

Except when a very low and clearly inadequate dosage of neuroleptic medication is used, studies consistently show that these drugs are substantially more effective than placebos in the treatment of schizophrenia. An overall summary would indicate that approximately 75% of drug-treated patients (compared with 25% of placebo-treated patients) improved significantly over a period of 6 weeks (Cole et al. 1964, 1965). In addition, it is important to emphasize that approximately 50% of the placebo-treated patients experience a worsening of symptomatology (Davis et al. 1989).

With regard to maintenance treatment trials, Table 6–1 provides data from 35 double-blind, random-assignment studies comparing relapse rates among placebo-treated patients with relapse rates among patients receiving maintenance medication. Of these 3,609 patients, 20% on medication

**Table 6–1.** Antipsychotic prevention of relapse

| Investigators | No. of patients | Percent relapse on placebo | Percent relapse on drug | Percent difference in relapse rate (placebo vs. drug) |
|---|---|---|---|---|
| Caffey | 259 | 45 | 5 | 40 |
| Prien | 762 | 42 | 16 | 26 |
| Prien | 325 | 56 | 20 | 36 |
| Schiele | 80 | 60 | 3 | 57 |
| Adelson | 281 | 90 | 49 | 41 |
| Morton | 40 | 70 | 25 | 45 |
| Baro | 26 | 100 | 0 | 100 |
| Hershon | 62 | 28 | 7 | 21 |
| Rassidakis | 84 | 58 | 34 | 24 |
| Melynk | 40 | 50 | 0 | 50 |
| Schauver | 80 | 18 | 5 | 13 |
| Freeman | 94 | 28 | 13 | 16 |
| Whitaker | 39 | 65 | 8 | 57 |
| Garfield | 27 | 31 | 11 | 20 |
| Diamond | 40 | 70 | 25 | 45 |
| Blackburn | 53 | 54 | 24 | 30 |
| Gross | 109 | 58 | 14 | 44 |
| Englehardt | 294 | 30 | 15 | 15 |
| Leff | 30 | 83 | 33 | 50 |
| Hogarty | 361 | 67 | 31 | 36 |
| Troshinsky | 43 | 63 | 4 | 59 |
| Hirsch | 74 | 66 | 8 | 58 |
| Chien | 31 | 87 | 12 | 94 |
| Gross | 61 | 65 | 34 | 31 |
| Rifkin | 54 | 83 | 14 | 61 |
| Clark | 35 | 78 | 27 | 51 |
| Clark | 19 | 70 | 43 | 27 |
| Kinross-Wright | 40 | 70 | 5 | 65 |
| Andrews | 31 | 35 | 7 | 28 |
| Westedt | 38 | 63 | 27 | 36 |
| Cheung | 28 | 62 | 13 | 48 |
| Levine, oral | 33 | 59 | 33 | 26 |
| Levine, I.V. | 34 | 30 | 18 | 12 |
| Kane | 28 | 41 | 0 | 41 |
| Zissis | 32 | 75 | 0 | 75 |
| Crow | 120 | 62 | 46 | 16 |

*Note.* Summary statistics: $P = 10^{-100}$.

*Source.* Reprinted with permission from Kaplan HI, Sadock BJ (eds): Comprehensive Textbook of Psychiatry/V, 5th Edition, Vol 2. Baltimore, MD, Williams & Wilkins, 1989, p. 1607.

and 53% on placebos experienced a relapse. When these findings are combined using the Mantel-Haenszel meta-analysis, this difference is highly significant ($P = 10^{-100}$).

It is clear that there is a degree of heterogeneity in outcome among both placebo- and drug-treated patients; despite this, however, the results are extremely consistent in supporting drug-placebo differences. In addition, the fact that various investigations may have utilized different methodologies in selecting and evaluating patients but were consistent in finding a significant drug effect is all the more impressive.

Even among patients who have been successfully maintained on neuroleptic medication for substantial periods of time, the risk of relapse following drug discontinuation remains high. Table 6–2 includes six studies focusing specifically on patients in good remission ranging from 6 months to 5 years in duration. Following drug discontinuation, these patients had an average relapse rate of 75% during the next 6 months to 2 years. This would indicate that remaining relapse-free on medication does not necessarily indicate diminished need for drug treatment. The fact that some patients may not relapse immediately following drug discontinuation has raised the possibility of utilizing intermittent treatment to capitalize on the feasibility of a lengthy drug-free interval. This issue will be reviewed subsequently and also discussed in Chapter 7.

Some critics of neuroleptic treatment in schizophrenia have pointed to the results from long-term naturalistic follow-up studies (Bleuler 1978; Ciompi 1980a, 1980b; Harding et al. 1986; Huber et al. 1979, 1980) to suggest that some patients appear to experience a chronic deteriorating course, whereas others may experience a much more benign outcome after 10 or 20 years. The heterogeneity of outcome, with the possibility for substantial improvement in some patients, does not diminish the need for (or efficacy of) antipsychotic drugs during the first several years of the ill-

**Table 6–2.** Relapse rate following drug discontinuation among patients in long-term remission

| Investigators | $n$ | Time in remission (years) | Length of follow-up off drug (months) | Relapse rate percentage |
|---|---|---|---|---|
| Hogarty et al. (1976) | 41 | 2–3 | 12 | 65 |
| Johnson (1976) | 23 | 1–2 | 6 | 53 |
| Dencker et al. (1980) | 32 | 2 | 24 | 94 |
| Cheung (1981) | 30 | 3–5 | 18 | 62 |
| Johnson (1979) | 60 | 1–4 | 18 | 80 |
| Wistedt (1981) | 14 | $\frac{1}{2}$ | 12 | 100 |

ness. Controlled studies have not been conducted for intervals of more than 2 years in a particular patient population, but the maintenance treatment trials referred to have included patients at various stages of the illness.

In addition, there is some indication that a delay in instituting neuroleptic medication following the onset of the schizophrenic illness may have a deleterious impact on the subsequent course. The only controlled trial that provided data to address this concern was conducted by May and his colleagues (May 1968, 1976; May et al. 1981). These investigators studied first-admission schizophrenic patients who were randomly assigned to five conditions: antipsychotic drug therapy plus psychotherapy, psychotherapy alone, medication alone, electroconvulsive therapy, and a control group (which received only milieu therapy). These patients were treated for at least 6 months. On a variety of outcome measures, those patients receiving psychotherapy plus medication or medication alone did significantly better than patients receiving psychotherapy alone or milieu therapy alone. Subsequent to the random assignment study, virtually all of the patients ultimately received antipsychotic medication and were followed for a period ranging from 3 to 5 years after discharge from their first hospitalization. During the follow-up interval, treatments were uncontrolled but most patients continued to receive medication. Interestingly, those patients who had initially not received antipsychotic medication experienced a substantially greater number of days of subsequent hospitalization than those patients who had received medication treatment.

There are several pharmacologic factors that should be considered in planning the treatment of an acute episode.

## Drug Type

Although we have seen the development of a variety of different antipsychotic medications and chemical classes of these compounds during the past three decades, there are at present no convincing data that, among those medications currently marketed in the United States, any one is more effective either in schizophrenia in general or in specific subtypes of the disorder, with the possible exception of clozapine in the treatment of patients who have failed to respond to other antipsychotics (Kane et al. 1988). It remains conceivable that other differences do exist but that appropriately designed and executed studies have not been initiated to address this issue. Very few studies provide generalizable data on differential treatment response to specific pharmacologic agents. The majority of the available information comes from comparisons of overall response rate in group data comparing one drug to another. Although a given sample of patients who are randomly assigned to one drug or another may experience a 70–80% proportion of at least moderate therapeutic response to either drug, this does not necessarily mean that a given individual would respond equally well to either drug. There are remarkably few studies (Gardos 1978) that have examined this issue, despite the enormous clinical importance in the day-to-day treatment of patients who fail to respond to an initial course of an antipsychotic drug. Despite clinical observation that some patients who show inadequate response to one drug might occasionally benefit from another drug, it is difficult to establish a cause-and-effect relationship in a specific single case, since other factors besides the change in medication (e.g., additional time on medication) could contribute to the improvement.

It is clear from preclinical investigations that antipsychotic drugs do differ considerably in their relative affinities for specific brain receptors (Hytell et al. 1985; Richelson 1985), including the dopamine receptors felt to mediate therapeutic response. These data also support the possibility that all medications do not have the same spectrum of therapeutic activity. At the same time, it has been suggested that the milligram potency of various antipsychotic drugs does correlate with receptor affinity in theoretically relevant binding assays (Creese et al. 1976). Antipsychotic medications do differ in their propensity to produce various adverse effects, and these differences may be important in choosing a medication for those individuals with a known sensitivity to a specific side effect. In addition, our knowledge of a patient's previous therapeutic response to a specific antipsychotic medication should be weighed heavily in choosing a specific drug.

One misconception that continues to be prevalent among some clinicians is that sedating drugs (e.g., chlorpromazine) are more effective in controlling highly agitated, excited, or hostile patients and that nonsedating drugs (e.g., haloperidol and trifluoperazine) are more appropriate for withdrawn or psychomotorically retarded patients. In addition, some clinicians believe that combinations of sedating and nonsedating are necessary to provide control of psychotic symptoms and to facilitate sleep. These relationships have never been established, and numerous studies suggest that high- and low-potency drugs are equally effective for all types of patients (Davis et al. 1989).

Clozapine, which has recently been marketed in the United States, is the first drug found to be significantly superior to comparison antipsychotic medications in the treatment of unresponsive schizophrenic patients. A trial conducted at 16 hospitals in the United States, including 268 patients, found clozapine to be superior to chlorpromazine plus benztropine (Kane et al. 1988). In order to be eligible for this study, patients had to meet DSM-III criteria (American Psychiatric Association 1980) for schizophrenia and the following criteria for treatment refractoriness: 1) at least three periods of treatment in the preceding 5 years with neuroleptic agents (from at least two different chemical classes) at dosages equivalent to or greater than 1,000 mg/day of chlorpromazine for a period of 6 weeks, each without significant symptomatic relief; and 2) no period of good functioning within the preceding 5 years. Eligible patients also had to have a total Brief Psychiatric Rating Scale (BPRS) score of at least 45 as well as a minimum Clinical Global Impressions Scale rating of 4 (moderately ill), with item scores of at least 4 (moderate) on two of the following four BPRS items: conceptual disorganization, suspiciousness, hallucinatory behavior, and unusual thought content. All patients who met both the historical criteria for treatment resistance and initial severity criteria and gave their informed consent entered a prospective treatment period with haloperidol of as much as 60 mg/day or greater (with benztropine mesylate) in order to confirm the lack of drug responsiveness.

Clozapine was found to be superior in both positive and negative symptom areas as well as global improvement. Using a priori criteria for "improvement," 30% of the clozapine patients were categorized as improved, compared with 4% of the chlorpromazine patients. Clearly, not all such patients benefit from treatment with this drug, but the fact that approximately one-third do is a major therapeutic opportunity.

Clozapine is associated with a higher incidence of agranulocytosis than that seen with other antipsychotic medications. Agranulocytosis is defined as a white blood cell count of fewer than 2,000 cells per $mm^3$, with fewer than 500 cells per $mm^3$ of polymorphonuclear leukocytes and relative lymphopenia. Agranulocytosis, if undetected, can cause death, so it requires immediate drug discontinuation. In the United States the incidence of agranulocytosis with clozapine has been between 1% and 2% with no fatalities, largely because of the careful monitoring of white blood cell counts and immediate discontinuation of the drug when the white blood cell count falls below 3,000. Because of this adverse effect, clozapine has been marketed for the treatment of those patients with a psychotic illness who are unresponsive to or who cannot tolerate available antipsychotic agents. Clozapine appears to produce almost no parkinsonian symptoms or dystonia and has rarely been associated with tardive dyskinesia. Therefore, clozapine may be helpful to those patients who have demonstrated an inability to tolerate other neuroleptics because of severe extrapyramidal side effects. The role of clozapine in the treatment of movement disorders remains unclear. Although some studies (see Chapter 5) have reported substantial improvement in abnormal involuntary movements when patients are treated with clozapine, it remains to be determined the extent to which this represents a suppression, a true therapeutic effect, or the passage of time off of prior neuroleptic treatment. Given clozapine's apparent reduced propensity to produce tardive dyskinesia, its use in the management of patients who require ongoing neuroleptic treatment, but have developed moderate or severe tardive dyskinesia, seems reasonable. The extent to which this indication is consistent with U.S. Food and Drug Administration labeling is open to interpretation; therefore, the clinician should be careful to document the considerations that took place prior to initiating such treatment.

A careful assessment of relative benefit and risk as well as the process of informed consent should also be evident in the medical record.

## Drug Dosage

Concern regarding tardive dyskinesia has served as an important impetus to clarify minimum dosage requirements for both the acute and maintenance treatment of schizophrenia. Although the relationship between cumulative neuroleptic dosage and the incidence of tardive dyskinesia is not clear-cut, there are data suggesting that dosage may be a factor in determining overall risk of tardive dyskinesia, along with a variety of other variables. Our ability to clearly delineate the relationship between cumulative dosage and the incidence of tardive dyskinesia is complicated by the fact that a minority of patients develops tardive dyskinesia, and any existing dosage effects would only be apparent in that subgroup. If better means were available to identify patients at high risk, then trials specifically designed to assess the impact of dosage would be much more revealing. In addition, oral dose may not reflect actual blood or central nervous system (CNS) levels, making correlations more difficult to detect.

We still have insufficient information regarding dose-response curves for antipsychotic drugs (the related issue of drug levels will be discussed subsequently). One of the difficulties in this area is that many studies of drug efficacy have not employed fixed-dose strategies. When flexible doses are employed, the clinician adjusts the dosage depending on clinical response. This can be misleading, however, in defining a dose-response relationship because a variety of factors may influence both dosage and clinical response. For example, if a patient receiving a given dose of an antipsychotic medication demonstrates little or no improvement after 10 days and the clinician decides to increase the dose, subsequent improvement might then be attributed to the higher dose when, in reality, improvement may have occurred solely because of the passage of additional time on the original dose. In addition, those studies that include patients who may be relative "placebo responders" would potentially obscure a dose-response relationship, as would those patients who may be refractory regardless of the dosage. In the latter group, the clinician would in all likelihood end up treating the patient with particularly high doses if a flexible schedule were used, and this would create an additional confound in any exploration of dose-response relationship.

The dosage issue can be conceptualized in terms of different dose-response curves. In the typical sigmoidal dose-response curve, when a very low dose is administered, there will be no clinical improvement. At a somewhat higher dose, the linear portion of the dose-response curve is reached, where an increase in dosage produces a proportionate increase in therapeutic response. When all of the therapeutic response that can occur has taken place, a point of diminishing return ensues, which is represented by the flat portion of the sigmoidal curve, where increasing the dose does not increase therapeutic response. The point of most interest in such a curve is the inflection point at which the linear portion changes to the flat part of the curve; at doses above this there is no further therapeutic gain, whereas there may be an increase in adverse effects. In the curvilinear dose relationship there is a point of dosage above which therapeutic response is impeded by further dosage increase. Although this has been suggested to be the case with a variety of psychotropic drugs, much work remains to be done to confirm this effect with antipsychotic medications. In many cases the appropriate validation strategy has not been pursued. This would require identifying patients whose dosage or blood level is above the putative therapeutic window and who have failed to respond clinically and then adjusting downward their dosage and/or blood level in order to demonstrate improved therapeutic response and confirm this relationship. By and large this has not been done, and it remains unclear as to what extent an increase in adverse effects (particularly those adverse effects that may be behaviorally manifest, such as akathisia) may play a role in the diminution of therapeutic response above a certain dosage level.

The relationship between neuroleptic dosage and the occurrence of tardive dyskinesia or acute drug-induced extrapyramidal symptoms is complicated. This should not be surprising, because not all patients will have the same vulnerability to developing these adverse effects and not all neuroleptics may have the same propensity to produce each of these effects. In addition, the dose-response relationship and the time of onset may be quite different in various reactions—for example, dystonia, akathisia, akinesia, and tardive dyskinesia. Prior neuroleptic exposure, bioavailability, age, sex, other manifestations of CNS dysfunction, and even genetic factors may play a role in the incidence and intensity of these neurologic side effects.

There are various sources of data that can be employed to suggest neuroleptic dose-response curves. Soon after the introduction of chlorpromazine, many low-dose, placebo versus chlorpromazine studies were done, and these data are summarized in Table 6–3. Virtually all of the studies employing dosages of 400 mg/day or more of chlorpromazine demonstrated it to be superior in efficacy to a placebo. A second source of data involves the many double-blind studies that compared different doses of the same drug. Table 6–4 summarizes all studies in which patients were randomly assigned to two different dosages. Approximately 30 such studies are included. When the lower dose employed was 300 mg or less in chlorpromazine equivalents, most studies showed this dose to be less effective than the higher dose. When the lower dose employed was 540–940 mg (chlorpromazine equivalents), all 10 such studies showed this to be equal in efficacy to a higher dose. It is important to note that when very high or megadoses were compared to high or moderate doses, the former were never shown to be unequivocally superior to the latter. This does not preclude the possibility that some patients may benefit from higher doses, but it suggests that some individuals represent a small subgroup and that better means of identifying appropriate candidates for high-dose treatment should be established. In general, the literature would suggest that doses of 400–900 mg/day of chlorpromazine or equivalents should be sufficient for the average patient. There had been a tendency to use particularly large doses of "high-potency" antipsychotics, because apart from parkinsonian side effects, high doses are generally well tolerated, but this practice should be discouraged unless it is clearly established that such doses are necessary for a specific patient.

## Dose Equivalents

With the appropriate increase in emphasis on establishing minimum effective dosage, a clear understanding of dose equivalency between antipsychotic medications is important. Chlorpromazine has usually been the standard against which equivalent doses are established. An ongoing problem, however, is that the customary method of determining dose equivalents is somewhat crude and unsystematic. The most common method has involved a double-blind clinical trial comparing two antipsychotic com-

**Table 6–3.**   Effectiveness of different dose levels of chlorpromazine

| Dose (mg) | Percentage of studies in which chlorpromazine was: | | | |
| | More effective than a placebo | Slightly more effective than a placebo | Equal to a placebo | N |
|---|---|---|---|---|
| 300 or less | 40 | 24 | 36 | 25 |
| 301–400 | 40 | 38 | 13 | 8 |
| 401–500 | 80 | 0 | 20 | 5 |
| 501–800 | 100 | 0 | 0 | 14 |
| 800 or more | 100 | 0 | 0 | 9 |

*Note:*  Reprinted with permission from Kaplan HI, Sadock BJ (eds): Comprehensive Textbook of Psychiatry/V, 5th Edition, Vol 2. Baltimore, MD, Williams & Wilkins, 1989, p. 1600.

pounds, with the clinician adjusting dosage as seen fit. At the end of the trial, comparisons are made of the dosages employed and a conversion ratio is suggested. In addition, results from drug-placebo comparisons may

**Table 6–4.**   Dose-response studies

| Investigators | Higher dose | Lower dose | Result | Status | |
|---|---|---|---|---|---|
| Quitkin | 100,000 | 2,500 | Fluphenazine | H = S | A |
| Wijsenbeck | 21,000 | 2,100 | Trifluoperazine | H = S | A |
| Donlon (1980) | 6,200 | 1,700 | Haloperidol | H = S | A |
| Dember | 2,700 | 1,360 | Thiothixene | H = S | A |
| Ericksen | 3,800 | 940 | Haloperidol | H = S | A |
| Donlon (1978) | 6,250 | 625 | Fluphenazine | H = S | A |
| Donlon (1978) | 2,700 | 625 | Fluphenazine | H = S | A |
| Coffman | 2,406 | 600 | Fluphenazine | H = S | A |
| Neborsky | 2,600 | 600 | Haloperidol | H = S | A |
| Fitzgerald | 1,600 | 300 | Haloperidol | H = S | A |
| Goldstein | 293 | 73 | Fluphenazine | H + | A |
| Anderson | 2,100 | 800 | Haloperidol | H = S | O |
| Slotnick | 1,900 | 300 | Haloperidol | H = S | O |
| Man | 2,200 | 300 | Haloperidol | H = S | O |
| Reschke | 875 | 230 | Haloperidol | H = S | O |
| Gerstenzang | 313 | 50 | Haloperidol | H = S | O |
| Rimon | 7,500 | 3,750 | Haloperidol | H = S | C |
| Itil (1970) | 67,000 | 2,500 | Fluphenazine | H = S | C |
| DeBuck | 67,000 | 1,700 | Fluphenazine | H = S | C |
| Bjordnal | 10,800 | 800 | Haloperidol | H = S | C |
| Itil (1971) | 3,300 | 800 | Fluphenazine | H = S | C |
| McCreadie | 6,250 | 600 | Fluphenazine | H = S | C |
| Prien (1969) | 2,900 | 540 | Trifluoperazine | H = S | C |
| Carscallen | 3,600 | 360 | Trifluoperazine | H = S | C |
| Prien (1968) | 2,000 | 300 | Chlorpromazine | H + | C |
| Clark (1970, 1972) | 600 | 300 | Chlorpromazine | H + | C |
| McClelland | 5,850 | 290 | Fluphenazine | H = S | C |
| Denker | 5,300 | 270 | Fluphenazine | H + | C |
| Gardose | 910 | 230 | Thiothixene | H = S | C |
| Lehmann | 2,600 | 230 | Fluphenazine | H + | C |
| Clark (1970, 1972) | 300 | 150 | Chlorpromazine | H + | C |
| Simpson | 440 + | 56 | Butaperazine | H + | C |

*Note.*   H = S indicates high dose equal to lower dose in efficacy; H + indicates higher dose is more effecacious than the standard dose; A indicates acute; C indicates chronic; O indicates acute study of first few hours of treatment.
*Source.*   Reprinted with permission from Kaplan HI, Sadock BJ (eds): Comprehensive Textbook of Psychiatry/V, 5th Edition, Vol 2. Baltimore, MD, Williams & Wilkins, 1989, p. 1599.

be combined to identify the clinically "effective" dosage range of a particular drug. The potential problems in assuming the validity of these results are numerous. It is particularly important to recognize the possibility that those conversion ratios that may be appropriate at the lower end of the dosage spectrum may not apply at higher dosage levels. It does appear from the literature that many clinicians are using dissimilar dosing practices with high-potency as compared to low-potency antipsychotics. Baldessarini et al. (1984) compared the findings of a survey of 110 private psychiatric hospital inpatients with the dosing practices as reported in surveys of nearly 16,000 U.S. Veterans Administration patients. The doses of high-potency drugs above the daily equivalent of 1 gram of chlorpromazine accounted for more than 40% of all prescriptions. The mean chlorpromazine equivalent dose of the two most potent antipsychotic agents (haloperidol and fluphenazine) was 3.54 times as high as the mean doses prescribed of chlorpromazine or thioridazine. As Baldessarini et al. (1984) suggested, the sedative and autonomic effects of low-potency drugs may limit their use in the higher dosage range, whereas it is feasible for clinicians to increase doses of high-potency antipsychotics without substantial increase in immediate adverse effects.

### Rapid Neuroleptization

One potential factor contributing to the use of higher doses is the increasing pressure on clinicians to reduce the length of hospital stays. This has in some cases fostered an approach utilizing rapid dosage increase frequently employing intramuscular preparations. The problem, however, is that the use of "rapid neuroleptization" and/or high-dose treatment has not been shown to shorten the time required for these drugs to exert their therapeutic effect or to improve clinical outcome in general (Neborsky et al. 1981). Virtually all investigators have consistently found that normal doses and high loading doses produce equal benefits (Davis et al. 1989). (The acute studies are indicated as such in Table 6–4.) Although the time course of response is unpredictable, with a degree of clinical improvement occurring rapidly in some patients and more slowly in others, our experience and the literature suggest that 4–6 weeks is usually necessary to begin to see the full therapeutic benefit, but in many cases even longer intervals are needed. Clearly, different patients will require different doses and the clinician should titrate the amount of medication prescribed for each patient based on his or her own response, both therapeutic and adverse.

### Drug Blood Levels

One of the difficulties in establishing dose-response relationships for either therapeutic benefit or the occurrence of adverse effects is the lack of high correlation between oral dosage and drug blood level. Since the recognition of considerable individual variability in absorption and metabolism of antipsychotic drugs and the availability of assays to measure levels of neuroleptics and blood (Curry and Marshall 1968), there has been considerable interest in attempting to determine the relationship between blood levels and clinical response. It was hoped that this strategy would provide important information that might help in explaining the enormous variability in drug response seen in schizophrenia. To a large extent these efforts have not met the original expectations, but blood levels may have some utility in specific clinical studies. In the last decade we have seen considerable advances in the laboratory technique available for measuring minute quantities of antipsychotic drugs in clinical specimens (e.g., plasma, cerebrospinal fluid, and red blood cells). Ironically, despite sophisticated technology, flaws in design and methodology of clinical trials employing blood levels have often limited the potential to draw meaningful conclusions. The importance of using a fixed-dose design in establishing correlations between dosage or blood level and clinical response has already been discussed. Relevant studies have been reviewed by Kane (1987), Volavka and Cooper (1987), and Van Putten et al. (1991). None of the studies conducted to date is ideal in addressing all of the potential methodologic concerns, but it is extremely difficult to carry out such investigations in the kinds of clinical settings where appropriate patients can be found.

The most frequently studied compound is haloperidol, and several of the aforementioned investigators have suggested a curvilinear relationship between blood level and clinical response or a putative "therapeutic window." Although these findings are intriguing, considerable further work is necessary to establish and define a therapeutic window. Most of the studies suggesting this phenomenon have had relatively few patients above the suggested upper limit and, more important, hardly any attempts have been made at the random assignment of those patients whose blood levels are out of the therapeutic range to a dosage necessary to manipulate the blood level into the therapeutic range or to remain at their current blood level (to control for continued time on the drug). Until this is done in a systematic, replicable fashion, conclusions must remain tentative. Volavka et al. (1990) reported preliminary data from a study in which patients who did not respond to an initial course of randomized doses and blood levels of neuroleptics were rerandomized to different blood levels. They did not find any relationship between blood levels and clinical response.

This concern is also important regarding the previous discussion of high-dose or megadose treatment. If patients were specifically selected because of their relatively low blood levels on standard doses of antipsychotics, then a substantial dosage increase might have a greater likelihood of being therapeutically beneficial. On the other hand, if studies using substantial dosage increases involve a heterogeneous group of drug nonresponders, then the likelihood of seeing a desired clinical effect may be reduced.

An additional issue of some importance in interpreting the suggestion of a therapeutic window is the possibility of those patients showing a poor or minimum clinical response at the higher blood levels in fact experiencing behaviorally manifest adverse effects that could alter or impede therapeutic response (Bolvig-Hansen et al. 1982). Although some investigators have suggested that an increase in adverse effects does not account for the lack of therapeutic effect seen at higher blood levels, this question requires further study. Behaviorally manifest adverse effects can be difficult to distinguish from psychopathology at times, and a patient who is experiencing a severe degree of psychopathology may not be able to articulate subjective feelings and sensations in a way that would contribute to a differential diagnosis.

The overall value of measuring blood levels of antipsychotic drugs remains far from clear, but the data that are available should emphasize to clinicians and investigators the importance of recognizing the potential problems of utilizing dosages that are too high, as well as the importance of appropriate clinical evaluation and research methodology in using or employing high-dose treatment in specific subgroups of schizophrenic patients.

The utilization of drug blood levels in assessing the relationship of antipsychotic drugs to tardive dyskinesia is discussed in Chapter 4.

## Maintenance Neuroleptic Treatment

The "acute" phase in the treatment of schizophrenia and other psychotic disorders involves an attempt to alleviate the signs and symptoms associated with an acute exacerbation. In general, antipsychotic drugs have a marked effect on the signs and symptoms of schizophrenia (e.g., delusions, hallucinations, and thought disorder) within 4–6 weeks, although improvement may continue well beyond that time period. The therapeutic gains achieved during this treatment phase will to some extent determine the rationale and expectations of any subsequent continuation or maintenance treatment.

We characteristically divide the pharmacological treatment of an illness with exacerbations and relative remissions into three phases: acute, continuation, and maintenance (or prophylactic). For those individuals who do achieve full or substantial therapeutic response during the acute treatment phase, the continuation phase begins when maximal improvement is reached, and its intent is to continue the treatment for a sufficient length of time to be sure that the episode for which the treatment was originally given is, in fact, over. After this interval has passed, then further pharmacological treatment would be intended to prevent the occurrence of a new episode rather than the reemergence of the original episode. This model has been applied more readily to affective illness, wherein episodes may be more discreet; however, in our view, it may be useful in schizophrenia as well. The specific delineation of these phases in the treatment of schizophrenia may be problematic, since, for example, some patients may not achieve a complete remission of psychopathology despite continuous pharmacotherapy. Although, as we have seen in results from clinical trials involving antipsychotic drug discontinuation, many of these patients would experience even more symptomatology without medication, in this instance pharmacotherapy may be viewed more as controlling or suppressing ongoing manifestations of the illness than as preventing a new episode. These patients, therefore, may be relatively poor candidates for drug discontinuation or substantial dosage reduction.

Maintenance antipsychotic drug treatment has proven to be of dramatic value in reducing the risk of psychotic relapse and rehospitalization. In the last 10 years we have witnessed the initiation of much more sophisticated long-term clinical trials that have focused not only on relapse rate and rehospitalization rate but on a variety of other factors that are relevant to assessing the overall benefits and risks of maintenance drug treatment.

It is clear that there is enormous variability in the relapse rates reported in the studies (see Table 6–1). Meaningful comparisons are complicated by differences in design and methodology, such as diagnostic criteria, level and duration of remission, patient selection and recruitment methods, and definition of relapse. In addition, not all of these reports have presented cumulative relapse rates or life-table analyses that allow for the appropriate handling of patients with incomplete data (e.g., those who dropped out of the study or those who are discontinued from the trial due to adverse effects). When cumulative relapse curves are presented, data from different studies can be contrasted even though investigators may have used different assessment intervals, conducted trials for different lengths of time, or experienced different drop-out rates.

Guaranteed medication delivery (i.e., the use of long-acting injectable neuroleptics) has played a major role in many of the largest maintenance medication studies in recent years, because it provides the investigator with the knowledge that relapse occurring in the context of long-term pharmacotherapy is not due to noncompliance in oral medication taking; therefore, the impact of other patient, treatment, or environmental factors can be considered and explored (Kane and Borenstein 1985).

In addition, the use of guaranteed medication delivery in clinical trials has made it quite clear that many patients continue to experience psychotic relapse despite medication, and this has underscored the importance of exploring other factors that might contribute to a poor outcome. At the same time, it is important to recognize that even though some patients may relapse despite continued neuroleptic treatment, this would not argue for withholding such treatment from this subgroup of patients. It is likely that relapses would be more frequent and more severe without any maintenance medication. At the present time, this assumption is based on clinical experience rather than systematic, random-assignment controlled trials involving patients who have demonstrated significant psychotic relapse despite continued maintenance medication.

The desire to reduce adverse effects—particularly tardive dyskinesia, but also behaviorally manifested parkinsonian side effects—has led to increasing interest in identifying minimum dosage requirements for the long-term treatment of schizophrenia as well as for acute treatment. This issue is reviewed in Chapter 7.

Ideally, we would benefit from having methods to enable us to identify specific patients who are best suited for a particular strategy on the basis of their propensity to relapse within a relatively short time following neuroleptic discontinuation. Pooled analyses from several large-scale collaborative studies suggest a constant rate of relapse among untreated patients ranging from 10% to 15% per month. This does not preclude the possibility that some predictors might be developed to identify those individuals at risk for rapid relapse following neuroleptic discontinuation. Various investigations have explored treatment history and demographic characteristics without deriving useful predictors. The work of Lieberman et al. (1984, 1987), using response to methylphenidate infusions as a potential predictor of relapse, is a logical extension of earlier work by Janowsky et al. (1973), Janowsky and Davis (1976), and Angrist et al. (1980, 1985). Lieberman's results suggest that those patients experiencing a transient exacerbation of psychotic signs and symptoms following 0.5 mg/kg of intravenous methylphenidate will relapse sooner (following discontinuance of an antipsychotic drug) than patients not responding to methylphenidate. This strategy is not necessarily intended to identify patients who can be maintained without medication on an indefinite basis, but in our experience this remains a very small subgroup.

### Conclusions

The efficacy of antipsychotic medication in the maintenance treatment of schizophrenia has been established in more controlled trials than most pharmacologic treatments in other areas of medicine. Nevertheless, there remain critics of long-term neuroleptic use. To some extent, these criticisms result from the complexity of the schizophrenic illness and the observations that a variety of factors may influence outcome and that for a given individual our ability to predict outcome is limited. Clinical judgments are based on the data available and on clinical experience; this body of knowledge has led to a strong consensus that the potential benefits of this treatment outweigh the potential risks. With current knowledge and currently available medications, the development of tardive dyskinesia in some patients is inevitable, even with the most judicious and careful use of these medications. The nature of schizophrenia, however, is such that without neuroleptic treatment many affected individuals remain severely symptomatic and disabled, leading to enormous personal suffering and the suffering of their families and friends. The suicide rate in schizophrenia has been shown to be 5–10% in long-term studies (Roy 1982), a consequence of the illness that is frequently overlooked.

There is no doubt that considerable gaps remain in our knowledge of this illness and the long-term impact of different treatment strategies. Data from controlled trials have usually been collected for 1- to 2-year periods, but most patients with this illness are affected for a substantially longer time. By the same token, various maintenance treatment trials have included a broad spectrum of patients, ranging from those recently recovered from their first episode (Crow et al. 1986; Kane et al. 1982) to those who have had multiple episodes over a decade or more, and the results remain consistent in demonstrating a highly significant drug effect regardless of the ages of the patients or the lengths of their illnesses.

The remaining unanswered questions should serve as an impetus for us to conduct additional research rather than to ignore or dismiss the vast body of data that has been accumulated. Debate regarding risks and benefits and a critical review of the knowledge base required to make rational decisions are both healthy and necessary.

## Treatment of Affective Disorders

Antipsychotic drugs are widely used in the treatment of acute mania, particularly during the earliest stages of such treatment. Although lithium is effective in alleviating the signs and symptoms of mania, neuroleptics may work more rapidly and be more effective in highly agitated or aggressive patients (Johnson et al. 1971; Platman 1970; Prien et al. 1972a, 1972b; Spring et al. 1970). Many clinicians combine lithium and neuroleptics during the initial days or weeks of the treatment of a manic episode. Unfortunately, we have far fewer data regarding dose-response relationships for antipsychotic medication in mania than we do for schizophrenia. In addition, there are no well-established guidelines for when neuroleptics should be discontinued, but most experts would advise relatively short-term use followed by a trial on lithium alone. The relative merits of antipsychotics and carbamazepine (or other anticonvulsants) as alternatives or adjuncts to lithium have not been well studied.

There are no long-term, random-assignment studies of neuroleptic treatment in disorders other than schizophrenia. This deficiency is particularly striking with regard to bipolar affective disorders and major depressive disorder with psychotic features.

Manic breakthrough remains an important problem in lithium-treated bipolar patients and may occur in as many as 40% of such patients (obviously relapse rates will vary depending on selection criteria, length of observation, relapse criteria, etc.). The only data available (Prien et al. 1974) suggest that those individuals who experience one manic relapse while receiving lithium do no better than placebo-treated patients after returning to the euthymic state. These patients were not randomly assigned to continue lithium or to be switched to placebo, however, so it is difficult to rule out the possibility that their subsequent course would have been even worse had they not continued lithium treatment. This study and one other (Dunner and Fieve 1974) also included samples of patients considered to be "rapid cyclers." Different criteria were employed in the two reports (i.e., four affective episodes per year or hospitalized three or more times for affective episodes during the 2 years preceding the study). The suggestion from both of these studies was that lithium is of relatively little value to such patients; however, this conclusion is not entirely justified by the data available.

We are not aware of any controlled clinical trials specifically assessing the efficacy of neuroleptic medication alone or combined with lithium in patients who experience breakthrough. Ahlfors et al. (1981) studied 162 patients who were switched from lithium to flupentixol decanoate for any of the following reasons: 1) unsatisfactory prophylactic effects; 2) doubtful tablet compliance; 3) troublesome side effects; 4) fear that continued lithium might be harmful. Patients received 20 mg of flupentixol decanoate every 3 weeks. The course during the flupentixol treatment (the average length of observation was 14 months) was compared to the course of illness during the 2 years preceding the start of flupentixol treatment. For the 85 bipolar patients who were observed for at least 6 months on flupentixol, the number of manic episodes per patient year and the percentage of time in a manic episode were reduced to a statistically significant degree. When the same measures were applied to depressive relapse, however, there was a significant worsening during flupentixol treatment. Unfortunately, those patients who had experienced affective relapse on lithium prior to entering the study were not analyzed separately from those patients who were noncompliant with lithium. In addition, the trial was not controlled but was "mirror image" in design.

Kielholz et al. (1979) reported that in a trial including 30 patients with "cyclic depression" who had experienced side effects with lithium, flupentixol decanoate (an average dose of 25 mg im every 3 weeks) produced a significant reduction in depressive episodes requiring hospitalization. These findings were based on a mirror-image comparison of the number of hospitalizations per year during a 2- to 7-year period prior to flupentixol and a 2- to 3-year open trial with flupentixol. It appears that only two bipolar patients were included in this sample. The authors suggested that flupentixol is equivalent to lithium in the prophylaxis of "cyclic" depression. Given the apparent higher morbidity and substantial risk of repeated hospitalizations in this group, the possibility that neuroleptics might have a therapeutic effect has been assumed by many clinicians but should be explored more systematically. At the same time, the potential for adverse effects must be examined, and the interaction between lithium and neuroleptics should be considered in terms of both therapeutic potential and potential for adverse effects (or possibly even for the diminution of specific adverse effects—i.e., concomitant lithium may reduce the risk of tardive dyskinesia associated with chronic neuroleptic treatment). Some animal studies (Pert et al. 1978) have suggested that lithium might prevent the development of dopamine receptor supersensitivity associated with neuroleptic drugs, and some clinical data support this relationship as well (Kane et al. 1986).

In the treatment of acute depressive episodes uncomplicated by psychotic symptoms, antidepressant medications or ECT are indicated. The use of antipsychotic drugs for typical cases of acute depression is probably not warranted unless alternative treatments have been found to be ineffective (Simpson et al. 1972).

The apparent continued widespread and frequently long-term use of preparations that combine antidepressants and antipsychotics seems hard to justify given the problems in titrating two medications provided in firm ratios of the two compounds, as well as the general lack of data supporting the advantages of the combination over antidepressants alone in long-term applications. Although several studies support the efficacy of these preparations as compared with placebos in heterogeneous groups of patients with mixed anxiety and depression (Diamond 1966; Hollister et al. 1966), these studies did not utilize methodology or diagnostic criteria that would now be considered state of the art. Although good epidemiologic studies of tardive dyskinesia have not been carried out among patients with anxiety and depression receiving low doses of neuroleptics, either alone or in combination with antidepressants, cases of tardive dyskinesia have been observed and reported among such individuals. We are unable to make firm statements regarding the relative risk of tardive dyskinesia in such cases as compared with patients receiving higher doses; however, this should still be viewed a risk when considering such treatment strategies.

In addition, the use of such preparations without prior adequate trials of each medication separately may lead to uncritical diagnostic evaluation of certain patients and potentially inappropriate long-term use of such combinations without consideration of alternatives. There are no controlled trials of such combinations in maintenance treatment.

Depressed patients with psychotic symptoms or severe agitation may benefit from antipsychotic medication; however, the relative benefits and risks of this strategy in contrast to ECT or antidepressant medications have not been well established in controlled clinical trials. There are studies that suggest that ECT is superior to tricyclic antidepressants alone in very agitated or delusional depressed patients (Sandifer et al. 1965; Simpson et al. 1976); however, we are not aware of any prospective random assignment studies comparing ECT, neuroleptics, and antidepressants (or a combination of neuroleptics and antidepressants). It is difficult at present to draw clear conclusions regarding the relative indications for neuroleptics in this context, and clinical judgment should include the careful weighing of all of the alternatives by the clinician. It should not be surprising that there are no data regarding the relative merits of these treatments in the long-term maintenance or prophylactic treatment of this subgroup of depressed patients. Given the fact that patients with affective illness may be at particular risk for developing tardive dyskinesia, it would be prudent wherever possible to limit neuroleptic exposure to the shortest possible duration. If a clinician identifies patients with whom clinical experience supports long-term administration of neuroleptics, because alternatives were ineffective, unacceptable, or contraindicated or produced intolerable adverse effects, then this set of conditions should be clearly documented in the medical record.

It is not unusual for controlled clinical research to follow rather than to precede the clinical use of specific pharmacologic treatments. It should, therefore, not be assumed that such use is dangerous or undesirable. Clinicians frequently employ treatments in individual cases in a thoughtful fashion with an attempt to balance demonstrated benefits against potential risks. Controlled clinical research may not yet provide compelling support for long-term uses in specific cases other than chronic schizophrenia, but it has not provided evidence that such uses are lacking in benefit or contraindicated. Clinicians must rely on their own evaluation of individual patients and their own clinical experience as further research data are generated and evaluated. Based on our own surveys and clinical experience, many patients with bipolar illness are treated with neuroleptic drugs, and in many cases this seems to be beneficial. It is important that clinicians use the minimum effective dose for the shortest duration possible and that other potentially less-toxic alternatives (e.g., carbamazepine) also be considered.

# Neuroleptic Use in the Elderly

As indicated by drug utilization reports, neuroleptic drugs are commonly used in the clinical management of a variety of conditions in the elderly. The indications for neuroleptics in the treatment of conditions that develop earlier but persist into late life would include schizophrenia, bipolar illness refractory to lithium, and depression with psychotic features unresponsive to antidepressants or ECT. It is important to recognize, however, that a variety of factors may be influenced by the aging process: The illness may not be as severe, dosage requirements may be lower, the risk of drug interactions may increase, and the incidence of tardive dyskinesia appears to be substantially higher. Therefore, continual review of the benefit-to-risk ratio should include these factors when neuroleptic drugs are continued into late life.

In addition, there are various conditions that may have their onset in late life, including dementia, psychoses, and major depressive episodes with psychotic features. Agitated behavior, extreme restlessness, and even assaultive behavior are common components of psychoses and depression among the elderly.

It is not uncommon for elderly individuals to experience various degrees of dementia, psychoses, and depression concurrently. Drugs are widely used to control agitation in this population. Several nonneuroleptic medications have been utilized, including benzodiazepines, beta-blockers, carbamazepine, and reserpine, but neuroleptics continue to be the most frequently prescribed class of medication. Those few comparative trials that have been carried out suggest that neuroleptics are more effective than benzodiazepines (Salzman 1987). Although beta-blockers, particularly propranolol, are being utilized by some clinicians, controlled clinical trials are lacking. The same applies to carbamazepine.

Several reviews have appeared on the use of antipsychotic drugs in the elderly (Salzman 1987; Satlin and Cole 1986; Sunderland and Silver 1988). The inherent difficulty in reviewing these studies is the variable inclusion criteria. Despite the methodologic shortcomings, the consensus has been that neuroleptic drugs are therapeutically useful in the treatment of agitation, restlessness, and hostility in elderly patients with a variety of diagnoses. Therefore, the indications are symptomatic rather than based on specific diagnostic categories, given our current state of knowledge. There remains enormous concern, however, about the potential for overutilization of neuroleptic drugs in this context, and further research is sorely needed to help clarify the benefit-to-risk ratio in this population. It is also important to emphasize that the overwhelming majority of the studies conducted in this population were 8 weeks or less in duration and, therefore, the relatively long-term indications for neuroleptic treatment in this population are far from clear.

It is also essential to appreciate, as Salzman (1987) concludes, that the overall therapeutic efficacy of these drugs is modest rather than striking. For some patients in fact, these drugs are not more therapeutic than placebo, and may even contribute to a worsening of behavior (Salzman 1987). This point is particularly worthy of emphasis, given the difficulty inherent in distinguishing akathisia from agitation in a psychotic or demented individual. At present, there are insufficient data to conclude that any particular neuroleptic or class of neuroleptics is more efficacious or safer in this population. Clearly, older individuals are more sensitive to and more in danger from sedation, orthostatic hypotension, and anticholinergic side effects. As we discussed in Chapter 4, it is also clear that the risk of tardive dyskinesia in the elderly is particularly high (Saltz et al. 1991). Adequate therapeutic effect may be achieved in this patient population, with doses substantially lower than those employed in younger individuals.

It is difficult to determine the extent to which these drugs are indicated and beneficial in all of the elderly patients receiving them, but at least for those elderly patients in whom the continuing need for antipsychotic medications has not been clinically established, a periodic, careful tapering and a trial without antipsychotic medication is indicated if no distinct and persistent worsening of the patient's clinical condition occurs.

## Disorders of Childhood and Adolescence

Neuroleptic drugs have been used at times to treat several psychiatric disorders occurring in childhood and adolescence, including schizophrenia, infantile autism, pervasive developmental disorder, Tourette's disorder, attention-deficit hyperactivity disorder, and conduct disorder, as well as some aggressive and nonspecific behavioral symptoms associated with mental retardation.

The use of neuroleptics in children and adolescents should be weighed very carefully and should be preceded by a thorough diagnostic evaluation and a complete discussion with the parents and child regarding the nature of the condition being treated, its course and prognosis (both with and without the recommended treatment), and the anticipated medication effects—including both therapeutic and potentially adverse effects. This information should be presented in a clear and understandable fashion, and questions and discussion should be elicited from parents and child. In addition, this process should be documented in the medical record (see Chapter 11).

It is also important that, as part of the diagnostic evaluation and pretreatment assessment, an examination for abnormal involuntary movements or stereotypic behavior occur. This is particularly important for autistic children and the developmentally disabled because of the high prevalence of preexisting abnormal movements. The presence and severity of such movements should be documented, ideally utilizing a rating instrument for this purpose (see Chapter 3).

## Schizophrenia

Schizophrenia in prepubertal children is a rare disorder. The incidence of this condition in children younger than 15 years is estimated at 0.08 per 1,000 (Babigian 1975). If one includes only prepubertal children, the incidence would be even lower. Chart reviews and studies of clinical services have documented that schizophrenia is rare in childhood (Green et al. 1984; Kydd and Werry 1982). There have been no studies of the efficacy of neuroleptics in the treatment of schizophrenia in children. Clinical experience indicates that neuroleptics are not as beneficial in children as in adolescents or adults with schizophrenia (Campbell 1985; Green 1984).

In adolescents with schizophrenia, one placebo-controlled study has been conducted. The efficacy of Loxitane and haloperidol was demonstrated in acute first-episode patients and those experiencing an exacerbation of chronic schizophrenia (Pool et al. 1976). Seventy-five inpatients (ages 13–18) were randomly assigned to Loxitane (a mean dose of 9.8 mg/day), haloperidol (a mean dose of 87.5 mg/day), or a placebo for a 4-week period. There was significant improvement as assessed on the BPRS and the Nurse's Observation Scale for Inpatient Evaluation. Haloperidol was found to be more sedating than Loxitane. (No comparison was made in responsiveness of the two patient subgroups.)

Realmuto et al. (1984) studied the efficacy of neuroleptics in adolescents with chronic schizophrenia. Thiothixene and thioridazine were compared in 21 patients for 4–6 weeks. Approximately one-half of the patients in both drug groups showed improvement. Thiothixene was more frequently associated with sedation. Neuroleptics are efficacious in adolescents with acute first-episode schizophrenia or those with an exacerbation of chronic schizophrenia; however, as with adults, positive symptoms generally respond better than negative symptoms.

The use of clozapine in adolescent schizophrenic patients refractory to other neuroleptics may be promising. One open clinical trial has demonstrated marked to moderate improvement in 80% of the 21 patients treated (Siefen and Remschmidt 1986). Clozapine has not been formally approved for use in adolescents; however, the physician should decide based on the literature and available clinical experience whether a therapeutic trial is warranted in carefully selected refractory patients. Clozapine is associated with a 1–2% incidence of agranulocytosis in adults, and the incidence in children or adolescents has not been established. Weekly complete blood counts are essential in any patient receiving this drug.

### Autistic Disorder and Pervasive Developmental Disorder

Several studies of the efficacy of neuroleptics in the treatment of autistic children have been conducted (Anderson et al. 1984; Campbell 1985; Campbell et al. 1984). The nomenclature for autistic disorder and pervasive developmental disorder has changed from DSM-III to DSM-III-R (American Psychiatric Association 1987). These disorders are characterized by a qualitative impairment or delay in social interaction, verbal and nonverbal communication, and developmental-appropriate activities and interests. The available studies of neuroleptics in autistic children did not use DSM-III-R criteria; therefore, the literature reviewed is based on the DSM-III criteria for infantile autism.

Neuroleptics have been shown to reduce symptoms of social withdrawal, hyperactivity, abnormal relatedness, and fidgetiness in young (ages 2–8) autistic children (Campbell et al. 1982). Clinical improvement in such areas would naturally be expected to render children more tractable in the classroom and presumably more amenable to an appropriate learning environment. Campbell et al. (1982) demonstrated that the administration of low doses of haloperidol to autistic children improved discriminatory learning in a laboratory task. Neuroleptics may be superior to certain types of behavior therapy in reducing specific symptoms in autistic children; the combination of neuroleptic and behavioral treatments has been found to be superior in facilitating the acquisition of adaptive functions (Campbell et al. 1978). Several studies have demonstrated that the less-sedating, high-potency neuroleptics decrease behavioral symptoms of autistic children (Fish 1970; Fish et al. 1966, 1969).

Haloperidol has produced short-term, beneficial effects as well as no reported adverse effects in autistic patients receiving the drug for 30–56 days (Anderson et al. 1989).

Currently, neuroleptics are the only pharmacologic agents with proven efficacy for decreasing behavioral symptoms of autistic children and may, therefore, be indicated for the treatment of this condition.

### Tourette's Disorder

Tourette's disorder is a psychiatric disorder composed of involuntary symptoms that include both motor and phonic tics. The syndrome most commonly has its onset in childhood and early adolescence. Obsessive-compulsive disorder and attention-deficit hyperactivity disorder are commonly associated with Tourette's disorder.

Haloperidol and pimozide are frequently effective in the treatment of Tourette's (Nee et al. 1980), and such pharmacotherapy is commonly used. In general, low doses of haloperidol (0.5–4 mg/day) or pimozide (1–10 mg/day) are efficacious in diminishing or eliminating motor and phonic tics (Shapiro and Shapiro 1984; Shapiro et al. 1973, 1989).

The adverse effects of haloperidol make compliance problematic. More than half of the patients discontinue medication because of haloperidol side effects. These reactions include extrapyramidal symptoms and "cognitive blunting." This term refers to a state of relative sedation, amergia, and dysphoria (Cohen et al. 1980).

The side-effect profile of pimozide is similar to that of haloperidol. Extrapyramidal effects and sedation are commonly reported but tend to be less severe in patients taking pimozide. Unusual anxiety and depressive symptoms and electrocardiogram (EKG) changes have been reported (Linet 1985; Shapiro and Shapiro 1984). Moldofsky and Sandor (1988) reviewed the cardiac effects of pimozide, and they are generally not clinically significant; however, baseline and follow-up EKG are recommended every 2 months (American Psychiatric Association 1989).

The only current alternative to neuroleptics for patients with Tourette's disorder is the alpha-adrenergic agonist clonidine. Clonidine may improve tics and some of the behavioral symptoms that can accompany this condition (Cohen et al. 1980; Shapiro et al. 1983). The major side effects of clonidine are sedation and hypotension. Clonidine requires further investigation with larger groups of patients, but it may prove to be a very useful treatment. Although therapeutic success with clonidine is less predictable, a favorable side-effect profile (compared with the neuroleptics) is an important consideration.

As always with neuroleptic treatment, the benefit-to-risk ratio should be carefully weighed. Neuroleptics suppress tic behavior, but they do not cure the illness. The decision to use neuroleptics is generally influenced by the severity of the symptoms. Patients with Tourette's disorder should not be treated with neuroleptics unless the tics are sufficiently severe and disabling, thereby causing the child or adolescent dysfunction and distress. Since the symptoms of this disorder may abate over time, drug-free periods should be instituted on a semiannual or annual basis.

### Attention-Deficit Hyperactivity Disorder

Although psychostimulants are the treatment of choice, neuroleptics also have therapeutic efficacy in the treatment of attention-deficit hyperactivity disorder (ADHD). Such stimulants as methylphenidate, pemoline, and amphetamine are indirect dopamine agonists, whereas the neuroleptics are dopamine receptor antagonists. Therefore, the efficacy of both presents a challenge to our understanding of potential mechanisms of action.

The stimulants (especially methylphenidate) are the most frequently prescribed psychoactive drugs for children. Such neuroleptics as thioridazine, chlorpromazine, and haloperidol are almost as effective as the psychostimulants in reducing locomotor hyperactivity and impulsive behavior in hyperactive children (Gittelman-Klein et al. 1976; Werry et al. 1976). Although clinical improvements in inattentiveness and distractibility may be noted in those who are treated with long-term neuroleptics (Gittelman-Klein et al. 1976), there are alternative data to suggest that behavioral improvement occurs without any demonstrable change in attention or cognition (Weiss et al. 1971). There is evidence from neuropsychological studies that shows an actual decrement in intellectual performance in neuroleptic-treated hyperactive children (Sprauge et al. 1970), although this may be a dose-related phenomenon (Gualtieri and Hicks 1985; Werry and Aman 1975).

A major problem in the management of the hyperactive child is how to treat the stimulant nonresponder. Tricyclic antidepressants are an effective second-line medication for the treatment of ADHD (Werry 1980). The utility of tricyclic antidepressants may be compromised by the development of tolerance (Quinn and Rapoport 1975) or by cardiovascular side effects (Gualtieri 1977). Clonidine may be another alternative; however, to date, positive controlled studies have not been published.

Neuroleptics should only be used in children with ADHD when psychostimulants, tricyclic antidepressants, clonidine, and psychosocial treatments have failed.

### Conduct Disorder

Conduct disorder is one of the most frequent reasons for referral to child psychiatry units. As described by the DSM-III-R, the disorder is characterized by a repetitive and persistent pattern of misconduct, with violations of rules and the rights of others. Conduct disorder in childhood is frequently associated with specific psychopathology in adult life (Rutter 1972). About 50% children with conduct disorder are subsequently diagnosed as adults with antisocial personality disorder (O'Neil and Robbins 1958).

Neuroleptics have demonstrated efficacy in a series of studies (Campbell et al. 1982, 1984). Chlorpromazine (100–200 mg/day) and haloperidol (1–6 mg/day) have been effective in reducing aggressive behavior. Patients receiving chlorpromazine reported excessive sedation compared with haloperidol. Campbell et al. (1984) found lithium (1,200–2,000 mg/day) to be efficacious in the treatment of inpatients with conduct disorder and observed fewer side effects (sedation and cognitive impairments). Ongoing studies of lithium have not observed the same results in outpatients with conduct disorder who were not as overtly aggressive (R. Klein and H. Abikoff, November 1991, personal communication). Methylphenidate has also been studied and found to be useful in children with both conduct disorder and ADHD (Abikoff et al. 1987).

## Miscellaneous Clinical Conditions

Mentally retarded children are subject to severe behavioral problems that are difficult to classify within existing nosology. These include stereotypy, self-injurious behavior, rumination, pica, destructive behavior, aggression, hyperactivity, and insomnia. As a general rule, these problems grow more severe in adolescence and adult life, especially in institutionalized individuals.

Although neuroleptics are used most frequently in retarded adults, the psychostimulants seem to be most frequently prescribed for retarded children. The presence of hyperactivity is the most common reason for prescribing psychotherapeutic drugs in this population (Gadow 1981).

In a recent study of mentally retarded young adults who developed tardive dyskinesia, most patients had begun neuroleptic treatment during childhood or early adolescence. The initiation of neuroleptic treatment in children is a particular concern for retarded individuals who are likely to remain on neuroleptics for most of their lives. Cumulative neuroleptic doses may play a role in the development of severe tardive dyskinesia in retarded individuals (Gualtieri et al. 1986).

Self-injurious behavior is a symptom that occurs most commonly in severely retarded individuals; a particularly devastating form occurs in Lesch-Nyhan syndrome. Treatment of self-injurious behavior usually requires intensive and creative forms of behavior management, which does not always produce sustained success. Sometimes, physical restraint is the only successful form of management (Schroeder et al. 1981).

Pharmacological approaches to self-injurious behavior have not been successful. Although neuroleptics are probably used more frequently than any other class of pharmacologic agents, there are hardly any systematic data available in the area (Lapierre and Reesal 1986).

## Neuroleptic Side Effects in Children

There is little difference between children and adults in the occurrence of most of the untoward effects of neuroleptic drugs. Hypotension, cholestatic jaundice, leukopenia, weight gain, seizures, constipation, and dysphoria have all been noted in greater or lesser degrees in children. Particularly troublesome side effects for children are coryza, which may be attributed to allergy or infection; photosensitivity, since children spend so much time outdoors; and urinary incontinence (especially with thioridazine). Sedation and cognitive impairment may interfere with classroom performance. Many patients with Tourette's disorder who are taking neuroleptics experience "cognitive blunting" and diminished energy.

The occurrence of acute extrapyramidal symptoms in children has been reviewed by Winsberg and Yepes (1978) and by Gualtieri and Hawk (1980).

The full range of extrapyramidal side effects to neuroleptic drugs may occur in children: dystonia, akathisia, and pseudo-parkinsonism. It would appear that the acute dystonias may be the most frequent and most troublesome extrapyramidal side effect and that children are especially sensitive even to low doses of high-potency neuroleptics in this regard (Gualtieri and Hawk 1980). In contrast, parkinsonian symptoms may be less frequent. Whether this pattern does indeed characterize the response of children to neuroleptics is an open question; it may be simply the consequence of patterns of reporting, the sensitivity of examiners, or the idiosyncrasies of a few clinical studies. The comparative sensitivity of adults and children has not been the focus of systematic study. It is tempting to predict that if such work were done, it would show an increased vulnerability to dystonia and diminished sensitivity to tremor, rigidity, and bradykinesia in children (Gualtieri and Hawk 1980). If, as Kane et al. (1984) suggested, early occurring extrapyramidal side effects may indicate increased vulnerability to tardive dyskinesia, then a different incidence or pattern of such effects in children may be of considerable importance.

## Neuroleptics in the Treatment of Personality Disorders

There has been relatively little research on the use of neuroleptics (or pharmacotherapy in general) in the treatment of personality disorders. The two conditions for which neuroleptics have been most frequently used are borderline personality and schizotypal personality. With recent nosologic revisions, it would appear that schizotypal personality may represent a diagnosis in the schizophrenia spectrum, implying a potential genetic relationship. In this context, therefore, it is not surprising that neuroleptics have been tried, but their use dates back to earlier diagnostic categories such as "pseudoneurotic schizophrenia" (Hedberg et al. 1971). Even more recent studies have frequently included both borderline and schizotypal personality disorder patients and, indeed, some patients who met criteria for both conditions simultaneously. Serban and Segel (1984) studied 52 inpatients with either schizotypal or borderline personality (DSM-III), with 36% having both disorders. Patients were also described as having "mild transient psychotic episodes." Subjects were randomly assigned to thiothixene (a mean daily dose of 9.4 mg) or haloperidol (a mean daily dose of 3.0 mg) for 12 weeks. Significant improvement was seen on all measures for both drugs, and 56% of the subjects were rated as markedly improved. The absence of a placebo group limits conclusions, however. Leone (1982) treated 80 outpatients who were considered "disruptive borderlines"—using Gunderson et al.'s (1981) criteria—with either loxapine (a mean daily dose of 14.5 mg) or chlorpromazine (a mean daily dose of 110 mg) for 6 weeks. Differences between the two drugs were minimal, but loxapine was slightly superior. Both groups experienced significant improvement on the Clinical Global Impressions Scale, but here too the lack of a placebo group is problematic. Goldberg et al. (1986) studied 50 symptomatic volunteer outpatients who met DSM-III criteria for borderline or schizotypal personality disorder (50% had both) and had one "psychotic symptom." (Presence of major depressive disorder was not an exclusion.) Patients were randomly assigned to thiothixene or a placebo for 12 weeks. The drug was superior to the placebo on some measures of illusions and ideas of reference, as well as factors involving psychoticism, obsessive-compulsive symptoms, and phobic anxiety on a self-administered checklist, but there were no significant differences on total borderline or schizotypal scores or on the Global Assessment Scale.

Soloff et al. (1986) studied 50 inpatients with borderline personality disorder (Gunderson et al. [1981] criteria) and with or without major depressive disorder who were randomly assigned to haloperidol (a mean daily dose of 7.2 mg), amitryptyline (a mean daily dose of 148 mg), or a placebo for 5 weeks. Haloperidol was superior to both amitryptyline and the placebo on overall severity. Amitryptyline was not superior to the placebo. The degree of response was described as modest but involving a broad range of symptoms. This is the most sophisticated study involving such patients, but clearly this would include a somewhat heterogeneous population. In addition, one could argue that the dose of haloperidol was adequate, but the dose of amitryptyline would be low by today's standards.

Interestingly, Gardner and Cowdry (1985) studied 12 borderline (DSM-III) patients randomly assigned to alprazolam (a mean daily dose of 4.7 mg/day) or a placebo for 6 weeks and reported a significantly greater incidence of "serious dyscontrol" with alprazolam.

These few studies point out the enormous gap in our knowledge with regard to the relative indications for and efficacy of neuroleptic drugs in the treatment of these personality disorders. There is reason to consider a therapeutic trial of such agents in cases where other pharmacologic and psychotherapeutic measures have failed. We emphasize the importance, however, of the concept of a therapeutic trial, which includes clear documentation of target signs and symptoms with ongoing assessment of their response during a finite period of time. It is also important to recognize that no long-term controlled trials have been carried out for these disorders. Given the obvious potential heterogeneity of these conditions, consideration as to the presence of affective and anxiety disorders is essential. The availability of antianxiety agents with a better benefit-to-risk ratio has placed the use of neuroleptics as tranquilizers on very shaky ground.

### Neurologic Conditions

The treatment of some neurologic conditions may also be an indication for acute and long-term neuroleptic use. Huntington's disease would be a specific example. Neuroleptics are frequently used to treat L-dopa-induced psychosis in patients with Parkinson's disease, although side effects are a particular problem. Clozapine may hold some promise in this regard because of its relative absence of pseudoparkinsonian side effects. In these conditions, careful differential diagnosis and, where appropriate, consultation with specialists should be emphasized.

## Summary and Conclusions

Neuroleptic drugs remain an important and effective treatment for a variety of disorders. These agents continue to be the primary pharmacologic treatment for acute psychotic states, particularly schizophrenia. They continue to be the most effective medications for maintenance treatment in schizophrenia. Neuroleptics are also effective in the acute manic phase of bipolar disorders, but lithium and carbamazepine are effective alternatives. Neuroleptics may also be indicated in the treatment of depression with psychotic features, but antidepressants and ECT may be effective alternatives.

In geriatric patients with psychiatric disorders, neuroleptics continue to be widely used in the treatment of agitated behavior, extreme restlessness, hostility, and assaultive behavior associated with psychotic states and dementias. The indications here are more symptomatic than diagnosis based, but ruling out reversible causes of dementia or psychoses in this population is critical, as is documenting the need for and benefit from neuroleptic drugs. Beta blockers and carbamazepine may prove to be alternatives, but too few data are currently available.

In the treatment of disorders occurring in childhood and adolescence, schizophrenia, infantile autism, pervasive developmental disorder, and Tourette's disorder are conditions that may benefit from neuroleptic drugs. In some cases of attention-deficit hyperactivity disorder, where other pharmacologic as well as psychosocial and cognitive behavioral treatments have failed, a trial of neuroleptics may be indicated. Neuroleptics may be indicated in the treatment of conduct disorder and may be symptomatically useful in controlling some aggressive, self-injurious, and other behavioral symptoms in children or adolescents with mental retardation.

In the treatment of personality disorders, neuroleptics may be helpful in some cases of schizotypal or borderline personality disorders, but the data base is extremely limited.

It is impossible to make blanket statements regarding indications for neuroleptic drugs, particularly in areas where few controlled trials have been carried out. It is essential, however, when considering the use of these compounds, that prior to their initiation and again before continuation or long-term maintenance (for more than a few months), the clinician should conduct: 1) a thorough diagnostic evaluation; 2) a review of alternative treatments and appropriate therapeutic trials if indicated; 3) a careful weighing of potential benefits and risks; and 4) a thorough discussion with the patient and family of the disease, its prognosis, its course (both treated and untreated), the potential benefits and risks of the treatment, and the methods for assessing outcome.

The importance of well-informed critical, clinical judgment regarding the individual patient cannot be overemphasized. This process of judgment and informed consent must be clearly evident in the medical record.

# References

Abikoff H, Gittelman R, Klass E: Methylphenidate in the treatment of conduct disordered children. Presented at the annual meeting of the American Academy of Child and Adolescent Psychiatry, Washington, DC, 1987

Ahlfors UG, Baastrup PC, Dencker SJ, et al: Flupenthixol decanoate in recurrent manic depressive illness: a comparison with lithium. Acta Psychiatr Scand 64:226–237, 1981

American Psychiatric Association: Diagnostic and Statistical Manual of Mental Disorders, 3rd Edition. Washington, DC, American Psychiatric Association, 1980

American Psychiatric Association: Diagnostic and Statistical Manual of Mental Disorders, 3rd Edition, Revised. Washington, DC, American Psychiatric Association, 1987

American Psychiatric Association: Treatments of Psychiatric Disorders: A Task Force Report of the American Psychiatric Association, Vol 1, Section 8. Washington, DC, American Psychiatric Association, 1989, pp 687–710

Anderson LT, Campbell M, Grega DM, et al: Haloperidol in infantile autism: effects on learning and behavioral symptoms. Am J Psychiatry 141:1195–1202, 1984

Anderson LT, Campbell M, Adams P, et al: The effects of haloperidol on discrimination learning and behavioral symptoms in autistic children. Journal of Autism and Developmental Disorders 19:227–239, 1989

Angrist B, Rotrosen J, Gershon SL: Responses to apomorphine, amphetamine and neuroleptics in schizophrenic subjects. Psychopharmacology 67:31–38, 1980

Angrist B, Peselow E, Rubenstein M, et al: Amphetamine response and relapse risk after depot neuroleptic discontinuation. Psychopharmacology 85:277–283, 1985

Babigian H: Schizophrenia: epidemiology, in Comprehensive Textbook of Psychiatry. Edited by Freedman AM, Kaplan HI, Sadock BJ. Baltimore, MD, Williams & Wilkins, 1975

Baldessarini R, Katz B, Cotton P: Dissimilar dosing with high-potency and low-potency neuroleptics. Am J Psychiatry 141:748–752, 1984

Bleuler M: The Schizophrenic Disorder: Long-Term Patient and Family Studies. Translated by Clemens SM. New Haven, CT, Yale University Press, 1978

Bolvig-Hansen LB, Larsen NE, Gulmann N: Dose-response relationship of perphenazine in the treatment of acute psychoses. Psychopharmacology 78:112–115, 1982

Breese GR, Baumeister AA, McCown TH, et al: Behavioral differences between neonatal and adult 6-hydroxydopamine-treated rats to dopamine agonists: relevance to neurological symptoms in clinical syndromes with reduced brain dopamine. J Psychopharmcol Exp Ther 231:343–353, 1984

Campbell M: Schizophrenic disorders and pervasive developmental disorders/infantile autism, in Diagnosis and Psychopharmacology of Childhood and Adolescent Disorders. Edited by Werry JM. New York, John Wiley, 1985, pp 114–150

Campbell M, Anderson LT, Meier M, et al: A comparison of haloperidol, behavior therapy and their interaction in autistic children. J Am Acad Child Psychiatry 17:640–655, 1978

Campbell M, Anderson LT, Small AM, et al: The effects of haloperidol and learning and behavior in autistic children. Journal of Autism and Developmental Disorders 12:167–175, 1982

Campbell M, Anderson LT, Deutsch SI, et al: Psychopharmacological treatment of children with the syndrome of autism. Pediatr Ann 13:309–316, 1984.

Cheung HK: Schizophrenics fully remitted on neuroleptics for three–five years: to stop or continue drugs? Br J Psychiatry 138:490–494, 1981

Ciompi L: Catamnestic long-term study on the course of life and aging of schizophrenics. Schizophr Bull 6:606–618, 1980a

Ciompi L: Three lectures on schizophrenia: the natural history of schizophrenia in the long-term. Br J Psychiatry 136:413–420, 1980b

Cohen DJ, Detlor J, Young JG, et al: Clonidine ameliorates Gilles de la Tourette's syndrome. Arch Gen Psychiatry 37:1350–1357, 1980

Cole JO, Goldberg SC, Klerman GL: Phenothiazine treatment in acute schizophrenia. Arch Gen Psychiatry 10:246–261, 1964

Cole JO, Goldberg SC, Davis JM: Drugs in the treatment of psychosis: controlled studies, in Psychiatric Drugs. Edited by Solomon P. New York, Grune & Stratton, 1965, pp 153–180

Creese I, Burt DR, Snyder SH: Dopamine receptor binding predicts clinical and pharmacological potencies on anti-schizophrenic drugs. Science 192:481–483, 1976

Crow TJ, McMillan JF, Johnson AL, et al: The Northwick Park study of first episodes of schizophrenia, II: a randomized controlled trial of prophylactic neuroleptic treatment. Br J Psychiatry 148:120–127, 1986

Curry SH, Marshall JHL: Plasma levels of chlorpromazine and some of its relatively non-polar metabolites in psychiatric patients. Life Sci 7:9–17, 1968

Davis JM: Overview: maintenance therapy in psychiatry, I: schizophrenia. Am J Psychiatry 132:1237–1245, 1975

Davis JM, Schaffer CB, Killian GA, et al: Important issues in the drug treatment of schizophrenia. Schizophr Bull 6:70–87, 1980

Davis JM, Barter JT, Kane JM: Antipsychotic drugs, in Comprehensive Textbook of Psychiatry. Edited by Kaplan HI, Sadock BJ. Baltimore, MD, Williams & Wilkins, 1989, pp 1591–1626

Dencker SJ, Lapp M, Malm U: Do schizophrenics well-adapted in the community need neuroleptics? a depot neuroleptic withdrawal study. Acta Psychiatr Scand 279 (suppl):64–76, 1980

Diamond S: Double-blind controlled study of amitryptyline-perphenazine combination in medical office patients with depression and anxiety. Psychosomatics 7:371–375, 1966

Dunner DL, Fieve RR: Clinical factors in lithium carbonate prophylaxis failure. Arch Gen Psychiatry 30:229–233, 1974

Fish B: Psychopharmacologic response of chronic schizophrenic adults as predictors of responses in young schizophrenic children. Psychopharmacol Bull 6:12–15, 1970

Fish B, Shapiro T, Campbell M: Long-term prognosis and the response of schizophrenic children to drug therapy: a controlled study of trifluoperazine. Am J Psychiatry 123:32–39, 1966

Fish B, Campbell M, Shapiro T, et al: Comparison of trifluperidol, trifluoperazine and chlorpromazine in preschool schizophrenic children: the value of less sedative antipsychotic agents. Curr Ther Res 11:589–595, 1969

Gadow KD: Prevalence of drug treatment of hyperactivity and other childhood behavior disorders, in Psychosocial Aspects of Drug Treatment for Hyperactivity. Edited by Gadow KD, Loney J. Boulder, CO, Westview Press, 1981, pp 13–76

Gardner DL, Cowdry RW: Alprazolam-induced dyscontrol in borderline personality disorder. Am J Psychiatry 142:98–100, 1985

Gardos G: Are antipsychotic drugs interchangeable? J Nerv Ment Dis 159:343–348, 1978

Gittelman-Klein R, Klein DF, Katz S, et al: Comparative effects of methylphenidate and thioridazine in hyperkinetic children. Arch Gen Psychiatry 33:1217–1231, 1976

Goldberg S, Schulz SC, Schulz PM, et al: Borderline and schizotypal personality disorders treated with low-dose thiothixene vs. placebo. Arch Gen Psychiatry 43:680–686, 1986

Green WH, Campbell M, Hardesty AS, et al: A comparison of schizophrenic and autistic children. J Am Acad Child Psychiatry 273:399–409, 1984

Gualtieri CT: Imipramine and children: a review and some speculations on the mechanism of drug action. Diseases of the Nervous System 38:368–375, 1977

Gualtieri CT, Hawk B: Tardive dyskinesia and other drug-induced movement disorders among handicapped children and youths. J Appl Res Ment Ret 1:55–69, 1980

Gualtieri CT, Hicks RE: The neuropharmacology of methylphenidate and a neural substrate for childhood hyperactivity. Psychiatr Clin North Am 8:875–892, 1985

Gualtieri CT, Schroeder SR, Hicks RE, et al: Tardive dyskinesia in young mentally retarded individuals. Arch Gen Psychiatry 43:335–340, 1986

Gunderson JG, Kolb JE, Austin V: The Diagnostic Interview for Borderline Patients. Am J Psychiatry 138:896–903, 1981

Harding CM, Brooks GW, Askihaga T, et al: The Vermont Longitudinal Study, II: long-term outcome of subjects who retrospectively met DSM-III criteria for schizophrenia. Am J Psychiatry 144:727–735, 1986

Hedberg DL, Houck JH, Glueck BC Jr: Tranylcypromine-trifluoperazine combination in the treatment of schizophrenia. Am J Psychiatry 127:1141–1146, 1971

Hogarty GE, Ulrichs RF, Mussare F, et al: Drug discontinuation among long-term successfully maintained schizophrenic outpatients. Diseases of the Nervous System 37:494–500, 1976

Hollister LE, Overall JE, Johnson MA, et al: Amitryptyline alone and combined with perphenazine in newly admitted depressed patients. J Nerv Ment Dis 142:460–469, 1966

Huber G, Gross G, Schuttler R: Verlaufs- und Sozialpsychiatriche langzeituntersuchunder an den 1945–1959, in Benn Hospitalizierten Schizophren Kranken. Monographien ans dem Gesamtgebiete der Psychiatrie 21:1–399, 1979

Huber G, Gross G, Shuttler R, et al: Longitudinal studies of schizophrenic patients. Schizophr Bull 6:592–605, 1980

Hytell J, Larsen JJ, Christensen AV, et al: Receptor-binding profiles of neuroleptics, in Dyskinesia: Research and Treatment. Edited by Casey DE, Chase TN, Christensen AV, et al. Berlin, Springer-Verlag, 1985, pp 9–18

Janowsky DS, Davis JM: Methylphenidate, dextroamphetamine and levamfetamine: effects on schizophrenic symptoms. Arch Gen Psychiatry 33:304–308, 1976

Janowsky DS, El-Yousef K, Davis JM, et al: Provocations of schizophrenic symptoms by intravenous administration of methylphenidate. Arch Gen Psychiatry 28:185–191, 1973

Johnson DAW: The duration of maintenance therapy in chronic schizophrenia. Acta Psychiatr Scand 53:298–301, 1976

Johnson DAW: Further observations on the duration of depot neuroleptic maintenance therapy in schizophrenia. Br J Psychiatry 135:524–530, 1979

Johnson G, Gershon S, Berdock E, et al: Comparative effects of lithium and chlorpromazine in the treatment of acute manic states. Br J Psychiatry 119:267–276, 1971

Kane JM: Treatment of schizophrenia. Schizophr Bull 13:147–170, 1987

Kane JM, Borenstein M: Compliance in the long-term treatment of schizophrenia. Psychopharmacol Bull 21:23–27, 1985

Kane JM, Lieberman JA: Maintenance pharmacotherapy in schizophrenia, in Psychopharmacology: The Third Generation of Progress: The Emergence of Molecular Biology and Biological Psychiatry. Edited by Meltzer HY. New York, Raven, 1987, pp 1103–1109

Kane JM, Rifkin A, Quitkin F, et al: Fluphenazine versus placebo in patients with remitted acute first episodes of schizophrenia. Arch Gen Psychiatry 39:70–73, 1982

Kane JM, Woerner M, Weinhold P, et al: Incidence of tardive dyskinesia: five-year data from a prospective study. Psychopharmacol Bull 20:39–40, 1984

Kane JM, Woerner M, Borenstein M, et al: Integrating incidence and prevalence of tardive dyskinesia. Psychopharmacol Bull 22:254–258, 1986

Kane JM, Honigfeld G, Singer J, et al: Clozapine for the treatment-resistant schizophrenic: a double-blind comparison versus chlorpromazine/benztropine. Arch Gen Psychiatry 45:789–796, 1988

Kielholz P, Terzoni S, Poldinscr W: The long-term treatment of periodical and psychlic depressions with flupenthixol decanoate. Int Pharmacopsychiatry 14:305–309, 1979

Klein DF, Davis JM: Diagnosis and Drug Treatment of Psychiatric Disorders. Baltimore, MD, Williams & Wilkins, 1969

Kydd RR, Werry JS: Schizophrenia in children under 16 years. Journal of Autism and Developmental Disorders 12:343–356, 1982

Lapierre TD, Reesal R: Pharmacologic management of aggressivity and self-mutilation in the mentally retarded. Psychiatr Clin North Am 9:775–754, 1986

Leone NF: Response of borderline patients to loxapine and chlorpromazine. J Clin Psychiatry 43:148–150, 1982

Lieberman JA, Kane JM, Gadaleta D, et al: Methylphenidate challenge as a predictor of relapse in schizophrenia. Am J Psychiatry 141:633–638, 1984

Lieberman J, Kane JM, Sarantakos S, et al: Prediction of relapse in schizophrenia. Arch Gen Psychiatry 44:597–603, 1987

Linet LS: Tourette's syndrome, pimozide and school phobia: the neuroleptic separation anxiety syndrome. Am J Psychiatry 142:613–615, 1985

May PRA: Treatment of Schizophrenia: A Comparative Study of Five Treatment Methods. New York, Science House, 1968

May PRA: When, what and why? psychopharmacology and other treatments in schizophrenia. Compr Psychiatry 17:683–693, 1976

May PRA, Van Putten T, Jenden DJ, et al: Chlorpromazine levels and the outcome of treatment in schizophrenic patients. Arch Gen Psychiatry 38:202–207, 1981

Moldofsky H, Sandor P: Pimozide in the treatment of Gilles de la Tourette, in Tourette's Syndrome and Tic Disorders: Understanding and Treatment. Edited by Cohen DJ, Bruun RD, Leckman JF. New York, John Wiley, 1988, pp 281–291

Neborsky R, Janowsky D, Munson E, et al: Rapid treatment of acute psychotic symptoms with high and low dose haloperidol. Arch Gen Psychiatry 38:195–199, 1981

Nee LE, Caine ED, Polinsky RJ, et al: Gilles de la Tourette's syndrome: clinical and family study of 50 cases. Ann Neurol 7:41–49, 1980

O'Neal P, Robins LM: The relation of childhood behavior problems to adult psychiatric status: a 30 year follow-up study of 150 patients. Am J Psychiatry 114:961–969, 1958

Pert A, Rosenblatt JE, Sivit C, et al: Long-term treatment with lithium prevents the development of dopamine receptor supersensitivity. Science 201:171–173, 1978

Platman S: A comparison of lithium carbonate and chlorpromazine in mania. Am J Psychiatry 127:351–353, 1970

Pool D, Bloom W, Mielke DH, et al: A controlled evaluation of loxitane and 75 adolescent schizophrenic patients. Curr Ther Res 19:99–104, 1976

Prien R, Caffey E, Klett C: A comparison of lithium carbonate and chlorpromazine in the treatment of mania: report of the Veterans Administration and National Institute of Mental Health Collaborative Study Group. Arch Gen Psychiatry 26:142–153, 1972a

Prien R, Caffey E, Klett C: A comparison of lithium carbonate and chlorpromazine in the treatment of excited schizoaffectives. Arch Gen Psychiatry 27:182–189, 1972b

Prien RF, Caffey EM Jr, Klett CJ: Factors associated with treatment success in lithium carbonate prophylaxis. Arch Gen Psychiatry 31:189–192, 1974

Quinn PO, Rapoport JL: One year follow-up of hyperactive boys treated with imipramine or methylphenidate. Am J Psychiatry 132:241–245, 1975

Realmuto GM, Erickson WD, Yellin AM, et al: Clinical comparison of thiothixene and thioridazine in schizophrenic adolescents. Am J Psychiatry 141:440–442, 1984

Richelson E: Neuroleptic affinities for human brain receptors and their use in predicting adverse effects. J Clin Psychiatry 45:331–336, 1985

Roy A: Suicide in chronic schizophrenia. Br J Psychiatry 141:171–177, 1982

Rutter ML: Relationships between child and adult psychiatric disorders. Acta Psychiatr Scand 48:3–21, 1972

Saltz BL, Woerner MG, Kane JM, et al: Prospective study of tardive dyskinesia incidence in the elderly. JAMA 266:2402–2406, 1991

Salzman C: Treatment of agitation in the elderly, in Psychopharmacology: The Third Generation of Progress. Edited by Meltzer HY. New York, Raven, 1987, pp 1167–1174

Sandifer M, Wilson I, Grambill J: The influence of case selection and dosage in an antidepressant drug trial. Br J Psychiatry 111:142–148, 1965

Satlin A, Cole JO: Pharmacologic treatment of dementia of the Alzheimer type, in Alzheimer's Disease: The Long Haul. Edited by Winograd C, Jarvik L. New York, Springer-Verlag, 1988, pp 59–79

Schroeder SR, Schroeder CS, Rohjahn J, et al: Self-injurious behavior: an analysis of behavior management techniques, in Handbook of Behavior Modification With the Mentally Retarded. Edited by Matson JL, McCartney JR. New York, Plenum, 1981, pp 61–115

Serban G, Siegal S: Response of borderline and schizotypal patients to small doses of thiothixene and haloperidol. Am J Psychiatry 141:1455–1458, 1984

Shapiro AK, Shapiro E: Controlled study of pimozide vs. placebo in Tourette's syndrome. J Am Acad Child Psychiatry 23:161–173, 1984

Shapiro AK, Shapiro E, Wayne HL: Treatment of Gilles de la Tourette's syndrome with haloperidol: review of 34 cases. Arch Gen Psychiatry 28:92–96, 1973

Shapiro AK, Shapiro E, Eisenkraft GJ: Treatment of Gilles de la Tourette's syndrome with clonidine and neuroleptics. Arch Gen Psychiatry 40:1235–1240, 1983

Shapiro E, Shapiro AK, Fulop G, et al: Controlled study of haloperidol, pimozide and placebo for the treatment of Gilles de la Tourette's syndrome. Arch Gen Psychiatry 46:722–730, 1989

Siefen G, Remschmidt H: Results of treatment with clozapine in schizophrenic adolescents. Kinder Jugen Psychiatr 14:245–257, 1986

Simpson GM, Angus JWS, Edwards JG, et al: Role of antidepressants and neuroleptics in the treatment of depression. Arch Gen Psychiatry 27:337–345, 1972

Simpson G, Lee J, Cuculic Z: Two dosages of imipramine in hospitalized andogenous and neurotic depressives. Arch Gen Psychiatry 33:1093–1102, 1976

Soloff PH, Anselm G, Nathan S: Progress in pharmacotherapy of borderline disorders: a double-blind study of amitriptyline, haloperidol and placebo. Arch Gen Psychiatry 43:691–697, 1986

Sprague RL, Barnes KR, Werry JS: Methylphenidate and thioridazine: learning reaction time, activity and classroom behavior in disturbed children. Am J Orthopsychiatry 40:615–628, 1970

Spring G, Schweid D, Gray G, et al: A double-blind comparison of lithium and chlorpromazine in the treatment of manic states. Am J Psychiatry 126:1306–1309, 1970

Sunderland T, Silver MA: Neuroleptics in the treatment of dementia. Int J Geriatr Psychiatry 3:79–88, 1988

Van Putten T, Marder SR, Wirshing WC, et al: Neuroleptic plasma levels. Schizophr Bull 17:197–216, 1991

Volavka J, Cooper TB: Review of haloperidol blood level and clinical response: looking through the window. J Clin Psychopharmacol 7:25–30, 1987

Volavka J, Cooper TB, Meisner M, et al: Haloperidol blood levels and effects in schizophrenia and schizoaffective disorder: a progress report. Psychopharmacol Bull 26:13–17, 1990

Weiss G, Minde K, Douglas N, et al: Comparison of the effects of chlorpromazine, dextroamphetamine and methylphenidate in the behavior and intellectual functioning of hyperactive children. Can Med Assoc J 104:20–25, 1971

Werry J: Imipramine and methylphenidate in hyperactive children. J Child Psychol Psychiatry 21:27–35, 1980

Werry JS, Aman MG: Methylphenidate and haloperidol in children: effects on attention, memory and activity. Arch Gen Psychiatry 32:790–795, 1975

Werry JS, Aman MG, Lampen E: Haloperidol and methylphenidate in hyperactive children. Acta Paedopsych Scand 42:26–40, 1976

Winsberg B, Yepes L: Antipsychotics, in Pediatric Psychopharmacology. Edited by Werry JS. New York, Brunner/Mazel, 1978, pp 274–283

Wistedt B: A depot neuroleptic withdrawal study. Acta Psychiatr Scan 64:65–84, 1981

Chapter 7

# Alternative Maintenance Treatment Strategies: Clinical Efficacy and Impact on Tardive Dyskinesia

The desire to reduce adverse effects, particularly tardive dyskinesia, but behaviorally manifested parkinsonian side effects as well, has led to increasing interest in identifying minimum dosage requirements for the long-term treatment of schizophrenia as well as for acute treatment.

Attempts to establish minimum dosage requirements have taken three major approaches: 1) exploration of the relationship between dosage and relapse in those reported clinical trials that allow such analyses; 2) conduct of prospective studies comparing patients undergoing gradual dosage reduction with control subjects maintained on stable doses of medication; and 3) assignment of patients randomly to different fixed dose levels, for comparison of dosage ranges or of an intermittent or targeted treatment strategy with standard dosage.

The first approach is limited because the dosage employed by clinicians using a flexible strategy may have been influenced by a variety of factors and cannot be assumed to be random. Dosage changes may not have been carried out in a systematic, objective, or reproducible fashion. In the second type of study, dosage reduction and time may be confounded. Even if patients discontinue medication completely, a psychotic relapse may not occur for several weeks or months. In a strategy that employs gradual dosage reduction, it is difficult to determine minimal dosage requirements given the unpredictable time frame in which a subsequent relapse may occur. Although the third strategy can minimize some of these concerns, setting a fixed dose or dosage range has generally been done on an arbitrary basis, given the lack of available data. Such designs do not necessarily identify the smallest effective dose for a given individual; rather, they provide a general guideline derived from group response data.

Given the accepted causal link between neuroleptic administration and tardive dyskinesia and the fact that not all patients who receive neuroleptic drugs develop tardive dyskinesia, the identification of characteristics of the treatment that either increase or decrease the risk is of obvious importance. Even more pressing is the resolution of the clinical dilemma facing patients, their families, and clinicians when tardive dyskinesia is identified: Should medication be continued and at what dosage? Most of the research on risk factors that increase or reduce tardive dyskinesia risk (see Chapter 4) deals with factors (e.g., age, sex, and diagnosis) that cannot be experimentally controlled.

In contrast, both the amount of medication administered and strategies for administration, such as "drug holidays" and methods for using medication on demand, are amenable to experimental manipulation. The ability to conduct clinical trials that test the effect of alterations in treatment schedule and dosage makes these factors particularly important, because such alterations are among the very few actions that can be taken clinically either to reduce risk of developing tardive dyskinesia or to try to change its course once it develops.

In the balance of this chapter, we first review the two strategies for which there are available data from clinical trials—dosage lower than conventional and intermittent or targeted treatment—in terms of their clinical effects on psychopathology and then examine the influence of these treatment strategies on development of tardive dyskinesia.

# Clinical Efficacy

### Low-Dose Treatment

Caffey et al. (1964) conducted the first controlled dosage-reduction study among hospitalized inpatients and found that patients whose dosage was reduced to three-sevenths of their original dosage experienced a 15% relapse rate within 4 months, compared with a 45% relapse rate for those patients receiving a placebo and a 5% relapse rate for those continuing on their original dose. The mean dose of either chlorpromazine or thioridazine that patients had been receiving for at least 3 months before the study began was 350–400 mg/day.

This study differs from the other later studies to be reviewed. It was carried out with inpatients rather than outpatients, it used oral medication, and it included a placebo comparison group.

Characteristics of the outpatient studies of low-dose treatment are presented in Table 7–1. Goldstein et al. (1978) studied the efficacy of two dose levels of fluphenazine enanthate, with and without crisis-oriented family therapy, in 104 recently discharged schizophrenic patients. These predominantly first-episode (69%) patients were randomly assigned to fluphenazine enanthate, received 25 mg or 6.25 mg im every 2 weeks, and were studied for 6 weeks following a brief 14-day hospitalization. Relapse was defined as the need to alter medication substantially or to rehospitalize the patient. Only 10% relapsed within the 6 weeks following discharge; 24% of those in the low-dose/no-therapy condition relapsed, compared with none of the high-dose/therapy patients. The low-dose/therapy and the high-dose/no therapy groups had relapse rates of 9% and 10%, respectively. Although this study involved a relatively brief period of controlled treatment, it is a classic study in suggesting the potential additive effects of medication and such psychotherapeutic strategies as crisis-oriented family therapy in a community setting.

Kane et al. (1983, 1985, 1986) reported results from a 1-year, random-assignment study of different dosage ranges of fluphenazine decanoate (a standard dose of 12.5–50 mg and a low dose of 1.25–5 mg every 2 weeks) of stable schizophrenic outpatients. At the end of 1 year, the cumulative relapse rate (determined by the psychotic items of the Brief Psychiatric Rating Scale) on the low dose was 56%, compared with 14% for the standard dose. An intermediate dose (2.5–10 mg every 2 weeks) was also studied and produced a cumulative relapse rate of 24%. Despite the significantly higher relapse rate among patients receiving the low-dose treatment, most

**Table 7–1.**   Maintenance low-dosage treatment studies

| Study | Goldstein et al. 1978 | Kane et al. 1983 | Marder et al. 1984 | Marder et al. 1987 | Hogarty et al. 1988 | |
|---|---|---|---|---|---|---|
| **Characteristics**[a] | | | | | | |
| Depot fluphenazine dose[b] | | | | | | |
| low | 6.25 | 1.25–5 | 5/10 | 5/10 | 5 | 4 |
| standard | 25 | 12.5-50 | 25/50 | 25/50 | 25 | 16 |
| $n$ | 104 | 125 | 50 | 66 | 70 | 48 |
| Duration (months) | 1.5 | 12 | 12 | 24 | 12 | 2nd 12 mos |
| Stabilization | 14 days | 4 weeks | > 2 months | > 2 months | X̄ 6 months | |
| **Study Results:** | | | | | | |
| Relapse % | | | | | | |
| Low dose | 16 | 56 | 22 | 41[c] | 22 | 30[d] |
| Standard dose | 6 | 7 | 20 | 33 | 14 | 24 |

[a] All studies used injectable long-acting fluphenazine.
[b] Injections administered biweekly in all studies.
[c] Increased exacerbations in low dose (69%) compared with high dose (36%).
[d] Increased minor episodes in low-dose, high–expressed emotion patients.

of the patients who did relapse were restabilized with temporary dosage increases and without requiring rehospitalization. On average, patients had returned to their baseline state within 9 weeks of resuming standard dose treatment.

Further, patients receiving the low dose were found to be performing better on some measures of psychosocial adjustment than the patients treated with the standard dose. Interestingly, patients receiving the low dose also showed less emotional withdrawal, blunted affect, tension, and psychomotor retardation. These statistically significant differences were not of such magnitude as to be obvious in individual patients; however, these findings emphasize the potential importance of the continuing presence of parkinsonian side effects, even during the maintenance phase of treatment, and highlight the complexity of assessing so-called negative symptoms.

Marder et al. (1984, 1987) studied 66 male veteran outpatients who were randomly assigned to 5 mg or 25 mg of fluphenazine decanoate administered every 2 weeks. Patients were followed for 2 years and were maintained on the assigned fixed dose of 5 or 25 mg as long as they "did well." The investigators defined three levels of unfavorable outcome, which could lead to a dosage change. When patients had an increase of three or more points on the Brief Psychiatric Rating Scale cluster scores for thought disturbance or paranoia, they were considered to have had a "psychotic exacerbation." These exacerbations were relatively mild and seldom led to rehospitalization, but the clinician was allowed to increase the dose to as much as 10 or 50 mg for the respective groups. When patients' symptoms could not be adequately controlled within this range, they were considered to have had a "relapse." The third level of outcome was rehospitalization. The results from this study highlight the importance of a long-term perspective. At the end of 1 year, the exacerbation rate was almost identical in the two treatment groups (35% on 5 mg and 43% on 25 mg). The relapse rates (shown in Table 7–1) were lower (22% vs. 20%) but also not different between the two groups. During the second year, however, the two doses produced different rates of exacerbation. Sixty-nine percent experienced an exacerbation on 5 mg, compared with only 36% on 25 mg. When the outcome of "relapse" is considered (indicating those patients who could not be controlled by the dosage increase), then the two treatments still produced similar results after 2 years: 44% relapsing on the lower dose and 31% on the higher dose.

Hogarty et al. (1988) reported on 70 stable schizophrenic outpatients living in high or low expressed emotion (EE) households who were randomly assigned, double-blind, to receive a standard dose of fluphenazine decanoate (mean dose 25 mg every 2 weeks) or a minimal dose representing 20% of the dose prescribed (mean dose 3.8 mg every 2 weeks).

At 1 year, the relapse rate for the patients receiving the standard dose was 14% and that for the minimal-dose group was 22%. After 2 years, the relapse rates were 24% and 30%, respectively. No significant differences between dose groups at either time point or between EE levels were observed. Within the standard-dose group, however, patients in high-EE households had a lower survivorship (43%) than patients in low-EE households (83%).

Four behavioral side effects and a total score, as well as 11 central nervous system side effects and a total score, were analyzed. At 1 year, minimal-dose recipients clearly experienced significantly fewer extrapyramidal side effects than did standard-dose recipients, although ratings for both groups were in the very mild range. At 2 years (except for nonsignificant trends on muscle rigidity and the total behavioral side effects scores favoring standard dose), however, all differences had disappeared. The investigators attributed this to the fact that standard-dose recipients received decreasing doses during the second year. Further, among 11 patients participating in the study who had evidence of tardive dyskinesia, relapse was not higher with the minimal dose than with the standard dose. The investigators also reported that at the end of 1 year, minimal-dose recipients were less emotionally withdrawn and psychomotorically retarded than were standard-dose recipients, in agreement with the report by Kane et al. (1983). In the second year, minimal-dose, high-EE household patients experienced more minor episodes. The minimal-dose patients had somewhat higher symptom levels—not surprising in view of the increased number of minor episodes—but they were rated as better socially adjusted, not only in their relationships with family members but in employment and overall adjustment.

Results from these studies suggest that dosage reduction is feasible for a large subgroup of stable schizophrenic outpatients and can lead to a diminution in adverse effects and improvement in some subjective and nonsubjective measures of well-being. The risk of psychotic exacerbation does increase earlier, however, with very low dosage and in the second year even with a moderately low dosage. Therefore, patients must be monitored and the clinician must be ready to increase medication when appropriate and on a temporary basis. This highlights the importance of viewing this approach as a strategy within the context of flexible, observant clinical management. In addition, there may be patients for whom dosage reduction is not feasible based on past attempts or potential dire consequences of psychotic relapse (e.g., history of serious suicide attempts or dangerousness).

## Intermittent or Targeted Treatment

The term *intermittent treatment* has been used in two ways. The first is to describe fixed medication-administration schedules that incorporate medication-free days (e.g., 3 days of each week; McCreadie et al. 1980). Generally, the goals of such fixed intermittent-treatment schedules are to simplify medication administration for nursing staff and patients and to reduce costs without reducing medication efficacy. A secondary goal may be to reduce side effects, such as tardive dyskinesia.

Intermittent or targeted treatment is also used to refer to the use of medication only during periods of incipient relapse or symptom exacerbation rather than continuously. The goals of this strategy include reduction of the risk of tardive dyskinesia by reducing long-term medication exposure for patients who are receiving maintenance treatment while limiting the risk of relapse. A secondary goal may be to improve social functioning through reduction of neuroleptic-induced side effects, such as akinesia and akathisia. Neuroleptic treatment only when "needed" is a long-term strategy that depends on both the existence of a prodromal period that allows for intervention with medication to prevent relapse and a strategy for careful clinical monitoring to detect prodromal symptoms so that medication can be introduced.

Targeted treatment is based on the assumption that patients require neuroleptic medication only during these times. According to this model, the advantage of continuous medication administration is that it ensures the availability of medication when the need arises. The logic according to which targeted or intermittent treatment reduces the risk of tardive dyskinesia is that it reduces total medication exposure over time.

The use of intermittent or targeted treatment depends on the accurate identification of times at which medication needs to be administered. In a retrospective study of newly hospitalized patients and their family members, Herz and Melville (1980) found that early signs of schizophrenic decompensation could be recalled. The questionnaire included items dealing with sleep disturbance, depression, reduced attention, changes in energy level, and some psychotic signs and symptoms. Patients and family members were able to describe signs and symptoms. Further, there was substantial agreement between them regarding the nature of these early signs. Herz and Melville suggested that these signs could be used prospectively as indicators of when medication needed to be administered.

The Early Signs Questionnaire developed by these investigators provides a systematic method for detecting periods when nonpsychotic signs and symptoms occur and, by implication, when medication should be introduced. Whether early signs inevitably lead to full episodes of symptom exacerbation or whether the waxing and waning of such early signs is a characteristic of schizophrenic illnesses that is not inevitably associated with relapse has not been systematically tested.

A second requirement for the use of a targeted medication strategy is the creation of a treatment structure that incorporates an ongoing therapeutic relationship for patient monitoring and support. Patients need to be educated regarding the nature of early signs and their implications. They must also be seen frequently in order to ensure that early signs of relapse are detected and medication is started before a major symptom exacerbation occurs. Family members and significant others also need to be aware of the variable course of schizophrenic illnesses, the nature of prodromal signs, and the importance of their identification in the targeted- or intermittent-treatment model. One of the points stressed by one of the groups working with this approach (Carpenter and Heinrichs 1983) is that it is not a no-medication strategy but a way of using medication.

Three groups have reported on this strategy. Table 7–2 summarizes the comparative design features of the studies and their results.

M. Herz and his colleagues have reported two studies of intermittent medication. The first (Herz et al. 1982) was an open pilot study of 19 schizophrenic patients who had been stable outpatients in remission for at least

**Table 7–2.** Maintenance targeted or intermittent treatment studies

| Study | Carpenter, et al. 1987, 1990 | Herz, et al. 1990 | Jolley, et al. 1989, 1990 |
|---|---|---|---|
| **Characteristics:** | | | |
| Patient population | Recently discharged | Outpatients | Outpatients |
| Stabilization | 8 weeks | 3 months | 6 months |
| Psychosocial support | Individual case managers | Weekly support groups | Monthly RN/ MD visits |
| Control features | Random/nonblind | Random/ double-blind | Random/ FPZ dec[a] double-blind |
| $n$ | 116 | 101 | 54 |
| **Results** | | | |
| Dosage | | | |
| Targeted | 1.0 | 150 | 298 |
| Continued | 1.7[b] | 290[c] | 1616[d] |
| 24-mo Relapse % | | | |
| Targeted | 62 | 36 | 54 |
| Continued | 39 | 17 | 14 |
| 1st 12-mo Relapse % | | | |
| Targeted | 55 | 29 | 22 |
| Continued | 33 | 10 | 9 |

*Note:* Treatment was 24 months in all studies.
[a] FPZ dec = fluphenazine decanoate.
[b] 1 = low, e.g., 300 mg chlorpromazine; 2 = moderate, e.g., 301–600 mg/day.
[c] Milligrams per day expressed in chlorpromazine equivalents.
[d] Mean total dose expressed in haloperidol equivalents.

6 months and had not shown suicidal or assaultive behavior during the preceding 2 years. Patients participated in weekly group therapy sessions led by a psychiatrist. Initial sessions focused on early signs of relapse, the need for medication during the prodromal phase, and monitoring of life events that might precipitate relapse. Families, when available, were enlisted to help monitor the patient's condition. Medication was gradually reduced throughout an 8-week period. Five patients could not be successfully withdrawn and were returned to medication. Of the 14 who were successfully withdrawn from medication, 5 remained stable off medication for at least 6 months, 5 experienced prodromal episodes but were returned to a medication-free state following brief neuroleptic treatment, and 3 could not be successfully treated without medication, although only 1 required hospitalization.

Based on these open pilot data supporting the feasibility of the strategy, Herz et al. (1991) have completed a large, double-blind study of intermittent treatment in 140 patients. Schizophrenic and schizoaffective-depressed patients who had been clinically stable and cooperative outpatients for 3 months and had a cooperative relative were openly withdrawn from medication over an 8-week period. Twenty percent experienced prodromal episodes during open withdrawal and did not enter the 2-year double-blind phase of the study. One hundred one patients were randomly and blindly assigned to reinstatement of medication (chlorpromazine, haloperidol, trifluoperazine, or fluphenazine decanoate) or matching placebos.

Patients were seen weekly in supportive group therapy sessions, and family members were invited to monthly open family meetings. The goal of these sessions was to educate patients and families about schizophrenia, the role of medication, and early signs of relapse. Attention was paid to the patient's own idiosyncratic signs of relapse, as well as common prodromal signs. Prodromal signs were monitored regularly. Prodromal episodes were treated by discontinuing double-blind medication and instituting known neuroleptic medication. Once the patient was restabilized, known medication was gradually decreased as double-blind medication was titrated upward. Intermittent-medication patients received significantly less medication, measured both as average daily dose (150 mg compared with 298 mg per day chlorpromazine equivalents) and as percentage of time on medication (27 mg compared with 100 mg).

Significantly more patients in the maintenance-medication group (72%) than in the intermittent group (38%) completed the 2-year study course. Intermittent-group patients experienced more and longer prodromal episodes. Although the total relapse and rehospitalization rates favored the maintenance group, neither of these differences was statistically significant. Life-table analyses using time to first prodromal episode and time to relapse were statistically significant, favoring the maintenance-medication group. Assessment of psychopathology, measures of side effects, and ratings by significant others showed few differences, but when differences did occur they favored the continuous-medication group.

The second group that has reported on this strategy, Carpenter et al. (1987), randomly assigned recently discharged and stabilized schizophrenic patients to either targeted medication in the context of psychosocial intervention ($n = 21$) or standard maintenance medication ($n = 20$) following a 28-day drug-free period. Treatment was not blind and continued for 2 years. All patients were seen weekly. Patients in the continuous-medication group were seen by nursing personnel and on alternate visits briefly by a pharmacotherapist. A minimum daily dosage of 300 mg (chlorpromazine equivalents) was administered. No systematic attempt to engage families was made. Patients in the targeted-medication group were assigned to a primary therapist who conducted weekly individual sessions designed to establish a close interpersonal bond and focused on individualized early prodromal signs and the role of environmental stress (Carpenter and Heinrichs 1983). Families and significant others participated with the patient in a 6-session program that reviewed the nature of psychosis, precipitants, stressors, strategies for stress reduction, and identification of early signs of relapse. Cooperation of families in prompt intervention was also emphasized. When prodromal signs were identified, patients received antipsychotic medication at therapeutic doses. As soon as the patient was restabilized, medication was discontinued.

Patients randomized to targeted treatment received medication 31% of the time and, as a result, received significantly less medication during the 2 years. Despite this significant dosage reduction, targeted medication recipients did not experience significantly more hospitalizations during the entire 2-year study course; however, they were significantly more likely to be hospitalized during the first 6 months of treatment. Assessments of psychopathology and psychosocial functioning at 1 and 2 years did not differ between the groups.

A second report based on 116 newly discharged patients has been completed by Carpenter et al. (1990). After a 4- to 8-week stabilization period and a 4-week medication discontinuation phase, patients were randomized to continuous-treatment and targeted-medication groups for 2 years. As in the first study, treatment was not blind. In this larger study, both groups received the enriched psychosocial treatment program described before. Treatment and assessment procedures were similar.

As in the first study, the significant reduction in dosage achieved with the targeted strategy reflected the reduction in proportion of days on medication—targeted patients received medication 52% of the time, and continuous patients received medication 90% of the time. Significantly more patients in the continuous-treatment group completed the full 2-year study. Further, patients on targeted treatment experienced significantly more clinical decompensations, even controlling for a shorter time in treatment. In general, patients in the continuous-medication group were less likely to be hospitalized during the 2-year period. Despite the significant differences in decompensation and hospitalization, cross-sectional comparisons of psychopathology at 1 and 2 years, although they favored the continuous-treatment group, were not statistically significant. For the reduced sample still in treatment after 2 years (targeted, $n = 21$; continuous, $n = 36$), extent of employment and quality of employment were significantly better among continuously treated patients. Assessments of side effects have not been reported.

The third group (Hirsch et al. 1987; Jolley et al. 1989, 1990) studied 54 schizophrenic outpatients who had been clinically stable for at least 6 months and had been on stable doses of injectable fluphenazine decanoate for at least 2 months. Under double-blind conditions, patients were randomly assigned either to continue medication or have placebo substituted for 2 years. Patients were seen every 4 weeks alternately by a psychiatrist in the clinic and a psychiatric nurse at a home visit. At the outset of the trial, patients and families participated in a 1-hour teaching session focused on schizophrenia and early signs of relapse. Prodromal signs or relapse were treated by the addition of open, oral haloperidol.

There were no differences in numbers of patients completing the first year of the trial in the two groups (Jolley et al. 1989). Significantly more patients in the intermittent-treatment group (76%) experienced prodromal episodes than in the continued-treatment group (27%). Relapse was also significantly more frequent in the intermittent-treatment group (using a one-tailed significance test), but the number of hospitalizations did not differ. Patients in the intermittent-treatment group received significantly less total medication, including fluphenazine injections and oral haloperidol. Extrapyramidal side effects—specifically akathisia, gait abnormality, parkinsonism, and nonliveliness—were significantly reduced in the intermittent-treatment group after 6 and 12 months.

The report of second-year outcome (Jolley et al. 1990) provides a somewhat different picture. Dosage administered was still lower in the intermittent-treatment group but both relapse and rehospitalization were significantly greater. Extrapyramidal side effects were significantly lower in the intermittent group, but the trend toward a lower rate of tardive dyskinesia observed at 1 year was not seen in the second year.

The work of these investigators is remarkably similar in goals, design, and execution. All experimental designs involved identification of stabilized schizophrenic outpatients or a period of prospective stabilization ranging from 8 weeks to 6 months. With the exception of the pilot study by

Herz et al. (1982), all use as comparison groups patients randomly assigned to continuation of medication. In both the Herz and Jolley trials, treatment was administered under double-blind conditions. Herz used four neuroleptic drugs, including fluphenazine decanoate; medication was restricted to fluphenazine decanoate in the Jolley study, thereby ensuring that relapse in the continuous medication group could not be due to covert noncompliance. The Carpenter studies were not blind and are subject to the criticism that patients in the targeted-medication group received greater surveillance and were therefore more likely to receive medication at the first indication of prodromal signs than patients who were known to be receiving active medication. This is less critical in the Carpenter et al. (1987) study, in which the level of psychosocial treatment and surveillance differed by design between the two groups. Their latter, larger study was designed to provide both groups with the same intensive psychosocial support. In this context, the question of whether there was a lower threshold for intervention in the targeted group has to be considered.

All of the studies included some psychosocial supports beyond those usual in the systems where the treatment was being delivered, and in all cases this involved attention to family members or other people in the patients' home milieu who were or could become sensitive to emerging symptomatology and the need for intervention with medication. The amount of psychosocial support varied: weekly group support sessions (Herz); weekly individual psychotherapy sessions (Carpenter); a single educational session for patients and families (Jolley).

All three groups studied treatment for a 2-year period. Length of treatment is of substantial importance in understanding the impact of dosage-reduction strategies in maintenance treatment of schizophrenia. For example, Marder et al. (1987) found no difference in psychotic exacerbations between 5- and 25-mg doses of fluphenazine decanoate in the first year, but they found a statistically significant and clinically meaningful difference after 2 years that favored the higher dose—36% of the patients who received the 25-mg dose experienced clinical exacerbations compared with 69% receiving the 5-mg dose.

The reports from Jolley and his colleagues with intermittent treatment are similar. In the first year there were no differences in rehospitalization, but there was a trend toward an increase in relapses ($P > .05$ but $< .10$). By the end of the second year, using life-table analysis, both relapse and rehospitalization were significantly greater in the intermittent-treatment group. Inspection of the life tables suggests that relapse and rehospitalization began to diverge toward the end of the first year and continued into the second year. Inspection of survival analyses from both the Herz and Carpenter groups suggests that the differences emerge earlier between the two treatments.

There are numerous characteristics of the studies that could account for these differences in results. First, the patients in the Jolley study received injectable fluphenazine decanoate (as did the patients in the Marder study of low dose), so covert noncompliance with treatment in the continued-medication group could not have influenced the results. Further, the time course of relapse following discontinuation of depot injectable medication may well be different from discontinuation of oral antipsychotic medication. Finally, patients in the Jolley study may have been more stable clinically or able to tolerate some period of time without medication; patients were referred by clinicians who "they thought might benefit from brief intermittent treatment approach" (Jolley et al. 1989, p. 986).

The results of these well-designed and carefully conducted studies suggest that intermittent-treatment strategies can be implemented in outpatient maintenance settings and do result in reduced dosages of medication and some reduction of side-effect burden. Particularly during an extended 2-year period, however, this strategy carries an increased risk of the expected prodromal episodes, relapses, and rehospitalizations. Further, there are no consistent benefits of intermittent treatment in terms of social functioning. As described in the section on tardive dyskinesia, the value of intermittent treatment in reducing either the prevalence or the development of tardive dyskinesia is unclear.

On balance, these studies serve to underscore the important role that antipsychotic medication plays in the long-term treatment of schizophrenic illnesses. Symptom exacerbation and relapse appear to be part of the course of such illnesses for many patients. The variable course makes it difficult to tease apart the interacting roles of medication and natural course in individual cases. Only when controlled treatment studies are carried out for a sufficient length of time and with sufficient numbers of patients can the influences of treatment be detected. In this case, it appears that intermittent-treatment strategies are not clinically viable for most maintenance treatment of schizophrenia.

### Clinical Efficacy Summary

The relative benefits and risks of maintenance pharmacotherapy in general, or alternative strategies in particular, will undoubtedly vary from patient to patient. In addition, it is likely that the relative desirability or efficacy of specific strategies may vary depending on the stage of illness that a given patient is experiencing. As previously discussed, the results from long-term, naturalistic follow-up studies emphasize the heterogeneity of outcome in this illness, with some patients appearing to experience a chronic deteriorating course and others experiencing a much more benign outcome after 10 or 20 years.

The observed variability in symptom pattern as well as drug responsiveness also argues for judgments with regard to individual treatment plans. The extent to which maintenance-medication treatment is actually prophylactic (i.e., preventing a new episode rather than suppressing continuously present symptomatology) may also vary from individual to individual. If this distinction could be made with any high degree of reliability, it would clearly be useful in establishing the most appropriate treatment strategy.

# Impact on Tardive Dyskinesia

The influence of the amount of neuroleptic medication that patients receive and the schedules for medication administration are two factors that have received extensive consideration in the study of risk for tardive dyskinesia. We review separately nonexperimental studies that parallel the more general literature on risk for tardive dyskinesia and then the studies that provide data from experimentally controlled studies. A third source of evidence is available regarding intermittent treatment—from animal studies of tardive dyskinesia. Although we do not review these in detail, we do comment on some studies that attempt to provide parallels to clinical administration strategies.

Drug-free intervals or drug holidays have been proposed as a factor that reduces the risk of developing tardive dyskinesia by reducing cumulative exposure to neuroleptic drugs and offers the potential advantage to patients with tardive dyskinesia of reducing the continued exposure to medication with the expectation that remission, or at least no progression of the dyskinetic symptomatology, would follow after reduction of neuroleptic drug exposure. Drug-free periods have, paradoxically perhaps, been implicated as a factor that increases the risk for tardive dyskinesia.

## Experimental Animal Studies

An intermittent treatment schedule following a drug-holiday model can be readily pursued in animals. Numerous such studies have been carried out. They provide some tantalizing clues, as long as the limits of interspecies generalization are recognized.

Bannet et al. (1980) compared four groups of mice that received haloperidol according to different treatment schedules and durations: 5 weeks continuous; 10 weeks continuous; 10 weeks alternating haloperidol and drug free weekly; 10 weeks drug free. Comparison of dopamine receptor binding among the four groups indicated that although all three haloperidol-treated groups showed significantly increased receptor binding compared with the group that received no haloperidol, there were no differences among the three groups.

Sant and Ellison (1984) compared three groups of rats. Two groups received haloperidol for 14 weeks; in one of these groups the drug was administered continuously while in the other group three 1-week drug-free intervals ("holidays") lengthened total exposure time to 17 weeks. A control group received no medication. Oral movements were measured periodically for 24 days after the conclusion of drug treatment. There is no indication of whether oral movements were quantified blind to treatment assignment. Both treated groups showed a significant increase of oral movements compared with the control group, but the patterns differed. The holiday group showed an earlier and ultimately greater increase in oral movements than the continuously treated group, but by 24 days oral movements in both groups had declined so that they were no longer significantly different from the control group.

Carey and DeVeaugh-Geiss (1984) also studied rats. Three groups received haloperidol either twice daily for 20 days, twice daily for 10 days, or every other day for 40 days. A control group was administered saline injections. Both spontaneous motor activity and homovanillic acid (HVA) were measured. Decreases in motor activity and HVA levels were used as indices of tolerance to the effects of haloperidol. The intermittent schedule of administration did not produce behavioral or biochemical tolerance. Continuous treatment for either 10 or 20 days produced the same levels of tolerance, suggesting that total dosage administered was not a factor within the range studied here.

These selected animal studies are far from conclusive. No two studies used the same indices of effect, and the schedules of drug administration and controls vary as well. There is some indication, however, that schedule of administration and total dosage or total length of exposure need to be considered. Extrapolation from such studies to clinical populations is difficult. First, all of these studies were carried out in animals with unimpaired dopaminergic function. Second, the treatment schedules used do not appear analogous to the treatment schedules or duration of treatment used clinically, even though they are identified as "holidays" or "intermittent" treatment. Third, the dependent measures used are ones that may be related to, but are not, tardive dyskinesia.

### Nonexperimental Clinical Studies

Numerous studies have examined the influence of drug-free periods on tardive dyskinesia, using several paradigms. In retrospective studies, the distinction between fixed-length drug holidays and targeted treatment cannot be made. When data are drawn from hospital records, it is usually not possible to determine whether breaks in neuroleptic treatment were of predetermined fixed length or depended on the course of illness. Further, it is often difficult to determine from records whether drug-free periods were in response to the development of tardive dyskinesia. Jeste et al. (1979) and Yassa (1985) specifically excluded drug-free periods from consideration if they followed the recorded appearance of tardive dyskinesia.

Crane (1974) surveyed a large chronically hospitalized population. He found no association of continuity of treatment with neuroleptics and presence of tardive dyskinesia; however, *continuous* was defined as more than 90% and *noncontinuous* was defined as less than 90%. In this study, total duration of treatment was related to presence of tardive dyskinesia.

In a prevalence study, Branchey and Branchey (1984) reported that both the number of drug-free episodes and their frequency were higher in the tardive dyskinesia than the no-tardive-dyskinesia group. They found no evidence in chart review that medication was discontinued in response to tardive dyskinesia development.

In a case-control study, Chien et al. (1982) found no difference between patients with and without tardive dyskinesia in terms of either number of medication-free periods or their length. Schizophrenic and affective disordered subjects were included in both studies. The patients studied by Chien et al. (1982) were substantially older (mean age 55 years) than those studied by Branchey and Branchey (1984; mean age 29 years).

Jeste et al. (1979) found that patients whose tardive dyskinesia persisted after withdrawal of medication were more likely to have experienced drug interruptions than those whose tardive dyskinesia remitted after withdrawal of medication. This finding was not due to longer total medication exposure.

Seeman (1981) reported on a prospective evaluation of 36 patients with tardive dyskinesia who were followed for 2 years with medication being discontinued whenever possible. Since no patients who were discontinued were maintained medication free for the full 2-year period, this strategy became, in effect, intermittent treatment. There were no differences in the course of tardive dyskinesia between those who had intermittent treatment and those who received medication continually throughout the 2-year period.

On balance, retrospective studies vary in finding a relationship between treatment pattern and presence of tardive dyskinesia or its nature. The finding of a relationship to course of tardive dyskinesia, as in the Jeste et al. (1979) study, is a much finer distinction than establishing a relationship to the presence of tardive dyskinesia in a prevalence study.

### Experimental Clinical Studies

As described earlier in this chapter and shown in Table 7–2, all three studies found that the group randomized to receive intermittent treatment did experience reduced medication exposure during the study period. At the end of 1 year of treatment, Jolley et al. (1989) found a reduction in the point prevalence of tardive dyskinesia ($P > .05 < .10$) in the intermittent group compared with the continuously treated group. At the end of 2 years, however, there was no difference between the two groups (Jolley et al. 1990). Herz et al. (1991) found no significant differences between the two groups in tardive dyskinesia movements at either 1- or 2-year cross-sectional evaluations, although inspection of the total Abnormal Involuntary Movement Scale (AIMS) scores reveals that the score remained stable for the maintenance group (3.0 at 1 year; 3.05 at 2 years) but was reduced in the intermittent group (2.33 at 1 year; 1.68 at 2 years).

Perhaps the most sophisticated analysis of the relationship of treatment schedule to development of tardive dyskinesia was carried out by Levine et al. (1990) of data from the Carpenter et al. (1990) study. First, in order to examine development of tardive dyskinesia, these investigators restricted their population to patients who did not have tardive dyskinesia at the beginning of the trial. Second, they set a criterion for tardive dyskinesia—two successive ratings of mild or greater on the global severity scale of the AIMS at any point during the 2-year trial. According to this criterion, there was no significant difference between the two treatment groups. Two other measures of tardive dyskinesia, indexing severity and persistence of abnormal movements during the 2-year period, also showed no significant differences between the groups. There was a significant relationship of dosage received to tardive dyskinesia in both groups: patients with tardive dyskinesia had received higher dosage. Further, within the group that received intermittent or targeted treatment, they found a relationship between the number of on-off cycles of medication and all three measures of tardive dyskinesia, such that the more cycles a patient experienced, the more likely he or she was to meet the diagnostic criterion and have more persistent and more severe tardive dyskinesia movements. Within the targeted group, an increased number of cycles and a higher dose combined to increase the likelihood that patients would develop tardive dyskinesia. The implications of these findings are that a targeted treatment strategy may reduce the risk of developing tardive dyskinesia in patients for whom the strategy "works"—that is, those who do not require repeated cycles of medication administration and who, therefore, actually receive substantially reduced dosages of medication.

Examination of the effects of a brief (6-week) fixed-length drug holiday in 31 schizophrenic patients by Shenoy et al. (1981) revealed no effect on tardive dyskinesia. These patients had been maintained for extensive periods on long-acting antipsychotic medications, so it is unclear whether the study period was long enough to detect changes in tardive dyskinesia–related movements. A 3-month discontinuation study by Levine et al. (1980), in which increases in tardive dyskinesia–associated movements were detected in patients discontinued from oral medication but not from long-acting injectable medication, supports this interpretation. To our knowledge there are no other controlled, fixed-length drug-holiday studies in the literature that specifically assessed tardive dyskinesia.

## Low-Dose Treatment

Table 7–1 presents the experimental studies of low-dose treatment that provide data regarding the efficacy of this strategy in terms of psychopathology and relapse reviewed earlier in this chapter. Of the four studies presented in the table, only the report by Kane et al. (1983) directly assessed tardive dyskinesia. They found significantly lower scores on the Simpson Dyskinesia Scale at the end of treatment exposure in the low-dose group. Hogarty et al. (1988) reported that patients with tardive dyskinesia were no more likely to relapse if treated with a "minimal" dose than if treated with a standard dose, but they did not report changes in tardive dyskinesia as a result of dosage reduction. S. Marder (July 1990, personal communication) found no difference in either total AIMS score or specific body areas between low and standard doses after either 1 or 2 years of treatment.

Although the finding by Kane et al. (1983) does not appear robust, in the absence of supporting data from other studies, it is unclear whether the lack of findings from other trials of low-dose treatment should be taken as an absence of effect or reflects the fact that other investigators have not yet examined their data. The low-dose group in the Kane et al. (1983) study received a substantially lower dose than the low-dose groups in the other trials. Finally, all of these studies used injectable fluphenazine decanoate; as we observed earlier, this agent may have properties that make withdrawal-emergent movements more difficult to detect.

## Summary of Impact on Tardive Dyskinesia

On balance, it appears that tardive dyskinesia or tardive dyskinesia–related movements show some sensitivity to manipulation of dosage or medication-administration schedules. If one were to hazard a clinical recommendation on the basis of the limited data available, it would be that although medication reduction or discontinuation may appear to be reasonable treatment approaches, both have significant risks. If medication must be started and stopped frequently in order to prevent clinical-symptom exacerbation, the effects on tardive dyskinesia may be worse than simply maintaining the patient on medication continuously. Clearly, more data and, in particular, more detailed analyses of existing data regarding dosage-reduction strategies are warranted.

# References

Bannet J, Belmaker RH, Ebstein RP: The effect of drug holidays in an animal model of tardive dyskinesia. Psychopharmacology 69:223–224, 1980

Branchey M, Branchey L: Patterns of psychotropic drug use and tardive dyskinesia. J Clin Psychopharmacol 4:41–45, 1984

Caffey EM Jr, Diamond LS, Frank TV, et al: Discontinuation or reduction of chemotherapy in chronic schizophrenics. J Chronic Dis 17:347–358, 1964

Carey RJ, DeVeaugh-Geiss J: Treatment schedule as a determinant of the development of tolerance to haloperidol. Psychopharmacology 82:164–167, 1984

Carpenter WT, Heinrichs D: Early intervention, time limited, targeted pharmacotherapy of schizophrenia. Schizophr Bull 9:533–542, 1983

Carpenter WT Jr, Heinrichs DW, Hanlon TE: A comparative trial of pharmacologic strategies in schizophrenia. Am J Psychiatry 144:1466–1470, 1987

Carpenter WT Jr, Hanlon TE, Heinrichs DW, et al: Continuous vs. targeted medication in schizophrenic outpatients: outcome results. Am J Psychiatry 147:1138–1148, 1990

Chien CP, Ross-Townsend A, Donnelly M: Past history of drug and somatic treatments in tardive dyskinesia, in Tardive Dyskinesia: Research and Treatment. Edited by Fann WE, Smith RC, Davis JM, et al. New York, SP Medical and Scientific Books, 1982, pp 297–308

Crane GE: Factors predisposing to drug-induced neurologic effects, in The Phenothiazines and Structurally Related Drugs. Edited by Forrest IS, Carr CJ, Usdin E. New York, Raven, 1974, pp 269–279

Goldstein MJ, Rodnick EH, Evans JR, et al: Drug and family therapy in the aftercare of acute schizophrenics. Arch Gen Psychiatry 35:1169–1177, 1978

Herz MI, Melville C: Relapse in schizophrenia. Am J Psychiatry 137:801–805, 1980

Herz MI, Szymanski HV, Simon JC: Intermittent medication for stable schizophrenic outpatients: an alternative to maintenance medication. Am J Psychiatry 139:918–922, 1982

Herz MI, Glazer WM, Mostert MA, et al: Intermittent vs. maintenance medication in schizophrenia: two year results. Arch Gen Psychiatry 48:333–339, 1991

Hirsch SR, Jolley AG, Manchanda R, et al: Early intervention medication as an alternative to continuous depot treatment in schizophrenia: preliminary report, in Psychosocial Treatment of Schizophrenia. Edited by Strauss J, Boker W, Brenner HD. Berne, Switzerland, Hans Huber, 1987, pp 63–72

Hogarty GE, McEvoy JP, Munetz M, et al: Dose of fluphenazine, familial expressed emotion, and outcome in schizophrenia. Arch Gen Psychiatry 45:797–805, 1988

Jeste DV, Potkin SG, Sinha S, et al: Tardive dyskinesia: reversible and persistent. Arch Gen Psychiatry 36:585–590, 1979

Jolley AG, Hirsch SR, McRink A, et al: Trial of brief intermittent prophylaxis for selected schizophrenic outpatients: clinical outcome at one year. Br Med J 298:985–990, 1989

Jolley AG, Hirsch SR, Morrison E, et al: Trial of brief intermittent neuroleptic prophylaxis for selected schizophrenic outpatients: clinical and social outcomes at two years. BMJ 301:837–842, 1990

Kane JM, Rifkin A, Woerner M, et al: Low-dose neuroleptic treatment of outpatient schizophrenics. Arch Gen Psychiatry 40:893–896, 1983

Kane JM, Rifkin A, Woerner M, et al: High dose versus low dose strategies in the treatment of schizophrenia. Psychopharmacol Bull 21:533–537, 1985

Kane JM, Woerner M, Sarantakos S: Depot neuroleptics: a comparative review of standard, intermediate, and low dose regimens. J Clin Psychiatry 47 (suppl):30–33, 1986

Levine J, Schooler NR, Severe J, et al: Discontinuation of oral and depot fluphenazine in schizophrenic patients after one year of continuous medication: a controlled study, in Long-Term Effects of Neuroleptics. Edited by Cattabeni F, et al. New York, Raven, 1980, pp 483–493

Levine J, Carpenter WT, Kirkpatrick B, et al: Targeted medication dosing and tardive dyskinesia. Presented at New Clinical Drug Evaluation Unit meeting, Key Biscayne, FL, May 1990

Marder SR, Van Putten T, Mintz J, et al: Costs and benefits of two doses of fluphenazine. Arch Gen Psychiatry 41:1025–1029, 1984

Marder SR, Van Putten T, Mintz J, et al: Low and conventional dose maintenance therapy with fluphenazine decanoate: two year outcome. Arch Gen Psychiatry 44:510–517, 1987

McCreadie RG, Dingwall JM, Wiles DH, et al: Intermittent pinozide versus fluphenazine decanoate as maintenance therapy in chronic schizophrenia. Br J Psychiatry 137:510–517, 1980

Sant WW, Ellison E: Drug holidays after onset of oral movements in rats following chronic haloperidol. Biol Psychiatry 19:95–99, 1984

Seeman MV: Tardive dyskinesia: two-year recovery. Compr Psychiatry 22:189–191, 1981

Shenoy RS, Sadler AG, Solomon C, et al: Effects of six week drug holiday on symptom status, relapse, and tardive dyskinesia in chronic schizophrenics. J Clin Psychopharmacol 1:141–145, 1981

Simpson GM, Lee JH, Zoubok B, et al: A rating scale for tardive dyskinesia. Psychopharmacology (Berlin) 64:171–179, 1979

Yassa R, Ghadirian AM, Schwartz G: Tardive dyskinesia: developmental factors. Can J Psychiatry 30:344–347, 1985

Chapter 8

# Alternatives to
# Neuroleptic Drug Therapy

Although neuroleptic drugs play an important role in the treatment of a variety of conditions (see Chapter 6), their association with tardive dyskinesia and other neurologic side effects (dystonia, pseudoparkinsonism, and akathisia) remains a limiting factor in their use. As a result, there have been continued efforts to develop alternatives to neuroleptic treatment.

Various other drugs, mainly available for other medical indications, have been claimed to have some efficacy in some psychiatric conditions in which neuroleptics are commonly used. None of these have, to date, shown consistent, reliable efficacy when given alone to schizophrenic patients, although occasional patients have shown improvement. A few drugs have limited evidence of efficacy in manic excitement or episodic violence, situations in which neuroleptics are often used; however, none of the widely diverse agents studied in the last 10 years has proven to be safe and effective alone in any other psychiatric condition in which neuroleptics are usually used. The possible exception is electroconvulsive therapy, where the short-term results in acute psychosis probably equal those achieved by neuroleptics. None of the alternative therapies have been more than tentatively studied as maintenance treatments. Attempts by a variety of drug companies to develop drugs effective in schizophrenia and free of typical neuroleptic side effects, other than clozapine, have not been successful to date, although some unusual compounds are in clinical trial. Reserpine and related drugs deplete dopamine rather than block dopamine receptors and have some efficacy in schizophrenia; they have been so little used in the last 20 years that their efficacy and, more important, their tardive dyskinesia risk are very unclear.

A wide variety of other drugs and drug classes have been studied briefly or extensively in conditions that are responsive to neuroleptic drugs—such as mania, schizoaffective excitement, and organic agitation—and some have been studied in brief 1- to 4-week trials in schizophrenia, either alone or in addition to a neuroleptic drug. These include carbamazepine, valpro-

179

ic acid, clonazepam, diazepam, lithium, propranolol, and clonidine. In this chapter we review the available evidence that supports the value of each of these drugs or drug classes in conditions for which neuroleptics are generally used. In these reviews, the possible mechanisms of action of these agents are considered only briefly, with the main focus being on clinical efficacy, side effects, and other limiting factors.

Depressive disorders and anxiety disorders are sometimes treated with antipsychotic drugs, but other classes of drugs are almost always adequate for these conditions, and physicians using neuroleptics in patients with these conditions or with borderline or other personality disorders must be prepared to justify such use adequately. A few such patients appear to respond uniquely and selectively to a neuroleptic and are not helped by or cannot tolerate more conventional tricyclic antidepressants or benzodiazepine treatment, but the general principle still holds. Alternative treatments for these conditions are beyond the scope of this review.

# Reserpine

## Schizophrenia

In the early 1950s both reserpine and chlorpromazine were used in the treatment of acute and chronic schizophrenia with considerable enthusiasm, but reserpine gradually fell out of favor, and during the past 10 years it has rarely been used in psychiatry except as a treatment for tardive dyskinesia. Since reserpine does not block dopamine receptors but acts by depleting brain stores of dopamine (and other biogenic amines), it is possible that it might not cause tardive dyskinesia. There are very few reported cases of dyskinesia in reserpine-treated psychiatric patients (Degkwitz 1969; Uhrbrand and Faurbye 1960; Wolf 1973), but probably many thousands of hypertensive patients received reserpine in low doses for years as a treatment for their hypertension without any of these patients having been reported, to our knowledge, as having developed tardive dyskinesia. If reserpine were widely used to treat acute and chronic psychosis, it is impossible to predict whether the risk of tardive dyskinesia in such patients would be less than if they were treated with standard neuroleptics.

If reserpine were reliably safer in terms of dyskinesia risk, would it be a generally effective, acceptable alternative to standard neuroleptics? Several reports, mainly involving chronic inpatients treated before standard neuroleptics were in general use, are enthusiastic about the degree and extent of improvement (Ayd 1959; Barsa and Kline 1956; Hollister et al. 1955; Kirkegaard 1959), whereas others report little effect. Some controlled studies are positive (Elkes 1960; Pearl et al. 1956), and some are negative (Gore et al. 1957; Somerness et al. 1955). The best large-scale study, carried out by the Veterans Administration (Lasky et al. 1962), showed reserpine at an average oral dose of 6 mg/day to be clearly less effective than chlorpromazine, thioridazine, or fluphenazine during an initial 8-week trial in recently readmitted DSM-II (American Psychiatric Association 1968) schizophrenic patients. Another elaborate trial, by Wirt and Simon (1959) and Simon et al. (1965), using newly admitted schizophrenic patients with an average oral dose of 6 mg/day, found reserpine less effective than chlorpromazine but more effective than a routine no-drug hospital treatment regimen. This study included a 1-year follow-up, however, at which point the reserpine group did particularly poorly. The positive, uncontrolled studies noted here mainly involved initial intramuscular doses of 5–10 mg of reserpine qd for as long as a month before shifting entirely to oral medication and report much better clinical response in chronic patients. A period of initial sedation, however, was often followed by a period of "turbulence," with overactivity and increased psychosis before general improvement appeared, usually several weeks later. Whether the "turbulence" was unrecognized akathisia is unclear. Reserpine used in this way produces as much pseudoparkinsonism and other extrapyramidal side effects (plus probably more drooling) as occur with standard neuroleptics.

There has been some study of reserpine in chronic or recurrently psychotic patients inadequately responsive to standard neuroleptics. Goldman (1966), in his work at a state hospital in Cincinnati, Ohio, found that of 127 chronic patients who had previously failed to improve on chlorpromazine, only 10 showed a good to excellent response to reserpine, whereas of 122 chronic patients who had failed to respond to reserpine, 32 showed a good to excellent response to chlorpromazine. However, 87 of 127 chlorpromazine failures showed some improvement on reserpine, and 102 of 122 reserpine failures showed some improvement on chlorpromazine. Braun (1960), using reserpine intramuscularly and orally in recently rehospitalized but treatment-resistant psychotic patients, obtained good to excellent improvement in 16 of the 28 patients studied. At the dose used of 5–10 mg im for 30 days followed by oral doses of 0.5–2 mg/day, only 25% developed neurological side effects, although most showed nasal stuffiness, dry mouth, sedation, and increased appetite. Subsequent to Braun's study, Bacher and Lewis (1978) reported benefit from adding 0.75–6 mg reserpine to prior neuroleptic therapy in chronically psychotic schizophrenic outpatients.

### Mania

There are no specific studies of the efficacy of reserpine in mania, although one assumes that in the early years when reserpine was widely used in schizophrenia, some patients who now would be considered bipolar were treated with reserpine and probably improved. Bacher and Lewis (1979) reported that six recurrently manic bipolar or schizoaffective outpatients who were poorly controlled on lithium plus a neuroleptic fared much better on a neuroleptic-reserpine combination.

The overall impression is that reserpine would be more useful than no medication at all in schizophrenia or mania and that more extensive work on the drug might lead to better, more rapidly effective, dosage regimens and better use of drugs to manage side effects. Reserpine is not an ideal alternative to a standard neuroleptic at this time, however. Other drugs with similar mechanisms of action—tetrabenazine and rescinnamine— exist, but there are not enough data to tell whether these have any advantages over reserpine.

### Reserpine and Tardive Dyskinesia

Only two clear cases of dyskinesia in patients exposed only to reserpine have been described (Degkwitz 1969; Uhrbrand and Faurbye 1960). A third report by Wolf (1973) was not available to us. There is extensive evidence that reserpine effectively decreases dyskinetic movements (Jus et al. 1979), especially in patients who do not have tardive dystonia (Fahn 1983). It is even proposed as the best of the available therapies in severe cases (Fahn 1983), although no clear controlled evidence for its superiority exists (Jeste and Wyatt 1982). The drug is usually given in gradually increasing doses, beginning with 0.25 mg/day (the only tablet size available in the United States) and increased by this dose every 1–7 days, watching for hypotension, oversedation, and akathisia until dyskinesia is controlled (as much as 6 mg/day given in divided doses). After the patient is relieved of dyskinesia for a number of weeks, the dose of reserpine can be gradually tapered to a low maintenance dose.

If reserpine has any advantage over standard neuroleptics in treating or not producing tardive dyskinesia, it could be because dopamine continues to be released into the synapse in small amounts, the dopamine receptor not being blockaded. Until a large group of psychiatric patients is treated only with reserpine for several years, it will be impossible to know whether it is really less likely to elicit dyskinesia than standard neuroleptics.

### Safety

Reserpine, at antipsychotic dosages, causes as many extrapyramidal side effects as the standard neuroleptics and may cause more drooling and nasal congestion. It may also aggravate a peptic ulcer and be more likely to cause hypotension than the high-potency neuroleptics. It has been associated with the emergence of depression in hypertensive patients, but predominantly in individuals with a prior history or a family history of depression.

# Benzodiazepines

## Schizophrenia

Although conventional wisdom suggests that benzodiazepines would not be useful in schizophrenia, except perhaps to reduce akathisia, there are now several studies, some controlled, that suggest that benzodiazepines sometimes are surprisingly effective, particularly in higher dosages. These studies have generally been only of a few weeks duration (Lingjaerde 1983).

In a 24-hour controlled study, Lerner et al. (1979), initially comparing parenteral diazepam with parenteral haloperidol, but shifting to oral medication at doses of 30–40 mg of diazepam and 20–35 mg of haloperidol per day, in newly admitted, acutely psychotic patients, found that the two drugs were essentially identical in efficacy and, overall, all patients improved substantially. In a much earlier crossover study involving 37 chronically hospitalized schizophrenic patients, Maculam (1964) found that improvement during 3 weeks on 20–60 mg of diazepam was essentially the same (59.2%) as after 3 weeks on 300–600 mg of chlorpromazine (46%) or after 3 weeks on 300–600 mg of chlorprothixene (53%). A placebo washout week was placed between each period on active drug. In an "own control" design by Kellner et al. (1975), in which neuroleptic-free schizophrenic patients were shifted from a week on chlordiazepoxide (15–300 mg/day) to a week on a placebo randomly during a 15-week period, 3 of 6 patients appeared to improve substantially on the benzodiazepine, 2 being free of psychotic symptoms during weeks on the active drug.

Haas (1983) described remarkable decreases in psychopathology on a high-dose diazepam regimen (100–400 mg/day) in most paranoid schizophrenic patients. He reported disinhibition, excitement, and worsening in all six schizoaffective patients studied. Psychopathology dropped rapidly in the paranoid patients, with marked improvement occurring by the end of the first week on diazepam. Sedation was a problem only initially. After a day or two, patients were generally not sedated and slept normally despite high daily doses of diazepam. Nestoros et al. (1982) reported a small double-blind study involving 12 carefully diagnosed, newly admitted paranoid schizophrenic patients, 6 initially treated for a week with diazepam in doses ranging from 70 to 400 mg/day and 6 treated with a placebo. After this initial week, all unimproved patients received 30 mg/day of haloperidol in addition to their double-blind medications. Five of the 6 diazepam patients showed a rapid decrease in ratings on the Brief Psychiatric Rating Scale (BPRS) the first week, compared with 1 of 6 placebo patients. Drug/placebo differences were highly significant. The diazepam response was much more rapid and complete than that occurring when haloperidol was added for the placebo patients. Sedation was only a problem in diazepam-treated patients after psychotic symptoms had markedly decreased. Most of the improvement in the diazepam patients had occurred by the third day of treatment. Vinar and Taussigova (1966) also found diazepam at 70 mg/day effective in 36 schizophrenic patients.

On the other hand, a series of well-controlled studies of low-dose chlordiazepoxide (30–40 mg/day) versus a placebo added to chlorpromazine (Michaux et al. 1966), thioridazine (Hanlon et al. 1969), or fluphenazine (Hanlon et al. 1970) in recently hospitalized psychotic patients at a state hospital found the benzodiazepine to result in a less favorable treatment response. Gundlach et al. (1967) compared diazepam (as much as 40 mg/day) with placebo in a mixed group of 100 outpatients, 63 of whom were schizophrenic, and found that more suicidal ideation and paranoid ideas developed in the diazepam-treated group. Lingjaerde et al. (1979) found 15 mg/day diazepam added to ongoing neuroleptic medication to be slightly better than a placebo in chronic, mainly schizophrenic, psychotic patients.

Others have added chlordiazepoxide to antipsychotics, in doses of 120–200 mg/day (Monroe and Wise 1965) and claimed that the benzodiazepine substantially improved the clinical status of hospitalized psychotic patients.

Jimerson et al. (1982) studied diazepam in 6 drug-free patients with chronic schizophrenia in a double-blind design in which the patients began on a placebo, were switched to diazepam, and were then switched back to the placebo. Two female patients who were able to tolerate 250–300 mg/day of diazepam were somewhat improved while 1 female patient was unchanged or slightly worse. Three male patients were unable to tolerate as much as 120 mg/day of diazepam and did not improve. In a crossover study, clonazepam of as much as 5 mg/day was no different from a placebo in 13 chronic schizophrenic patients, and 4 patients became violent, mainly when coming off clonazepam.

These limited studies of benzodiazepines in schizophrenic patients are intriguing. All in all, they suggest that at least some schizophrenic patients are moderately to markedly improved on moderate to high doses of diazepam or chlordiazepoxide, but they are not helped by dosages more commonly used in anxiety disorders. In some studies, improvement is rapid and substantial, but there are no data on longer-term administration and it is impossible to tell whether the effect can be maintained for the prolonged periods often required in chronic psychotic illnesses. Physical dependence would undoubtedly occur with prolonged, high-dose benzodiazepine therapy. This approach deserves further study, but it is far from being a generally safe and effective alternative to standard neuroleptic therapy.

## Mania

In mania, for which neuroleptic therapy is often given for weeks during acute episodes, there is limited evidence that benzodiazepines may be useful with or without lithium as alternatives to neuroleptic use. Chouinard et al. (1983) reported on a double-blind crossover study in 12 newly hospitalized manic patients who received clonazepam or lithium for an initial 10-day period, then the other drug for the next 10 days. Both drugs brought about some improvement, with clonazepam being a bit more effective, especially on motor overactivity and logorrhea. Haloperidol was given in prn dosages to 4 patients during clonazepam phases and to 7 patients during lithium phases, mainly for only a few days. An average of 4.2 mg of clonazepam was given on the first study day, increasing to 10.4 mg by the 10th day, with a maximum dose of 16 mg/day. Sedation and ataxia occurred in 7 and 4 patients, respectively, but were not major problems. The authors reported that sedation was not correlated with the observed therapeutic effects of clonazepam.

Modell et al. (1985) reported the use of lorazepam as an adjunct to lithium in four newly hospitalized, drug-free, manic patients with good results. Only three patients during the first few days required maximum doses in the 20–30 mg/day range. Again sedation and ataxia were not major problems. The patients were doing well on 2–4 mg/day of lorazepam plus lithium by the end of the 11-day study period.

## Other Disorders

Benzodiazepines have also been described as useful in irritable, violent personality disorders. Lion (1979) reported that oxazepam (120 mg/day) was superior to both chlordiazepoxide (100 mg/day) and a placebo in a 1-week double-blind outpatient study. When the doses were doubled for a second week, sedation became a problem. Both drugs were superior to the placebo. Griffith (1985) described two epileptic patients with frequent explosive rage or anxiety attacks who were able to control these with prn doses of triazolam or clorazepate; chronic benzodiazepine medication was not helpful. On the other hand, Gardner and Cowdry (1985) found alprazolam to increase serious acting-out behavior in borderline outpatients.

This all reinforces the notion that benzodiazepines may be as, or more, effective than neuroleptics in nonpsychotic or even psychotic patients for whom short-term sedation to control anger or agitation is needed (Cole 1985).

## Tardive Dyskinesia

Although there is a general clinical presumption that benzodiazepines have some modest antidyskinetic effect in patients with tardive dyskinesia, this has rarely been explicitly tested. There are a few case reports of favorable effects from oral diazepam (Singh 1976), clorazepate (Itil et al. 1974), and clonazepam (O'Flanagan 1975; Sedman 1976), but none of these is conclusive. One controlled study (Bobruff et al. 1981) compared clonazepam with phenobarbital but not a placebo and showed both drugs to mildly reduce dyskinetic movements.

Clinical experience suggests that clonazepam's effects are limited by its strong sedative properties. Occasional patients claim moderate to marked benefit from benzodiazepines, but slight effects are more common. Some patients, perhaps because of the antianxiety or sedative effects of the drugs, believe that they are better even though the movements appear essentially unchanged to the observing clinician.

### Safety

Benzodiazepines alone are relatively safe. Respiratory depression is a potential problem if large doses are given intravenously. Persisting sedation and ataxia occur with large oral or parenteral doses but seem much less of a problem in the few high-dose studies than would have been expected. If the drugs were effective and used in acute schizophrenia or mania, maintenance therapy could become a problem. Several months of treatment with 10–20 mg of lorazepam or 100–200 mg of diazepam would surely lead to physical dependence and possibly serious withdrawal symptoms if the drug were stopped abruptly.

# Lithium

### Schizophrenia

After 40 years of clinical experience with the use of lithium salts in psychotic patients, several extensive reviews (Cole et al. 1984; Delva and Letemendia 1982), and a variety of double-blind studies, it is still difficult to make precise statements about the value of lithium therapy in schizophrenia. Part of the problem lies in the difficulty in precisely defining and diagnosing schizoaffective disorder versus atypical bipolar disorder versus "true" schizophrenia versus schizophreniform disorder.

A reasonable interpretation of the available evidence is that lithium, alone, in chronic schizophrenia is not usually an adequate therapy but may reduce excitement or impulsive, angry outbursts; when added to neuroleptics, it can provide further benefit in perhaps half of the patients treated and is superior to a placebo. This difference is probably independent of the schizoaffective versus schizophrenic differentiation, although most clinicians expect schizoaffective patients to respond more substantially. In one open study, 7 of 9 schizophreniform patients improved, whereas 15 schizophrenic patients were unimproved on lithium alone (Hirschowitz et al. 1980). The NIMH collaborative study of lithium versus chlorpromazine showed that schizoaffective patients improved on chlorpromazine, irrespective of degree of excitement, whereas lithium was as useful as chlorpromazine only in the less excited half of the diagnostic group (Prien et al. 1972a, 1972b).

## Mania

Tyrer (1985) noted four double-blind, placebo-controlled studies, all confirming lithium's efficacy, with an overall improvement rate of 76%. He noted that lithium takes 6–10 days to have an appreciable antimanic effect and strongly endorsed the need to add another drug, usually a neuroleptic, to achieve early control of the mania. Tyrer also expressed the hope that lithium-carbamazepine combinations might be rapidly effective in mania, citing four small sets of case reports, totalling eight patients in all, in which drug efficacy was noted in 2–5 days. In the one available study comparing the lithium plus haloperidol combination with haloperidol alone, the combination had no advantage in severely manic patients. This study, which had only seven patients in each treatment group, included a lithium-only group showed no improvement.

## Other Disorders

There is reasonable evidence (Shader et al. 1974; Sheard 1984; Tupin et al. 1972) that lithium can be useful in impulsively, episodically violent personality disorders and probably some brain-damaged individuals.

## Tardive Dyskinesia

Cole et al. (1984) and Jeste and Wyatt (1982) reviewed the use of lithium in tardive dyskinesia. There are 10 relevant studies that show, overall, a 27% improvement rate. This varies widely from study to study; occasional patients probably benefit, whereas other patients have tardive dyskinesia induced or aggravated by lithium. It is not a reliable antidyskinesia medication.

## Safety

Lithium has been in use for many years, and its toxicities are well known. Chronic interstitial nephritis with decreased glomerular function is rare but possible. Polyuria, polydipsia with nephrogenic diabetes insipidus, is more common, although still only an occasional problem. Weight gain, skin reactions, tremor, nausea, and diarrhea are more common, although generally not serious. Serious toxicity can occur at elevated serum levels.

In summary, lithium is not an effective substitute for neuroleptics in most patients with schizophrenia, although it might reduce the required dose of neuroleptic. Some manic patients, generally those with less severe, nonparanoid manias will respond, albeit slowly, to lithium alone and may not require a neuroleptic if adequate time is allowed. Lithium may also be superior to neuroleptics in treating impulsive violence in personality disorders.

The current status of lithium as a replacement for neuroleptics is, thus, still not entirely clear. It can certainly be used to replace neuroleptics in mania some of the time.

# Carbamazepine

### Schizophrenia

There is no direct evidence that carbamazepine alone is effective in the treatment of schizophrenic disorders, although some studies report good response in some schizoaffective patients. Carbamazepine has, however, been shown to be more effective than a placebo when added to haloperidol in a rehospitalized mixed group of manic and schizophrenic patients who had responded inadequately to neuroleptics in previous admissions (Klein et al. 1984).

DeVogelaer (1981) described good response to carbamazepine in hospitalized patients with "psychotic and behavioral disorders" with agitation who have shown moderate to marked extrapyramidal side effects during neuroleptic drug treatment but without EEG abnormality or a history of epilepsy. Twenty of these patients (presumably selected from a larger sample), already stable on carbamazepine, were placed in a double-blind, placebo-controlled crossover study in which all patients received their old carbamazepine dose for 2 weeks and a placebo for 2 weeks. Eleven patients were better during the 2 weeks on active drug, whereas only two were better on the placebo. From the case reports it appears that some may have been on concomitant neuroleptic therapy.

Hakola and Loulumaa (1984), in contrast, studied carbamazepine only in schizophrenic patients with EEG abnormalities who had repeated violent outbursts despite massive doses of neuroleptics or lithium. Carbamazepine was added to the neuroleptic medication and led to good to moderate overall improvement in 11 of 18 patients. Violent episodes were reduced in 1 patient and disappeared in 14 patients during an average of 2.6 years of carbamazepine therapy. Neppe (1982) studied a probably similar group of mainly (8 of 11) schizophrenic, treated, nonresponsive, psychiatric inpatients with temporal lobe abnormality on EEG. The patients were maintained on their prior neuroleptic dose in a "15-week double-blind crossover controlled study" comparing 600 mg of carbamazepine per day with a placebo. Eight of the 11 patients were judged clinically better on carbamazepine. The 6 "aggressive" patients all showed less of this on active drug treatment. Luchins (1984) confirmed both studies in a mixed group of mainly schizophrenic patients selected for an open carbamazepine trial because of "violent" behavior on chronic psychiatric wards. Seven patients with normal EEGs showed improvement on carbamazepine, compared with a 6-week period before and after the drug. In a second trial in the same setting, 11 patients with normal EEGs and 8 patients with abnormal EEGs were observed for 6 weeks before carbamazepine and 6 weeks on carbamazepine. Although both groups improved by a decrease in violent behavior and verbal hostility, only the group with normal EEGs showed a decrease in need for prn medication. Overall, the normal EEG patients tended to show a bit more improvement.

## Mania

There are now several double-blind studies comparing carbamazepine with chlorpromazine in the treatment of acute mania. One Japanese study (Okuma et al. 1979) involved 63 patients, whereas the others, one Indian (Sethi and Tiwari 1984) and one Italian (Grossi et al. 1984), involved smaller numbers. All three showed the two drugs to be essentially equivalent in efficacy. Post and Uhde (1985) found that 10 of 17 mainly resistant manic patients had a good response to carbamazepine; however, Lerer et al. (1985) found carbamazepine inferior to lithium in a small double-blind study involving 15 acutely manic patients. There is also a subgroup of patients in whom the combination of lithium and carbamazepine is superior to either drug alone in mania (Grof 1983; Lipinski and Pope 1982).

There is also growing evidence that carbamazepine has some value as a prophylactic treatment in the longer-term prevention of recurrences in bipolar patients (Cole et al. 1986).

## Other Disorders

Carbamazepine has also been reported (Garbutt and Loosen 1983; Hermann and Melyn 1984; Tunks and Demer 1977) to be useful in suppressing episodic behavioral disturbances that may have violent or paranoid components or manifest as severe anxiety. These case reports describe patients with and without other evidence of epilepsy or EEG abnormality. Uhde et al. (1984) reported amelioration in the intensity of panic attacks and the associated "help-seeking" behavior of panic patients during the carbamazepine phase of a small placebo-controlled crossover trial. Cowdry and Gardner (1983) reported that carbamazepine improves stability and impulsivity in patients with borderline personality disorder. Carbamazepine also can reduce hyperactivity in severely retarded patients (Reid et al. 1981) who may have shown manic features.

In the only large uncontrolled study of carbamazepine in 34 well-characterized, nonpsychotic psychiatric inpatients with rage outbursts, Mattes (1984) briefly noted improvement in "most" patients with a marked decrease in mean physical assault scores. None of a variety of EEG, neurological, or diagnostic features was related to degree of improvement.

### Tardive Dyskinesia

Of the many drugs reviewed in this chapter, carbamazepine is the only one that has not been claimed to improve tardive dyskinesia. No comment has been located in the many papers reviewed on changes in (or even the presence of) any preexisting tardive dyskinesia. Our own clinical experience is equally unhelpful; numerous patients with tardive dyskinesia have received carbamazepine without the treating clinician being impressed by either favorable or unfavorable change in the dyskinesia.

### Safety

The one available study that compared ongoing side effects in 20 patients, each on lithium or carbamazepine, reports roughly comparable incidences of treatment-emergent symptoms (Placidi et al. 1984). Generally, sedation is the most common subjective side effect, although ataxia and diplopia can occur. Skin rashes may also be a problem. Uhde et al. (1984) assessed the drug as "well tolerated and safe" on the basis of their group's experience at NIMH. Aplastic anemia and agranulocytosis have been reported but may or may not be more common than agranulocytosis is with chlorpromazine. Occasional patients show a tendency toward both anemia and leukopenia and, generally, regular blood counts are done every 2 weeks for the first few months. Impairment of liver function can also occur. The drug is widely used in seizure disorder patients.

### Summary

If carbamazepine is to replace neuroleptic drugs at all, it would be by serving as a potentially effective antimanic agent, alone or in combination with lithium or by offering a potentially better alternative to neuroleptics in impulsive, occasionally violent, unstable nonpsychotic patients who often receive neuroleptics as prns or as maintenance medication. Adjunctive carbamazepine may also be helpful as an alternative to high-dose neuroleptic therapy in neuroleptic-resistant schizophrenic patients for whom a neuroleptic plus carbamazepine may be better than the neuroleptic alone.

# Valproic Acid

Valproic acid (Depakene) and divalproex sodium, a stable enteric coated combination compound of sodium valproate and valproic acid (Depakote), are available in the United States. Valproic acid amide, also called dipropylacetamide, is available in Europe and appears to be converted entirely to valproic acid in the body in humans. There is some debate over whether the recommended "therapeutic" serum levels of 50–100 ng/ml are valid (Lautin et al. 1980). The half-life is said to be 8–15 hours in adults without liver disease.

## Schizophrenia

There are two contradictory studies in drug-free schizophrenic patients. Gundurewa et al. (1980) gave valproic acid to 10 nonexcited patients with "paranoid-hallucinatory syndrome" for 20 days in doses up to 2,100 mg/day. One patient worsened, 1 became delirious, and 1 refused the medication. Six of the other 7 patients improved, with significant decreases in the paranoid and hallucinatory symptoms and the thought-disorder cluster of the BPRS, but there was no significant drop in BPRS total score. Lautin et al. (1980) gave sodium valproate for as many as 31 days in 7 drug-free patients with chronic schizophrenia recently readmitted to Bellevue Hospital in New York. The dose was increased to 2,000–3,000 mg/day. One patient was minimally improved while all others worsened rather markedly with irritability and agitation with or without markedly increased psychotic symptoms.

Linnoila et al. (1976), in a study designed to test the effect of sodium valproate on tardive dyskinesia in 31 mixed geriatric chronic psychotic patients, added the drug at 900 mg/day to ongoing neuroleptic medication in a placebo-controlled, double-blind crossover study, 2 weeks each on the drug and on a placebo. They found a significant decrease in BPRS total score, greatest after 2 weeks on the sodium valproate.

## Mania

Emrich et al. (1984) and Brennan et al. (1984) described placebo-controlled crossover trials in, respectively, 5 and 8 acutely manic patients, using sodium valproate in doses of 900–3,800 mg/day, with good results in 10 of the 13 patients.

Lambert (1984) and Lambert et al. (1975) appear to have treated almost 400 patients with valpromide (dipropylacetamide) since 1965. Lambert finds it generally more useful than lithium as a maintenance therapy in bipolar disorder but seems to use it with lithium or with neuroleptics in the treatment of acute mania, mainly in doses of 900 mg/day. Neuroleptics, antidepressants, or lithium are added as needed in some patients. Puzynski and Klosiewicz (1984) treated 15 bipolar or schizoaffective patients with the amide for 2–4 years as maintenance therapy, with about a 60% decrease in manic episodes. The results from bipolar patients were slightly better than those from schizoaffective patients. Most patients received only valproic acid amide.

### Tardive Dyskinesia

In the Linnoila et al. (1976) study, 900 mg of sodium valproate (compared with a placebo) significantly reduced akinesia, rigidity, akathisia, and dystonic spasms in these neuroleptic-maintained patients. Fourteen of the 31 patients showed improvement in tardive dyskinesia while on the active drug, but 5 improved only after sodium valproate was stopped and a placebo begun and 8 of the patients who improved on valproate continued to improve on the placebo, making for a lack of drug/placebo difference. Gibson (1978) gave sodium valproate at 900 mg/day to 25 dyskinetic patients in an open study, recording the dyskinesia on videotape. Only 8 of the 25 patients were judged less dyskinetic while on valproate, whereas 3 were judged better on a placebo. Nagao et al. (1979) reported improvement in 3 of 7 dyskinesia patients on 600 mg of dipropylacetamide per day.

### Safety

Sedation and nausea are the most common side effects. The latter is reduced if valproic acid itself is not used. Enteric coated Depakote, in the United States, is likely to have fewer gastrointestinal side effects. Hair loss, weight gain, and confusion are rare side effects. Vencovsky et al. (1984) claimed that maintenance dipropylacetamide caused undesirable side effects in only 8% of 38 patients, compared with a possible 60% rate in lithium-treated patients. The problem of serious hepatic toxicity exists, but the prevalence is unclear (probably low). Nevertheless, it warrants repeated laboratory and clinical monitoring for changes in liver function.

### Summary

There is modest but reasonable evidence from two partially controlled studies that valproic acid has efficacy alone in acute mania. It is probably not useful alone in schizophrenia, but it might yet be shown to have a role as an adjunctive treatment in schizophrenic patients. It could decrease neuroleptic use either in acute mania or by averting future manic episodes in bipolar or schizoaffective patients. Some schizoaffective patients may be stable on valproic acid alone, although this is far from certain.

# Summary and Conclusions

It appears that proven safe and effective alternatives for neuroleptic treatment in the acute and long-term treatment of schizophrenia have not emerged, despite clinical studies employing a varied array of pharmacologic agents.

Although subgroups of patients may at times benefit from nonneuroleptic medications, we are unable to identify these individuals prior to appropriate treatment trials. Therefore, neuroleptic drugs continue to remain the treatment of choice for patients with schizophrenia unless there are specific contraindications or clear evidence that such agents are not helpful. The treatment of those patients who fail to benefit adequately from available neuroleptics continues to present a challenge to clinicians, and in this context, a variety of "unproven" or experimental treatments might be indicated.

Alternatives to neuroleptic treatment are, however, well established in a variety of conditions other than schizophrenia, and the use of neuroleptics in that context must be carefully weighed and fully justified.

# References

Ayd F: Prolonged use of reserpine in schizophrenia, in Psychopharmacology Frontiers. Edited by Kline NS. Boston, MA, Little, Brown, 1959, pp 33–38

Bacher N, Lewis H: Addition of reserpine to antipsychotic medication in refractory chronic schizophrenic outpatients. Am J Psychiatry 135:488–489, 1978

Bacher N, Lewis M: Lithium plus reserpine in refractory manic patients. Am J Psychiatry 136:811–814, 1979

Barsa J, Kline N: Use of reserpine in disturbed psychotic patients. Am J Psychiatry 112:684–691, 1956

Bobruff A, Gardos G, Tarsy D, et al: Clonazepam and phenobarbital in tardive dyskinesia. Am J Psychiatry 138:189–193, 1981

Braun M: Reserpine as a therapeutic agent in schizophrenia. Am J Psychiatry 116:744–745, 1960

Brennan M, Sandyk R, Borsook D: Prophylactic effect of dipropylacetamide in patients with bipolar affective disorder, in Anticonvulsants in Affective Disorders. Edited by Emrich N, Okuma T, Muller A. Amsterdam, Excerpta Medica, 1984, pp 56–65

Chouinard G, Young S, Annable L: Antimanic effect of clonazepam. Biol Psychiatry 18:451–466, 1983

Cole J: Medication and seclusion and restraint. McLean Hosp J 10:37–53, 1985

Cole JO, Gardos G, Rapkin R, et al: Lithium carbonate in tardive dyskinesia and schizophrenia, in Tardive Dyskinesia and Affective Disorders. Edited by Gardos G, Casey D. Washington, DC, American Psychiatric Press, 1984, pp 50–73

Cole JO, Chiarello RJ, Merzel APC: Long-term pharmacotherapy of affective disorders. McLean Hosp J 11:106–138, 1986

Cowdry R, Gardner D: Carbamazepine in borderline disorder: implications for possible limbic dysfunction. Presented at the Annual Meeting, American College of Neuropsychopharmacology (ACNP), Puerto Rico, Dec 16, 1983

Degkwitz R: Extrapyramidal motor disorders following long-term treatment with neuroleptic drugs, in Psychotropic Drugs and Dysfunction of the Basal Ganglia (U.S. Public Health Service Publication No. 1938). Edited by Crane GE, Gardner R Jr. Washington, DC, U.S. Government Printing Office, 1969, pp 22–32

Delva N, Letemendia F: Lithium treatment in schizophrenia and schizoaffective disorders. Br J Psychiatry 141:387–400, 1982

DeVogelaer J: Carbamazepine in the treatment of psychotic and behavioral disorders. Acta Psychiatr Belg 81:532–541, 1981

Elkes C: Rauwolfia alkaloids and reserpine in the treatment of the chronic psychiatric patient. J Mental Science 103:464–474, 1960

Emrich H, Dose M, von Zerssen D: Use of sodium valprote in the management of affective disorders, in Anticonvulsants in Affective Disorders. Edited by Emrich H, Okuma T, Muller A. Amsterdam, Excerpta Medica, 1984, pp 45–55

Fahn S: Treatment of tardive dyskinesia: use of dopamine-depleting agents. Clin Neuropharmacol 6:151–158, 1983

Garbutt JC, Loosen PT: Is carbamazepine helpful in paroxysmal behavior disorders? Am J Psychiatry 140:1363–1364, 1983

Gardner D, Cowdry R: Alprazolam–induced dyscontrol in borderline personality disorder. Am J Psychiatry 142:98–100, 1985

Gibson A: Sodium valproate and tardive dyskinesia. Br J Psychiatry 133:82, 1978

Goldman D: Drugs in treatment of psychosis, in Psychiatric Drugs. Edited by Solomon P. New York, Grune & Stratton, 1966, p 136

Gore CP, Egan GP, Walton D: The place of reserpine in the treatment of the chronic patient. Am J Psychiatry 114:333–337, 1957

Griffith J: Treatment of episodic behavioral disorders with rapidly absorbed benzodiazepines. J Nerv Ment Dis 173:312–315, 1985

Grof P: Response to long-term lithium treatment: research studies and clinical implications, in Affective Disorders. Edited by Davis JM, Maas JW. Washington, DC, American Psychiatric Press, 1983, pp 357–366

Grossi E, Sachetti E, Vita A, et al: Carbamazepine vs chlorpromazine in mania: a double-blind trial, in Anticonvulsants in Affective Disorders. Edited by Emrich H, Okuma T, Muller A. New York, Elsevier, 1984, pp 177–187

Gundlach R, Engelhardt DM, Hankoff L, et al: A double-blind outpatient study of diazepam (Valium) and placebo. Psychopharmacologia 9:81–92, 1967

Gundurewa M, Beckman H, Zimmer R, et al: Effect of valproic acid on schizophrenic syndromes. Arzneimittel Forschung 30:1212–1213, 1980

Haas S: Treatment of schizophrenia with benzodiazepines: experiences with high-dose diazepam, in Benzodiazepines: From Molecular Biology to Clinical Practice. Edited by Costa E. New York, Raven, 1983, pp 383–388

Hakola H, Loulumaa V: Carbamazepine in violent schizophrenics, in Anticonvulsants in Affective Disorders. Edited by Emrich H, Okuma T, Muller A. Amsterdam, Excerpta Medica, 1984, pp 204–207

Hanlon TE, Ota KY, Agallianos DD, et al: Combined drug treatment of newly hospitalized, acutely ill psychiatric patients. Diseases of the Nervous System 30:104–116, 1969

Hanlon TE, Ota KY, Kurland AA: Comparative effects of fluphenazine, fluphenazine-chlordiazepoxide and fluphenazine-imipramine. Diseases of the Nervous System 31:171–176, 1970

Hanssen T, Heyden T, Sundberg I, et al: Propranolol in schizophrenia. Arch Gen Psychiatry 37:685–690, 1980

Hayes P, Schulz SC: The use of beta-adrenergic blocking agents in anxiety disorders and schizophrenia. Pharmacotherapy 3:101–117, 1983

Hermann B, Melyn M: Effects of carbamazepine on interictal psychopathology in TLE with ictal fear. J Clin Psychiatry 45:169–171, 1984

Hirschowitz J, Casper J, Garver D, et al: Lithium response in good prognosis schizophrenia. Am J Psychiatry 137:916–920, 1980

Hollister L, Krieger G, Kringel A, et al: Treatment of chronic schizophrenic reactions with reserpine. Ann NY Acad Sci 61:92–100, 1955

Itil TM, Unverdi C, Mehta D: Clorazepate dipotassium in tardive dyskinesia. Am J Psychiatry 131:1291, 1974

Jeste D, Wyatt R: Therapeutic strategies against tardive dyskinesia. Arch Gen Psychiatry 39:803–816, 1982

Jimerson D, Post R, Stoddard F, et al: Preliminary trial of the noradrenergic agonist clonidine in psychiatric patients. Biol Psychiatry 15:45–57, 1980

Jimerson D, van Kammen D, Post R, et al: Diazepam in schizophrenia: a preliminary double-blind trial. Am J Psychiatry 139:489–491, 1982

Jouvent R, Lecrubier Y, Puech A, et al: Antimanic effect of clonidine. Am J Psychiatry 137:1275–1276, 1980

Jus A, Jus K, Fontaine P: Long-term treatment of tardive dyskinesia. J Clin Psychol 30:73–79, 1979

Kellner R, Wilson R, Muldawer M, et al: Anxiety in schizophrenia: the response to chlordiazepoxide in an intensive design study. Arch Gen Psychiatry 32:1246–1254, 1975

Kirkegaard A: Clinical experiences with reserpine, in Psychopharmacology Frontiers. Edited by Kline NS. Boston, MA, Little, Brown, 1959, pp 49–52

Klein E, Bental E, Lerer B, et al: Carbamazepine and haloperidol v placebo and haloperidol in excited psychosis. Arch Gen Psychiatry 41:165–170, 1984

Lambert P: Acute and prophylactic therapies of patients with affective disorders using valpromide, in Anticonvulsants in Affective Disorders. Edited by Emrich N, Okuma T, Muller A. Amsterdam, Excerpta Medica, 1984, pp 33–44

Lambert P, Carraz G, Borselli S, et al: Dipropylacetamide in treatment of manic-depressive psychosis. L'Encephale 1:25–31, 1975

Lasky JJ, Klett JC, Caffey EM, et al: Drug treatment of schizophrenic patients. Diseases of the Nervous System 23:698–705, 1962

Lautin A, Angrist B, Stanley M, et al: Sodium valproate in schizophrenia. Br J Psychiatry 137:240–244, 1980

Lerer B, Moore N, Meyendorff E, et al: Carbamazepine and lithium: different profiles in affective disorders? Psychopharmacol Bull 21:18–22, 1985

Lerner Y, Lwow E, Levitin A, et al: Acute high dose parenteral haloperidol treatment of psychosis. Am J Psychiatry 136:1061–1064, 1979

Lingjaerde O: Benzodiazepines in the treatment of schizophrenia, in Benzodiazepines: From Molecular Biology to Clinical Practice. Edited by Costa E. New York, Raven, 1983, pp 369–381

Lingjaerde O, Engstrand E, Ellingsen P, et al: Antipsychotic effect of diazepam when given in addition to neuroleptics in chronic psychotic patients. Curr Ther Res 26:505–514, 1979

Linnoila M, Vinkar M, Hietala O: Effect of sodium valproate on tardive dyskinesia. Br J Psychiatry 129:114–119, 1976

Lion J: Benzodiazepines in the treatment of aggressive patients. J Clin Psychiatry 40:70–71, 1979

Lipinski JF, Pope HG: Possible synergistic action between carbamazepine and lithium carbonate in the treatment of three acutely manic patients. Am J Psychiatry 139:948–949, 1982

Luchins D: Carbamazepine in violent non-epileptic schizophrenics. Psychopharmacol Bull 20:569–571, 1984

Maculam GA: Comparison of diazepam, chlorprothixene and chlorpromazine in chronic schizophrenic patients. Diseases of the Nervous System 25:164–168, 1964

Mattes J: Carbamazepine for uncontrolled rage outbursts. Lancet 2:1164–1165, 1984

Michaux MH, Kurland AA, Agallianos DD: Chlorpromazine-chlordiazepoxide and chlorpromazine-imipramine treatment of newly hospitalized acutely ill psychiatric patients. Curr Ther Res 8 (suppl):117–152, 1966

Modell J, Lenox R, Weiner S: Inpatient clinical trial of lorazepam for the management of manic agitation. J Clin Psychopharmacol 5:109–113, 1985

Monroe R, Wise S: Combined phenothiazine, chlordiazepoxide and primidone therapy for uncontrolled psychotic patients. Am J Psychiatry 122:694–698, 1965

Nagao T, Oshimo T, Mitsunobu K, et al: Cerebrospinal fluid monoamine metabolites and cyclic nucleotides in chronic schizophrenic patients with tardive dyskinesia or drug-induced tremor. Biol Psychiatry 14:509–523, 1979

Neppe V: Carbamazepine in the psychiatric patient (letter). Lancet 2:334, 1982

Nestoros J, Suranyi B, Spees R, et al: Diazepam in high doses is effective in schizophrenia. Prog Neuropsychopharmacol Biol Psychiatry 6:513–518, 1982

O'Flanagan PM: Clonazepam in the treatment of drug-induced dyskinesia. Br Med J 1:269–270, 1975

Okuma T, Inanaga K, Otsuki S, et al: Comparison of antimanic efficacy of carbamazepine and chlorpromazine: a double-blind controlled study. Psychopharmacology 66:211–217, 1979

Pearl D, Vanderkamp H, Olson AL, et al: The effects of reserpine on schizophrenic patients. Am J Psychiatry 112:936, 1956

Placidi G, Lenzi A, Rampello E, et al: Long-term double–blind prospective study on carbamazepine versus lithium in bipolar and schizoaffective disorders: preliminary results, in Anticonvulsants in Affective Disorders. Edited by Emrich H, Okuma T, Muller A. Amsterdam, Excerpta Medica, 1984, pp 188–197

Post RM, Uhde TW: Carbamazepine in bipolar illness. Psychopharmacol Bull 21:10–17, 1985

Prien R, Caffey E, Klett C: A comparison of lithium carbonate and chlorpromazine in the treatment of excited schizoaffectives. Arch Gen Psychiatry 27:182–189, 1972a

Prien R, Caffey E, Klett C: Comparison of lithium carbonate and chlorpromazine in the treatment of mania. Arch Gen Psychiatry 26:146–153, 1972b

Puzynski S, Klosiewicz L: Valproic and amide in the treatment of affective and schizoaffective disorders. J Affective Disord 6:115–121, 1984

Reid A, Naylor G, Kay D: A double-blind placebo controlled crossover trial of carbamazepine in overactive severely mentally handicapped patients. Psychol Med 11:109–113, 1981

Sedman G: Clonazepam in the treatment of tardive oral dyskinesia. Br Med J 2:583, 1976

Sethi B, Tiwari S: Carbamazepine in affective disorders, in Anticonvulsants in Affective Disorders. Edited by Emrich H, Okuma T, Muller A. New York, Elsevier, 1984, pp 167–176

Shader RI, Jackson AH, Dodes LM: The antiaggressive effects of lithium in man. Psychopharmacologia 40:17–24, 1974

Sheard MH: Clinical pharmacology of aggressive behavior. Clin Neuropharmacol 7:173–183, 1984

Simon W, Wirt AL, Wirt RD, et al: Long term follow-up study of schizophrenic patients. Arch Gen Psychiatry 12:510–515, 1965

Singh MM: Diazepam in the treatment of tardive dyskinesia. Int Pharmacopsychiat 11:232–234, 1976

Somerness MD, Lucero RJ, Hamlon JS, et al: A controlled study of reserpine on chronically disturbed patients. Arch Neurol Psychiatry 74:316–319, 1955

Tunks ER, Demer SW: Carbamazepine in the dyscontrol syndrome associated with limbic system dysfunction. J Nerv Ment Dis 164:56–63, 1977

Tupin JP, Smith DB, Clanon TL, et al: The long term use of lithium in aggressive prisoners. Compr Psychiatry 13:533–537, 1972

Tyrer S: Lithium in the treatment of mania. J Affective Disord 8:251–257, 1985

Uhde T, Post R, Ballenger J, et al: Carbamazepine in the treatment of neuropsychiatric disorders, in Anticonvulsants in Affective Disorders. Edited by Emrich H, Okuma T, Muller A. Amsterdam, Excerpta Medica, 1984, pp 111–131

Uhrbrand L, Faurbye A: Reversible and irreversible dyskinesia after treatment with perphenazine, chlorpromazine, reserpine and electroconvulsive therapy. Psychopharmacologia 1:408–418, 1960

Vencovsky E, Soucek K, Kabes J: Valproic acid amide as a prophylactic agent in affective and schizoaffective disorders, in Anticonvulsants in Affective Disorders. Edited by Emrich H, Okuma T, Muller A. Amsterdam, Excerpta Medica, 1984, pp 66–67

Vinar O, Taussigova D: Therapeutic effects of diazepam in psychotics. Act Nerv Super (Praha) 8:441–444, 1966

Wirt RD, Simon W: Differential Treatment and Prognosis in Schizophrenia. Springfield, IL, Charles C Thomas, 1959

Wolf SM: Reserpine: cause and treatment of oral-facial dyskinesia. Bull Los Angeles Neurological Soc 38:80–84, 1973

Chapter 9

# Are There Behavioral Analogues of Tardive Dyskinesia?

I t has been suggested that prolonged neuroleptic administration might result in neuropharmacologic changes producing alterations in behavior in an analogous fashion to tardive dyskinesia. This possibility was first clearly delineated by Davis and Rosenberg (1979). In fact, at least three such syndromes have been postulated. Of these, *supersensitivity psychosis* (Chouinard et al. 1978; Cole et al. 1984) is the most commonly discussed. The possibility of a *tardive dysmentia* has also been proposed in psychiatric patients, and *tardive dysbehavior* has been described in children and adolescents.

The general concept has a seductive face validity. Neuroleptic drugs could cause an alteration in dopamine receptors in the limbic area—or some other relevant brain area involved in emotion or psychosis—which might parallel the changes in the dopamine receptor function in the basal ganglia suspected of causing tardive dyskinesia. If neuroleptics did this, then one might see some of the variegated psychiatric phenomena described in papers on supersensitivity psychosis or tardive dysmentia.

The main and unavoidable problem is that tardive dyskinesia is a relatively unique though heterogeneous set of abnormal movements not usually seen as a concomitant of psychosis. If an individual with schizophrenia shows grimacing, tongue protrusion, chewing, and choreoathetoid arm movements, it is relatively unlikely that this cluster of dyskinesias is due to the psychosis. If the same patient shows worsening of psychotic symptoms when coming off of neuroleptics or despite increasing doses of neuroleptics, it is impossible to prove that this is an adverse consequence of prolonged antipsychotic drug treatment. The course of psychosis is variable enough to make any outcome or shift in clinical status entirely plausible. If a psychotic patient worsens, there is no compelling reason to assume that the increase in symptoms is due to dopaminergic supersensitivity in relevant brain regions.

Unfortunately, it is equally difficult to prove that any worsening in psychosis is not due to some increase in dopaminergic activity in the brain. The dopamine hypothesis of schizophrenia remains very tenable, at least for a large subgroup of patients with this illness. The theory may, in fact, be correct, but empirical data proving dopaminergic overactivity in untreated psychosis are lacking or weak. The strongest evidence that dopamine excess "causes" schizophrenia lies in the high correlation between the potency of neuroleptics in blocking dopamine receptors and their usual effective clinical dosage in patients with schizophrenia. Indirect dopamine agonists, such as *d*-amphetamine or methylphenidate, sometimes (but by no means always) aggravate psychosis—some schizophrenics even improve on stimulant drugs (Chiarello and Cole 1987). The effects of direct dopamine agonists (e.g., apomorphine, L-dopa) in psychosis are even less clear.

In this chapter we review the characteristics of the proposed syndromes and the available evidence for and against their existence.

One, tardive dysmentia, assumes a chronic condition accompanying prolonged neuroleptic use, possibly resembling a long-standing persistent tardive dyskinesia. The second, tardive dysbehavior, is equally clearly a withdrawal phenomenon resembling a withdrawal dyskinesia that develops in children and adolescents as neuroleptics are discontinued, which peaks in intensity in a few weeks and diminishes within 16 weeks. Supersensitivity psychosis in psychiatric patients falls in between. It mainly describes the development of florid psychotic symptoms in psychiatric patients during neuroleptic withdrawal or discontinuation but also sometimes includes the need for steadily increasing doses of neuroleptics over time to maintain the same degree of control over psychotic symptoms. Thus it could resemble either a transient withdrawal dyskinesia or a tardive dyskinesia worsening slowly despite attempts to suppress it with dopamine-blocking drugs.

## Supersensitivity Psychosis

The main contributor to the literature on supersensitivity psychosis is G. Chouinard, who has authored at least five papers on the topic (Chouinard 1982; Chouinard and Jones 1980; Chouinard et al. 1978, 1982, 1986). Although the details of his ideas about the condition have shifted somewhat over time, the main points are constant. The syndrome is characterized by the following:

1. A rapid return of psychotic symptoms during or following antipsychotic withdrawal or dose reduction. He suggests 6 weeks after stopping an oral neuroleptic or 3 months after the last injection of a depot preparation as the outer limits.
2. Psychotic exacerbations consisting only of positive symptoms of schizophrenia.

3.   Tolerance to neuroleptic drugs as manifested by a need for increasing dosages over time to keep psychotic symptoms under control.

Chouinard also suggests that patients with supersensitivity psychosis are likely to show dramatic, rapid improvement when antipsychotic drugs are readministered. Supersensitivity psychosis is more likely to occur if the patient has been on high-potency neuroleptics (e.g., fluphenazine or haloperidol instead of chlorpromazine or thioridazine) and is more likely in patients whose original psychotic symptoms were in full remission before neuroleptic dosage was reduced or stopped. Chouinard also believes that life stresses tend to precipitate the acute psychosis, making the condition more evident in outpatients than in inpatients.

Chouinard et al. (1986) surveyed 234 schizophrenic patients attending an aftercare clinic for evidence of supersensitivity psychosis, meaning a need for increasing an antipsychotic dose over time and a clear tendency to relapse rapidly when the dose is tapered or stopped. He restated this as "a greater relapse rate during continuous neuroleptic treatment than when not continuously treated." Borderline cases either relapsed more slowly (see criterion 1, above) or had only shown definite drug tolerance without relapse when medication was decreased. By these standards, 22% of his patients had "definite supersensitivity psychosis" and 21% were borderline cases. There was no correlation between the psychotic phenomena and the existence of tardive dyskinesia. Patients with supersensitivity psychosis were on higher neuroleptic dosages than patients without it—not surprising, given the tolerance requirement—and tended to have high prolactin levels and be more likely to have good-prognosis characteristics.

No other papers describe more than a few probable cases. There does not appear to be any strong association between the presence of tardive dyskinesia and the occurrence of supersensitivity psychosis.

Surprisingly, during the period since 1978 when Chouinard first described the concept of supersensitivity psychosis in a widely read journal, there has been only a handful of case reports describing cases that may constitute examples of supersensitivity psychosis. Chouinard and Jones (1980) mainly described patients on maintenance depot neuroleptics followed as outpatients who tended to have increases in psychotic symptoms just before the next injection and, as a result, received steadily increasing dosages up to, for example, 150 mg of fluphenazine decanoate or its equivalent every week, with only partial relief of symptoms. Csernansky and Hollister (1982) described a similar patient, a paranoid schizophrenic whose dosage requirements escalated over 22 years from 800 mg of chlorpromazine per day to 200 mg of trifluoperazine plus 160 mg of thiothixene per day. Attempts to taper this massive dose led to a recurrence of psychosis. Both of these reports show increasing tolerance with a rapid return of symptoms, although it is less clear that the symptoms were worse than or different from those shown in the patient's initial psychosis.

Three other cases reported may fit a somewhat different but related hypothesis. Does prolonged use of neuroleptics lead to a withdrawal psychosis in patients who had not previously been psychotic? One elderly woman, after many years on reserpine for hypertension, developed a manic state when reserpine was withdrawn (Kent and Wilber 1982); mania cleared rapidly when reserpine was reinstituted. A schizoid young woman who had received chlorpromazine for obsessive-compulsive symptoms as a child developed a prolonged schizophrenic psychosis after receiving chlorpromazine briefly again for anxiety (Sale and Kristall 1978). A patient with obsessive-compulsive disorder received trifluoperazine for 6 years in dosages up to 60 mg/day. When severe tardive dyskinesia developed, neuroleptics were stopped and a florid schizophrenic psychosis evolved and persisted for 2 years off of all medication. The psychosis, but not the dyskinesia, improved on low-dose neuroleptics without evidence of tolerance development during the next 3 years (Cole et al. 1984).

There is one additional case of a man with recurring manic episodes who relapsed floridly 3 days after his fluphenazine dose was decreased from 5 mg/day to zero. He recompensated rapidly on fluphenazine and then tolerated a more gradual dosage-reduction regimen uneventfully (Witschy et al. 1984).

The only recent cases involve relapse after clozapine withdrawal, which may well be a quite different phenomenon. Five patients have been reported in two articles (Ekblom et al. 1984; Perenyi et al. 1985). Four of the five became floridly psychotic within 1–3 days after moderate to low clozapine doses were abruptly stopped for clinical reasons. The fifth relapsed 3 days after his dose was reduced from 150 mg/day to 75 mg/day. None of these patients had shown tolerance, and none recovered rapidly when standard antipsychotics or even clozapine was readministered. J. Cole (September 1990, personal communication) reported that of 35 patients treated with clozapine over the years at McLean Hospital, 1 patient showed a similar phenomenon. After 8 years of freedom from psychosis on clozapine with gradually decreasing dosages, she became severely psychotic with manic features 2 days after stopping her 50 mg/day dosage. It took 3 weeks for her psychosis to clear on 300 mg/day of clozapine. J. Kane and J. Lieberman (September 1990, personal communication) observed 7 clozapine-treated patients who underwent abrupt discontinuation following the development of agranulocytosis and did not see an unusually rapid or florid pattern of relapse.

Three studies have explicitly looked for something resembling supersensitivity psychosis. Borison et al. (1988) followed up the reports of sudden psychotic relapses in patients suddenly taken off clozapine. They studied 12 chronic patients stable on various neuroleptics who had their medication abruptly stopped. After a week off medication, they were treated with clozapine at 200 mg/day for 8 weeks. The clozapine was then abruptly stopped. Six of the 12 patients showed a much more dramatic worsening of psychosis in the week after clozapine discontinuation than they had shown in the preclozapine drug-free week. This tends to confirm the possibility that clozapine discontinuation can lead to a rapid increase in psychotic symptoms independent, presumably, of any general tendency to supersensitivity psychosis. The difference could simply be pharmacokinetic, however—clozapine's effect in the brain may wear off more rapidly than that of other, more conventional neuroleptics. (This is supported to some extent by a study by Hartvig et al. [1986] employing positron-emission tomography of $^{11}$C-clozapine binding in the rhesus monkey striatum, suggesting that clozapine is more loosely bound to dopamine receptors in the striatum than N-methylspiperone.)

Another study, by Weinberger et al. (1981), concerned changes in psychosis after withdrawal of antipsychotic medication in 20 patients with chronic schizophrenia. Patients were studied for 4 weeks off medication. Ten worsened to some degree (5 rather markedly), and 3 improved. Four patients showed a course suggestive of initial worsening followed by improvement.

Chouinard et al. (1986) criticized the study because too many patients were on low-potency neuroleptics; they argued that autonomic withdrawal symptoms caused by these drugs (i.e., cholinergic rebound) can obscure the emergence of supersensitivity psychosis. Some patients apparently did become more psychotic off medication, but the data are not detailed enough to determine whether Chouinard's criteria of tolerance—rapid exacerbation and the emergence of new, more severe symptoms with rapid improvement when a drug is restarted—were met.

The third study, by Schooler et al. (1982), involved 67 schizophrenic patients who had participated in a 1-year study comparing oral fluphenazine with fluphenazine decanoate. Patients were then randomly assigned to continued medication or to a placebo, with the majority of the patients assigned to a placebo. Two-thirds of the patients then on benztropine had this drug stopped by placebo substitution at the time of the change if they were placed on placebo fluphenazine. The oral fluphenazine patients who were withdrawn from medication had a 59% relapse rate over 15 weeks (compared with 33% in those patients remaining on the oral drug), with most of the relapses occurring in the first 3 weeks. Relapse rates were lower and occurred more slowly in patients who had been on depot fluphenazine. There was a positive, though modest, correlation between relapse and the emergence of dyskinetic movements. The results of the study are compatible with the existence of some type of dopaminergic sensitivity; the concomitant discontinuation of the antiparkinsonian medication complicates the picture.

The review by Cole et al. (1984) suggests that such rapid relapse following drug withdrawal was rarely observed in other earlier studies.

## Tardive Dysmentia

Wilson et al. (1983) postulated the syndrome of tardive dysmentia, based on Wilson's clinical observations while doing a naturalistic study of tardive dyskinesia in a public mental hospital. He noted that certain chronic schizophrenic subjects with severe tardive dyskinesia presented with behavior resembling that of hypomania as well as schizophrenia. The patients tended to be loquacious and to speak in a loud voice. They showed thought disconnection and were generally circumstantial and aimless in conversation. Disassociated, inappropriate statements were common. The prevailing mood was generally one of euphoria, but unheralded, inexplicable, explosive changes in affect occurred as good humor changed rapidly to explosive hostility or sullen petulance. Social withdrawal and autistic preoccupation were punctuated by episodes of overactive behavior when the subject talked loudly, often close to the observer's face, and was quite intrusive and invasive of the privacy of others.

These chronic patients had not had these schizoaffective features earlier in the course of their illnesses. Therefore, it was hypothesized that a central dopaminergic hyperactivity analogous to that presumed in tardive dyskinesia might be causing this "dysmentia." It was suggested that five phenomena—euphoria, labile mood, loud speech, approach to examiner, and excess words—rated on 100 mm lines, should correlate with each other and with the severity of dyskinesia as measured by the Abnormal Involuntary Movement Scale (AIMS) in 29 patients in a chronic ward with a history of at least 2 years of continuous neuroleptic therapy. The five concepts did intercorrelate significantly and three—loud speech, labile mood, and approach to examiner—correlated significantly (but not impressively) with dyskinesia (AIMS) scores.

This study cannot, of course, prove the existence of the syndrome or prove that the syndrome, if real, is new and would not have been found in equally chronic patients prior to the existence of antipsychotic drug therapy.

Mukherjee (1984) critiqued the Wilson et al. (1983) study on a variety of issues. He judged that the behavior described would fit better with the term *dyscontrol* than with *dysmentia*. More important, he noted that in his study of tardive dyskinesia (in a cohort of 131 bipolar outpatients) he found no evidence of behavior resembling tardive dysmentia in his patients during periods of remission from affective episodes and that this casts doubt on the likelihood that tardive dysmentia could be a general neurotoxic consequence of antipsychotic drug therapy. This point is reinforced by Goldberg's (1985) analysis of the tardive dysmentia syndrome. He noted marked similarities between the behaviors described and behavioral disinhibition seen in frontal lobe lesions, especially those of the frontal-orbital/mediobasal surfaces, and anticipates the recent surge of research interest in the possibility that schizophrenia is associated with preexisting deficits in the frontal lobes.

These two papers, taken together, suggest that the behaviors observed by Wilson et al. (1983) could be specific to chronic schizophrenia and could be due to a preexisting frontal lobe deficit in schizophrenic patients, perhaps aggravated by neuroleptic therapy. None of this is proven but, as with supersensitivity psychosis, tardive dysmentia is an intriguing subject on which to base elaborate theoretical debates. What is really needed, however, are more relevant clinical data.

## Tardive Dysbehavior

Gualtieri et al. (1984) described a withdrawal-induced acute behavior deterioration that comes on fairly rapidly after neuroleptics are stopped in children or adolescents who have been on maintenance neuroleptics for months or years. The behaviors can include insomnia, hyperactivity, aggression, screaming, running, and agitation. The syndrome was diagnosed only when these behaviors were clearly different from those that led to the original treatment. In one anterospective study of 41 patients who were taken off neuroleptics, 4 developed this picture. All remitted within 8 weeks.

One other case of new psychotic symptoms occurring 4 weeks after haloperidol at 50 mg/day had been discontinued in a 15-year-old patient with long-standing Tourette's disorder has been described (Caine et al. 1978). The psychotic picture persisted for 5 weeks and appeared to be intensifying. Haloperidol was then reinstituted with good results, leaving moot the question of whether the picture would have cleared spontaneously over a longer time period.

## Drug Discontinuation

There is no doubt that schizophrenic patients relapse while antipsychotic medication is being tapered or after drug discontinuation. Except for the Weinberger et al. (1981) and Diamond and Borison (1980) studies, however, no published study was carried out with supersensitivity psychosis in mind.

The largest relevant body of data was reported by Prien et al. (1971), combining data from two large double-blind multihospital studies of drug therapy in chronic schizophrenic patients. The placebo groups totaled 301 patients, who were placed on a placebo for 24 weeks. The relapse rates were 37% of the 199 patients in the first study and 50% of the 102 patients in the second study.

Relevant to the Chouinard concept of supersensitivity psychosis, only 12% of relapsing patients did so in the first 5 weeks, whereas 73% relapsed between weeks 6 and 16. The type of relapse was, in fact, mainly in the form of positive symptoms, as described. Patients on moderate to high preplacebo neuroleptic dosages (more than 300 mg in chlorpromazine equivalents) were substantially more likely to relapse. In a report on the second study (Prien et al. 1969), relapses were analyzed separately for patients initially on high-potency or low-potency neuroleptics; no differences were found.

If one looks at older relevant studies in which a placebo was substituted for an antipsychotic, one finds that all of the studies involved only chronically hospitalized patients. Several give inadequate information on which to even consider any of the characteristics of supersensitivity psychosis. Two small studies of patients previously on perphenazine (Whitaker 1963) or trifluoperazine (Hershon et al. 1972) found frequent relapses in the first 6 weeks off medication; three studies, two of chlorpromazine withdrawal (Andrews et al. 1976; Freeman 1962), found less in the way of early relapse, with most relapses occurring presumably later than 6 weeks. One study (Diamond and Marks 1960) included equal numbers of patients initially on trifluoperazine and on chlorpromazine but reported no differential relapse rate; 8 of the 11 relapses occurred in the second 3 months of the 6-month placebo period.

These studies do not comment on the rapidity with which clinical improvement occurs when drug therapy is resumed; nor is initial neuroleptic dose described. Two studies describe higher relapse rates in patients taken off all medication than in those receiving a placebo (Olson 1962; Whitaker 1963).

## Discussion

There is currently no foolproof way of proving that supersensitivity psychosis or tardive dysmentia does or does not exist. Clearly, some psychotic patients relapse rapidly and floridly when neuroleptic drugs are tapered or discontinued, and some chronic psychotic patients may show different behavior patterns over the years. Fortunately or unfortunately, the patterns of care for chronic psychosis have changed radically during the last 20 years; many more patients are maintained in the community, and many more patients are treated with high-potency antipsychotics, which permit very high dosages to be administered with little increase in serious side effects. No large and systematic body of data is available with which to assess the likelihood that patients similar to those described by Chouinard (1982), Chouinard and Jones (1980), Chouinard et al. (1978, 1982, 1986), and Wilson et al. (1983) could have been readily found before neuroleptics were used or when low-potency neuroleptics were mainly employed.

It is even difficult to conceive of an anterospective study that could settle either question at all definitively. If supersensitivity psychosis is really a transient rebound phenomenon and not a permanent condition, then maintaining a series of patients who appear to manifest supersensitivity psychosis off oral neuroleptics for, perhaps, 16 weeks would tell whether any substantial proportion does better off neuroleptics in the long run. Even the occurrence of remissions in, say, half the patients, however, might only demonstrate the variability in the course of untreated psychosis.

The fact that these phenomena have been principally or only described by a few investigators during the past several years leads to the weak conclusion that the syndromes are either relatively rare or hard to identify amid the general clinical vagaries of the course of treated psychosis.

# References

Andrews P, Hall J, Snaith R: A controlled trial of phenothiazine withdrawal in chronic schizophrenic patients. Br J Psychiatry 128:451–455, 1976

Borison RL, Diamond BI, Sinha D, et al: Clozapine withdrawal rebound psychosis. Psychopharmacol Bull 24:260–263, 1988

Caine E, Margolin D, Brown G, et al: Gilles de la Tourette's syndrome, tardive dyskinesia and psychosis in an adolescent. Am J Psychiatry 135:241–243, 1978

Chiarello RJ, Cole JO: The use of psychostimulants in general psychiatry. Arch Gen Psychiatry 44:286–295, 1987

Chouinard G: Neuroleptic-induced supersensitivity psychosis, in Tardive Dyskinesia. Edited by DeVeaugh-Geiss J. Boston, MA, John Wright PSG, 1982, pp 109–115

Chouinard G, Jones B: Neuroleptic-induced supersensitivity psychosis: clinical and pharmacologic characteristics. Am J Psychiatry 137:16–21, 1980

Chouinard G, Jones B, Annable L: Neuroleptic induced supersensitivity psychosis. Am J Psychiatry 135:1409–1410, 1978

Chouinard G, Creese I, Boisvert D, et al: High neuroleptic plasma levels in patients manifesting supersensitivity psychoses. Biol Psychiatry 17:707–711, 1982

Chouinard G, Annable L, Ross-Chouinard A: Supersensitivity psychosis and tardive dyskinesia: a survey of schizophrenic outpatients. Psychopharmacol Bull 22:891–896, 1986

Cole J, Gardos G, Gelernter J, et al: Supersensitivity psychosis. McLean Hosp J 9:46–72, 1984

Csernansky J, Hollister L: Probable case of supersensitivity psychosis. Hosp Formulary 17:395–399, 1982

Davis K, Rosenberg G: Is there a limbic equivalent of tardive dyskinesia? Biol Psychiatry 14:699–703, 1979

Diamond B, Borison R: Basic and clinical studies of neuroleptic-induced supersensitivity psychosis and dyskinesia. Psychopharmacol Bull 22:900–905, 1986

Diamond LS, Marks JB: Discontinuance of tranquilizers among chronic schizophrenic patients receiving maintenance dosage. J Nerv Ment Dis 131:247–251, 1960

Ekblom B, Eriksson K, Lindstrom L: Supersensitivity psychosis in schizophrenic patients after sudden clozapine withdrawal. Psychopharmacology 83:293–294, 1984

Freeman LS, Alson E: Prolonged withdrawal of chlorpromazine in chronic patients. Diseases of the Nervous System 23:522–525, 1962

Goldberg E: Akinesia, tardive dysmentia and frontal lobe disorder in schizophrenia. Schizophr Bull 11:255–263, 1985

Gualtieri C, Quade D, Hicks R, et al: Tardive dyskinesia and other clinical consequences of neuroleptic treatment in children and adolescents. Am J Psychiatry 141:20–23, 1984

Hartvig P, Eckernas SA, Lindstrom L, et al: Receptor binding of N-(methyl-[11]C) clozapine in the brain of rhesus monkey studied by positron emission tomography (PET). Psychopharmacology 89:248–252, 1986

Hershon HL, Kennedy PF, McGuire RJ: Persistence of extrapyramidal disorders and psychiatric relapse after withdrawal of long-term phenothiazine therapy. Br J Psychiatry 120:41–50, 1972

Kent T, Wilber R: Reserpine withdrawal psychosis. J Nerv Ment Dis 170:502–504, 1982

Mukherjee S: Tardive dysmentia: a reappraisal. Schizophr Bull 10:151–152, 1984

Olson G, Peterson D: Intermittent chemotherapy for chronic psychiatric inpatients. J Nerv Ment Dis 134:145–149, 1962

Perenyi A, Kuncz E, Bagdy G: Early relapse after sudden withdrawal or dose reduction of clozapine. Psychopharmacology 86:244, 1985

Prien R, Levine J, Cole J: High dose trifluoperazine therapy in chronic schizophrenia. Am J Psychiatry 126:305–313, 1969

Prien R, Levine J, Switalski R: Discontinuation of chemotherapy for chronic schizophrenics. Hosp Community Psychiatry 22:20–23, 1971

Sale I, Kristall H: Schizophrenia following withdrawal from chronic phenothiazine administration: a case report. Aust N Z J Psychiatry 12:73–75,1978

Schooler N, Severe J, Levine J, et al: Der abruck der neuroleptischen behandlung bei schizophrenen patienten and dessen einfluss auf ruckfalle and auf symptome der spatdyskinesi, in Ergebnisse der Psychiatrischen Therapieforschung. Edited by Kryspin-Exner K, Hinterhuber H, Schubert H. Stuttgart, Germany, F K Schattauer Verlag, 1982

Weinberger D, Bigelow L, Klein S, et al: Drug withdrawal in chronic schizophrenic patients: in search of neuroleptic-induced supersensitivity psychosis. J Clin Psychopharmacol 1:120–123, 1981

Whitaker CB, Hoy RM: Withdrawal of perphenazine in chronic schizophrenia. Br J Psychiatry 109:422–427, 1963

Wilson I, Garbutt J, Lanier C, et al: Is there a tardive dysmentia? Schizophr Bull 9:187–192, 1983

Witschy J, Malone G, Holden L: Neuroleptic withdrawal psychosis in a manic depressive patient. Am J Psychiatry 141:105–106, 1984

Chapter 10

# Clinical-Legal Issues

Litigation is a pervasive concern in contemporary American society, both inside and outside medicine. Because of this concern, the task force's discussion of clinical-legal issues in the use of antipsychotic medication is addressed more extensively than in the first Tardive Dyskinesia Task Force report (1979). In this section we address general issues of liability for the prescribing psychiatrist and treatment team, with a particular emphasis on informed consent to antipsychotic medication. We do not discuss other medical-legal issues, such as the drug manufacturer's liability, or deal with problems related to the development and approval of psychotropic medications. This discussion is not meant to provide legal advice or to recommend how to tailor clinical practices to existing legal requirements. The legal standards vary from state to state and continue to evolve. Thus practitioners who are concerned about these legal issues can seek consultation with lawyers who are knowledgeable about the area.

## Psychopharmacology Litigation

The prescription of psychoactive medication exposes the psychiatrist to significant professional liability claims (Brackins 1985; Dukes and Swartz 1988; Wettstein 1985). Indeed, improper medication was the most common allegation against psychiatrists insured with the American Psychiatric Association professional liability insurance program from 1973 to 1984 (Slawson 1989). The psychiatrist's prescription liability pertains largely to two areas, *negligence* and *informed consent.*

A negligence (or "tort") action against a psychiatrist is successful when the plaintiff proves by a preponderance of the evidence (the plaintiff's case is more convincing than that of the defendant) that: 1) the psychiatrist had a legal duty to care for the patient in a way that meets the prevailing standard of care, 2) the psychiatrist violated that duty either through an omission or commission in the care of the patient, and 3) the patient suffered a physical or emotional injury as a result of the psychiatrist's violation of the standard of care.

Prescribing psychiatrists risk negligence liability in a variety of areas when they prescribe psychoactive medication. These include the following (Wettstein 1983, 1988):

1. Failure to take an adequate history.
2. Failure to obtain an adequate physical examination.
3. Failure to obtain an adequate laboratory examination.
4. Lack of indication for a prescription.
5. Contraindication for a prescription.
6. Prescription of an improper dosage.
7. Prescription for an improper duration.
8. Failure to recognize, monitor, and treat medication side effects.
9. Failure to abate drug reactions and interactions.
10. Failure to consult with other physicians.

### Tardive Dyskinesia Case Examples: Negligence

An indeterminate amount of litigation regarding tardive dyskinesia has occurred in the United States since tardive dyskinesia became recognized as an iatrogenic disorder. Suits have been brought against nonpsychiatric physicians, psychiatrists, hospitals, and manufacturers. In the absence of any national centralized reporting system for tort cases, it is not possible to ascertain the true number of cases, their allegations, or their outcomes. Few such legal cases are published in the legal literature, which largely contains those that have been tried and then appealed by the losing party. Those that are settled out of court are usually sealed from disclosure by the settlement agreement. Information about some cases can also be obtained from the litigants, the attorneys, or expert witnesses in the cases. The following cases are, therefore, intended only to illustrate some of the potential negligence litigation for tardive dyskinesia.

In *Collins v. Cushner* (1980), a 56-year-old housewife consulted a family practitioner for treatment of anxiety. The physician diagnosed "spastic colon" and prescribed low doses of trifluoperazine for 6 years between 1969 and 1975. For a 29-month period, the patient was not seen by the defendant physician but received renewals of her prescription by telephone. The patient developed abnormal movements in her arms and hands and the defendant discontinued the medication for 2 months but then reinstituted it within a month and doubled the dose. Six months later, the physician prescribed benztropine to treat the patient's involuntary movements of the face. In the lawsuit, the plaintiff charged that the defendant continued to prescribe antipsychotic medication despite product information warnings regarding its use in the treatment of anxiety as well as warnings about tardive dyskinesia in long-term treatment of females in the patient's age bracket. She further alleged that treatment with benztropine had aggravated rather than relieved her condition. The litigation was settled for $125,000.

In *Clites v. Iowa* (1980), the parents of a mentally retarded male at a state residential facility sued the state for negligence and for treating without obtaining adequate informed consent (see below). The patient had been treated with a variety of antipsychotic medications since age 18 for "aggressive behavior" under the auspices of several physicians. Medication continued for 5 years before tardive dyskinesia of the face and extremities was diagnosed.

The trial court determined that medication had been inappropriately used for the staff's convenience and not for the patient's treatment and that evidence of the severe aggression and self-destructiveness required to justify such use of antipsychotic medication was lacking. The court also ruled that the patient was improperly monitored because he was not "regularly visited" by a physician and physical examinations had not been conducted for a 3-year period; the staff, without justification, "ignored the known risks of uninterrupted use of major tranquilizers"; the medical staff failed to react to the patient's symptoms of tardive dyskinesia and alter the drug-treatment program accordingly; and the attending physician, being unfamiliar with tardive dyskinesia, failed to obtain consultation. The court further stated that polypharmacy was not warranted by the patient's status and the particular drugs involved. The trial court ruled for the plaintiff and awarded $385,165 for future medical expenses and $375,000 for past and future pain and suffering. The district court's ruling was subsequently upheld in the Iowa Court of Appeals (1982).

In *Hedin v. U.S.* (1985), after a 2-month psychiatric hospitalization for treatment of alcohol abuse, the plaintiff was treated with thioridazine and then chlorpromazine as an outpatient. He continued to take 600 mg of chlorpromazine daily for nearly 4 years before his physicians noted his movement disorder and discontinued the medication. The patient had been aware of the movements, which involved the face, mouth, trunk, and extremities, but testified that he was unaware that they were due to the medication. The defendant (the U.S. Veterans Administration) admitted that it had been negligent in prescribing excessive amounts of medication for a prolonged period of time without proper supervision. Damages of nearly $2.2 million were awarded to the plaintiff, who had become functionally disabled because of the tardive dyskinesia.

These and other legal cases illustrate patient-plaintiff allegations of psychiatrists' failures to properly prescribe and monitor treatment with antipsychotic medication and then make a timely diagnosis of tardive dyskinesia (Mills et al. 1986; Wettstein 1985). In addition, claims may also allege that tardive dyskinesia, as a medical disorder in itself, has not properly been treated.

# Informed Consent

Since the early 1900s, physicians in the United States have been required to obtain the consent of their patient before proceeding with a proposed procedure or treatment. Only in the last 30 years, however, have physicians also been legally required to provide information to the patient about the proposed intervention prior to proceeding (Tietz 1986). These dual elements, consent and information disclosure, serve to promote the patient's self-determination and autonomy in health care decision making (Faden and Beauchamp 1986). In fact, the legal doctrine of informed consent to health care has been adopted to various degrees by many English-speaking countries throughout the world. From a clinical perspective, adequate informed consent, which includes patient participation in medical decision making, can help to maximize the patient's compliance with treatment and improve the psychiatrist-patient alliance.

## Elements of Informed Consent

Informed consent to medical care consists of three elements: information, competency, and voluntariness of decision making. It is information disclosure with which we are primarily concerned in the present context.

According to the legal doctrine of informed consent, certain information must be provided to the patient before a valid informed consent to medical care can be said to exist. This applies both to diagnostic evaluation procedures as well as treatment. This information includes the following (Rozovsky 1990):

1. The nature or diagnosis of the patient's condition.
2. The nature of the proposed intervention.
3. The purpose of the proposed intervention.
4. The benefits of the proposed intervention.
5. The risks of the proposed intervention, including incidence, severity, and significance.
6. The possible alternatives to the proposed intervention, including no treatment.
7. The benefits of the alternative interventions.
8. The risks of the alternative interventions, including incidence, severity, and significance.

The extent of the information to be disclosed is ordinarily governed by state law, whether statute or case law. One of two general standards of information disclosure applies, the physician standard and the patient standard. Under the physician standard, the extent of disclosure is dictated by what physicians in the community disclose to their patients about a particular intervention. Under the patient standard, the extent of disclosure is dictated by what information a hypothetical patient, or even the particular patient in question, would need to make the health care decision. It is generally assumed that information disclosure in a patient-standard jurisdiction should exceed that in a physician-standard jurisdiction, since many patients desire more information than physicians think it is necessary to provide to them, but this is not invariably the case (Faden et al. 1981; Strull et al. 1984). Generally, information about the risks of treatment warrant disclosure when the risks are frequent, significant, or severe (e.g., death).

In a legal action based on informed consent, the plaintiff must prove that the psychiatrist failed to disclose some information that should have been disclosed according to the prevailing standard. He must also prove that had he, or any hypothetical reasonable person, been properly informed, he would have refused that particular procedure or treatment. Finally, he must prove that his injury resulted from the procedure or treatment that was administered, not that the procedure or treatment was itself negligently administered.

### Exceptions to Informed Consent

Although different states have different rules, as a general matter there are four exceptions to the consent and disclosure requirements of informed consent: 1) emergency, 2) waiver, 3) therapeutic privilege, and 4) incompetence.

In a psychiatric *emergency*, when treatment is immediately necessary and the need for consent or information disclosure would be impractical or cause such a delay that the patient or others would be harmed, consent need not be obtained from the patient and information need not be disclosed to the patient.

The patient may *waive* his or her right to decide about the proposed intervention and ask that the physician or others decide for him or her. In addition, the patient may waive his or her right to information disclosure and inform the psychiatrist that he or she does not wish to be told some information.

Information need not be disclosed to a patient about a proposed intervention when that information is likely to be substantially detrimental to the patient's condition. This is referred to as the *therapeutic privilege* and includes situations in which the patient's disorder is likely to worsen following information disclosure. The psychiatrist is not, however, justified in withholding information because the patient is likely to refuse the proposed treatment.

Informed consent to health care need not be obtained from a person who is legally *incompetent* either because of status (young age) or because he or she has been given a guardian (e.g., because of developmental disability or dementia). Informed consent in such cases must be obtained from a legally authorized person, such as a parent or personal guardian. In the case of a patient who is legally competent but appears decisionally incapacitated (e.g., catatonic, psychotic denial of illness, delusional misperception about the proposed intervention, indecisive due to anxiety or paranoia, or inattentive due to thought disorder), applicable law may require that a substitute decision maker be designated or appointed by a court prior to deciding to initiate treatment.

### Empirical Studies of Informed Consent

There is a relatively small body of clinical research regarding informed consent to psychopharmacological treatment in the chronically mentally ill. These studies generally reveal that, in many cases, psychiatrists often do not inform their patients and, to a lesser extent, their patients' families of their diagnoses; patients do not know the nature or diagnosis of their condition; and patients do not know the names, purposes, or side effects of medication except for the particular side effects that they have personally experienced (Beck 1988; Benson 1984; Berg and Hammitt 1980; Geller 1982; Green and Gantt 1987; Grossman and Summers 1980; Jaffee 1981, 1986; Lidz et al. 1984). When clinician-researchers have attempted to educate their mentally ill patients about side effects to treatment (e.g., tardive dyskinesia), these efforts, whether short-term or long-term, have been only partially successful (Ganguli and Raghu 1985; Irwin et al. 1985; Kleinman et al. 1989; Munetz and Roth 1985). Research has also indicated that physicians are especially poor at disclosing treatment alternatives and the benefit-risk profiles of the alternatives (Lidz et al. 1984). Informed consent to treatment practices appears to be particularly deficient in the nursing-home setting with geriatric patients (Gurian et al. 1990).

### Application of Informed Consent to Tardive Dyskinesia

Given the incidence, prevalence, and potential irreversibility of tardive dyskinesia in patients treated with prolonged antipsychotic medication, it is a sufficiently significant or material risk of prolonged treatment to merit disclosure to the patient or legal guardian under either the professional medical standard or the patient-centered standard of disclosure. Tardive dyskinesia is neither too infrequent nor too insignificant a risk of treatment to avoid disclosure. Disclosure about the risk of tardive dyskinesia should occur as soon as clinically feasible. In addition, since tardive dyskinesia may be a risk when medication in a previously treated patient is resumed, redisclosure may be necessary in this case prior to resumption. Disclosure about tardive dyskinesia is especially important if the patient already has tardive dyskinesia and the psychiatrist is considering resuming medication. With the prolonged course of treatment typical of the use of antipsychotic medication, it is unlikely that the psychiatrist could successfully assert the therapeutic-privilege exception to informed consent and claim that informing the patient about tardive dyskinesia would worsen the patient's condition, although this is possibly justifiable with short-term treatment of a disorganized patient.

Should the psychiatrist suspect or diagnose tardive dyskinesia in a patient under consultation or treatment, then the patient should be informed of the diagnosis. As tardive dyskinesia is a disorder in itself, the psychiatrist must then discuss the available evaluation and treatment alternatives, and their risks and benefits, with the patient. Referral to a specialist in tardive dyskinesia may also be necessary for consultation or continued care.

### Clinical Concerns With Regard to Informed Consent

There appear to be several barriers to obtaining meaningful informed consent to antipsychotic medication from psychiatric patients, particularly with regard to tardive dyskinesia. These originate in the psychiatrist, clinic or hospital, mental health system, and patient (Lidz et al. 1983).

Psychiatrists fear noncompliance and decompensation should patients be told about tardive dyskinesia (Munetz 1985). Psychiatrists also fear that such information will encourage litigation. There are few data regarding these concerns, and physicians must apply and document their clinical judgments in this context (Munetz and Roth 1985).

Clinics and hospitals also fear patient noncompliance, decompensation, and litigation if patients are told about tardive dyskinesia. Staff members are also concerned about the need for a secure environment, which could be jeopardized if patients refuse medication. Again, there are no data to support or refute the claim that informing patients about tardive dyskinesia will lead to wide-scale treatment refusal. Clearly, the nature of the information presented with regard to the benefits of neuroleptic treatment and the risk of tardive dyskinesia is likely to influence patient compliance.

Finally, some patients are limited in their ability to comprehend and use information that is provided to them because of cognitive dysfunction, denial of illness or tardive dyskinesia (Caracci et al. 1990), and externalization of decision-making responsibility.

### Obtaining Informed Consent to Antipsychotic Medication

Informed consent to psychiatric treatment is properly conceptualized as a process that occurs over a period of time rather than an event at a single time point (Appelbaum et al. 1987; Lidz et al. 1988). This is an especially useful notion for mental health professionals who treat the chronically ill population for extended periods of time, in contrast to much of the acute-care, hospital-based medical practice, where the legal doctrine of informed consent originated.

Psychiatrists and the mental health treatment team have many means and opportunities to provide information about antipsychotic medication and tardive dyskinesia to their patients. Some recommended procedures include the following:

1.  Information about medication and tardive dyskinesia should be periodically reviewed and discussed with the patient throughout the course of treatment, rather than on a single occasion. This allows the patient many opportunities and additional time to absorb the relevant information. When more than one psychiatrist is involved in the patient's care, whether simultaneously or consecutively, each has an obligation to obtain a valid informed consent to treatment.

2.  The psychiatrist should not simply recite the benefits and risks of treatment but should encourage patient participation in decision making. This means attempting to stimulate a discussion with the patient rather than providing a lecture. The psychiatrist should encourage the patient to express his or her thoughts and decisions about the treatment alternatives. The psychiatrist can assist the patient in weighing and assessing this information, help the patient to clarify his or her values and expectations, and put the treatment risks into perspective for the patient. The psychiatrist can also share his or her own views about the relevant issues with the patient.

3.  Patients should be encouraged to ask questions about their treatment, and the psychiatrist should allow adequate time to respond to these questions.

4.  Patients should be encouraged to monitor themselves for side effects, including tardive dyskinesia, and report changes in symptoms and side effects to the treatment team.

5.  The presentation and format of information about medication and tardive dyskinesia should be individualized according to the patient's needs, interests, and cognitive abilities. This also permits the psychiatrist to discover erroneous or unrealistic ideas that the patient may have about his or her illness and its treatment and to correct any misunderstandings.

6.  As a matter of sound clinical practice, medication counseling can be provided by pharmacists and nurses as well as the psychiatrist. This can be conducted on an individual or a group basis, whether in the hospital or the community (Eng and Emlet 1990). Such counseling can be incorporated into existing social-skills-management training programs (Eckman et al. 1990).

7. Written medication information can be made available. This includes information sheets, brochures, and pamphlets, whether privately drafted or commercially produced. These can be separate documents or portions of a hospital or clinic newsletter.
8. Information about antipsychotic medication and its side effects can be audiotaped or videotaped, and the tapes can be made available to patients and interested others.
9. Pharmacists can provide a warning label about involuntary movements on prescription bottles upon the psychiatrist's instruction or independently by the pharmacist. This can include a patient instruction to report tardive dyskinesia to the psychiatrist (Brown et al. 1988).
10. Psychiatrists and mental health treatment facilities should have policies and procedures regarding the use of antipsychotic medication, informed consent to antipsychotic medication, and the detection and monitoring of patients for tardive dyskinesia. Consent policies and procedures should be consistent with applicable legal requirements. The use of a facility or individual protocol, in conjunction with training to implement the protocol, will help to ensure that these areas are properly addressed in clinical practice (Dixon et al. 1989; Guidry et al. 1988; Kalachnik 1985; Kalachnik and Slaw 1986).
11. Each facility should implement a quality-assurance program to monitor the use of antipsychotic medication, the occurrence of adverse medication effects, and the compliance with relevant policies and procedures.

### Decision-making Incapacity

When treating a patient who is legally incompetent whether by age or guardianship, the psychiatrist must obtain the informed consent of the legal guardian. In this case, there should be little hesitation to provide complete information to the guardian, given that there is less likely to be decision-making incapacity in the guardian than in the patient. Nevertheless, legal guardians often have difficulty making decisions for their wards and are instructed to use a "best medical interests" approach or a "substituted judgment" approach, depending on the jurisdiction and guardianship order. The psychiatrist may be helpful to the guardian by sharing his or her knowledge of the patient's history and values with the guardian. Even though the patient has been adjudicated legally incompetent, the psychiatrist should attempt to inform the patient about the treatment and facilitate the patient's cooperation with it.

When a legally competent patient appears to have significant decision-making incapacity regarding treatment (e.g., catatonic, psychotic denial of illness, delusional misperception about the proposed intervention, indecisive due to anxiety or paranoia, or inattentive due to thought disorder), some states require that a substitute decision maker be designated. This may require a court order for guardianship. By contrast, in other states it is common practice in this situation for the psychiatrist to meet with family members or significant others to review the proposed treatment and its risks and benefits. Treatment decisions are then made with the joint participation of patient and family.

Even if the patient is able to make his or her own treatment decisions, it may be useful to involve family members in discussions and decision making regarding antipsychotic medication and tardive dyskinesia, although actual decisions will be left to the patient. Family members may be able to provide additional information to the treatment team about the patient's functioning and behavior. Family members may also be helpful to the patient in decision making, since they may be better able to judge the patient's need for medication and may be more capable of weighing the benefits and risks of treatment than the patient.

### Tardive Dyskinesia Case Examples: Informed Consent

A plaintiff may allege that not only was the psychiatrist negligent in the diagnosis of the patient's condition and in the prescription of medication, but informed consent to treatment was not properly obtained. Thus, in *Clites v. Iowa* (1980, 1982), discussed before with regard to negligence, the trial court also ruled that the patient's parents, his legal guardians, "were never informed of the potential side effects of the use, and prolonged use, of major tranquilizers, nor was consent to their use obtained," thus violating the "standard that requires some form of informed consent prior to the administration of major tranquilizers." Since the parents had not been informed of the risks attendant to the treatment program, the trial court rejected the defendant's argument that the parents had implicitly consented to the treatment.

In *Barclay v. Campbell* (1984), the defendant psychiatrist admitted that he had failed to disclose the risk of tardive dyskinesia to a young male schizophrenic patient. At the trial, the court directed a verdict for the psychiatrist, which was upheld on appeal, on the basis that the psychiatrist was justified in not disclosing this risk because it was not "medically feasible" to do so and that the patient was not a "reasonable person." This was reversed on appeal to the Texas Supreme Court (1986) on the grounds that the psychiatrist could not use the therapeutic-privilege exception to the informed-consent disclosure requirement. The court also ruled that the smallness of the risk of tardive dyskinesia due to the patient's young age did not negate the psychiatrist's duty to disclose tardive dyskinesia. At the trial, the jury found that the defendant had not informed the plaintiff of the risk of tardive dyskinesia but that he would have consented to the treatment anyway. The case was subsequently settled out of court.

# Tardive Dyskinesia Monitoring

Screening for tardive dyskinesia should occur before starting treatment with antipsychotic medication. Screening should also occur before restarting treatment, after a medication-free period. After treatment has begun, the patient must be monitored for the development of tardive dyskinesia, paying particular attention to any manifestations that could be disabling to the patient (e.g., gait, blepharospasm, dystonia, or respiratory). Assessment for tardive dyskinesia should occur for a period of time after medication has been discontinued, whatever the reason for its withdrawal.

The frequency of tardive dyskinesia monitoring will vary with the nature of the patient population, the extent of use and dose of medication, and the base rate of tardive dyskinesia. No single monitoring procedure or frequency will be appropriate for all patients treated with antipsychotic medication in a wide variety of clinical settings. A monitoring procedure will be judged as having met the legal standard of care according to the appropriateness of the clinical monitoring of the particular patient under the circumstances. This is likely to be judged according to a national standard, rather than a local one. Of course, patients with severe and disabling tardive dyskinesia will require more frequent evaluation than those who have never had involuntary movements. But even this latter patient group must be seen on a routine basis to detect tardive dyskinesia symptoms.

Various rating scales and instruments are available to the psychiatrist to help identify, assess, measure, and monitor the presence of involuntary movements, including tardive dyskinesia (see Chapter 3 and Appendix). Clinical personnel should be trained in their proper use (Kalachnik 1985; Kalachnik et al. 1988). The use of a structured examination will minimize the psychiatrist's opportunity to overlook abnormal movements and ensure a reliable examination over time.

Although the prescribing psychiatrist is responsible for evaluating and monitoring the patient's involuntary movements, many mental health clinics delegate this responsibility to nonphysicians on the treatment team, such as nurses, social workers, and pharmacists (Munetz and Benjamin 1990). Trainees, such as residents and students, also become involved in this task. Regardless of who actually performs the monitoring procedures, the prescribing psychiatrist will be held responsible for ensuring the adequacy of the monitoring, as well as for being aware of the results.

# Documentation

Documentation is an important and underappreciated component of health care service. Record keeping is as much a part of providing health care as the underlying care activity itself. Medical records are legal as well as clinical documents. They provide the only contemporaneous and objective account of the patient's condition, the services offered and administered, and the patient's response to treatment. Litigation typically occurs many months to years after the treatment has been rendered; the lapse in time distorts the memories of patient, family, and treatment staff. Few psychiatrists will recall the details of clinical events, especially psychiatrist-patient conversations that occurred long ago.

The psychiatrist need not document every event that occurred during the course of treatment—only the most significant ones. Documentation need not be lengthy—only concise; the psychiatrist should document the treatment events with an awareness that others may later review the record in the course of litigation. Courts and juries will frequently operate under the assumption that if something is not appropriately recorded, then it did not in fact occur, even though the psychiatrist may state otherwise at the time of deposition or trial.

A medical record documenting informed consent should include each of the aforementioned elements. At least in outline form, the psychiatrist should indicate how and what he or she told the patient about his or her condition and its treatment; what the patient said and understood about it, including any questions that the patient may have asked; and how they came to a decision about the course of treatment. When possible, the record should quote the patient's exact words. When the patient has questionable capacity to consent to treatment, then data about the patient's decision-making capacities and incapacities should also be included.

The following is a sample progress note for a schizophrenic outpatient on long-term antipsychotic medication who has tardive dyskinesia:

> Mr. Jones was seen for his quarterly medication appointment today for 30 minutes. Individual therapy notes were also reviewed. He reports that he is living in a halfway house, rarely drinks alcohol, is no longer using marijuana, and is compliant with his haloperidol 8 mg/day (the staff allows him to manage it himself). He continues to have distracting auditory hallucinations, which keep him awake at night.

> Exam: Alert, oriented ×3, guarded, blunted affect, marginal grooming, without evident thought disorder or delusions. Good attention, concentration. There is mild depressed mood, no vegetative signs, and no suicide ideation, intention, or lifetime attempts.

> Side effects: Patient denies weight gain, constipation, blurred vision, or restlessness. No tremor, akinesia, dystonia on exam. AIMS (Abnormal Involuntary Movement Scale) testing today showed "moderate" on lips, tongue, and face for spontaneous movements (AIMS rating form in chart). No involvement of eyes, extremities, neck, trunk, respiratory, or gastrointestinal by history or exam.

I again discussed the movements with the patient, who is aware of them but not distressed by them. He is aware that they are caused by his antipsychotic medications, have been present for the last 1.5 years, and have not worsened in severity or distribution. We also discussed reducing his dosage or switching to a prn dosing strategy, since he is fairly stable and there is a risk of tardive dyskinesia progression or irreversibility, but he is afraid to risk an exacerbation at this time.

Plan: Continue the haloperidol 8 mg/day, see the patient q 3 months, monitor his psychotic symptoms and his tardive dyskinesia, see if we can reduce his dosage, and continue to discuss it with him. Patient has already attended several medication groups and understands his disorder and treatment, so there is no need to refer him back for more group work. He will continue to see his individual therapist. The patient was given copies of our two information sheets on antipsychotic medication and tardive dyskinesia.

### Consent Forms

Written consent forms for antipsychotic medication have been used as an alternative or addition to the progress note in the patient's medical record. Consent forms may be short documents that do not themselves detail any information about the proposed treatment or its benefits and risks but simply state that such information has been provided to the patient. Longer consent forms actually provide information about the proposed treatment (Rozovsky 1990). Although written consent forms, when signed by the patient, may provide some evidence that consent to treatment was obtained and information was provided, their value in this regard is limited and they present additional risks. A patient who signs a form may later allege that he or she did not understand what he or she was signing, that he or she did not understand the information that was disclosed, that there was no opportunity for discussion with the psychiatrist, and that he or she only signed the form because he or she was told to do so.

Further, there is a risk that consent forms introduce a detrimental adversarial element to the psychiatrist-patient relationship, since patients view consent forms as defensive measures for the psychiatrist rather than as a benefit to themselves. As has been the result in much of medicine, there is a danger that written consent forms substitute for the psychiatrist-patient discussion about treatment, rather than serve as only the documentation of that discussion. Medical consent forms have too often been written at the graduate-student level (Grundner 1980; Morrow 1980), and more effort should be made to assure they are written in such a manner as to be easily understood.

Written consent forms for nonexperimental medications are not generally used in medical practice, especially in the chronic-care setting. Given the perceived clinical risks of their use and their uncertain benefits, written consent forms for antipsychotic medication are not recommended by the task force. They may, however, serve some legal purposes and, indeed, may be required by hospital policy or state law. Thus a psychiatrist should determine the status of these matters before making an individual decision. In any event, when such forms are used, clinicians should be careful to avoid allowing them to substitute for talking with the patient and family about medication and tardive dyskinesia, both before and after the consent form has been signed. Having the patient sign the written consent form does not end the psychiatrist's ethical or legal obligation to obtain and renew a valid consent to treatment. Consent forms will also be required in psychopharmacological research protocols.

# References

Appelbaum PS, Lidz CW, Meisel A: Informed Consent: Legal Theory and Clinical Practice. New York, Oxford University Press, 1987

Barclay v Campbell, 683 SW2d 498 (Tex 1984); 704 SW2d 8 (Tex 1986)

Beck JC: Determining competency to assent to neuroleptic drug treatment. Hosp Community Psychiatry 39:1106–1108, 1988

Benson PR: Informed consent: drug information disclosed to patients prescribed antipsychotic medication. J Nerv Ment Dis 172:642–653, 1984

Berg A, Hammitt KB: Assessing the psychiatric patient's ability to meet the literacy demands of hospitalization. Hosp Community Psychiatry 31:266–268, 1980

Brackins LW: The liability of physicians, pharmacists, and hospitals for adverse drug reactions. Defense Law Journal 34:273–344, 1985

Brown CS, Solovitz BL, Bryant SG, et al: Short- and long-term effects of auxiliary labels on patient knowledge of precautionary drug information. Drug Intelligence and Clinical Pharmacy 22:470–474, 1988

Caracci G, Mukherjee S, Roth SD, et al: Subjective awareness of abnormal involuntary movements in chronic schizophrenic patients. Am J Psychiatry 147:295–298, 1990

Clites v Iowa, Law #46274, Iowa District Court, Pottawattamie County, August 7, 1980; Clites v Iowa 322 N.W.2d 917 (Iowa 1982)

Collins v Cushner, Montgomery County, Maryland, Circuit Court, Number 48751, October 20, 1980

Dixon L, Weiden PJ, Frances AJ, et al: Management of neuroleptic-induced movement disorders: effects of physician training. Am J Psychiatry 146:104–106, 1989

Dukes MNG, Swartz B: Responsibility for Drug-Induced Injury. Amsterdam, Elsevier, 1988

Eckman TA, Liberman RP, Phipps CC, et al: Teaching medication management skills to schizophrenic patients. J Clin Psychopharmacol 10:33–38, 1990

Eng K, Emlet CA: SRx: a regional approach to geriatric medication education. Gerontologist 30:408–410, 1990

Faden RF, Beauchamp TL: A History and Theory of Informed Consent. New York, Oxford University Press, 1986

Faden RF, Lewis C, Becker C, et al: Disclosure standards and informed consent. J Health Politics, Policy and Law 6:255–284, 1981

Ganguli R, Raghu U: Tardive dyskinesia, impaired recall, and informed consent. J Clin Psychiatry 46:434–435, 1985

Geller JL: State hospital patients and their medication: do they know what they take. Am J Psychiatry 139:611–615, 1982

Green RS, Gantt AB: Telling patients and families the psychiatric diagnosis: a survey of psychiatrists. Hosp Community Psychiatry 38:666–668, 1987

Grossman L, Summers F: A study of the capacity of schizophrenic patients to give informed consent. Hosp Community Psychiatry 31:205–206, 1980

Grundner TM: On the readability of surgical consent forms. N Engl J Med 302:900–902, 1980

Guidry J, Rinck W, Rinck C: Persons with developmental disabilities and tardive dyskinesia: a historical perspective and an examination of state policies responding to litigation questions. J Psychiatry Law 16:625–659, 1988

Gurian BS, Baker EH, Jacobson S, et al: Informed consent for neuroleptics with elderly patients in two settings. J Am Geriatr Soc 38:37–44, 1990

Hedin v US, No. 5-83 CIV 3 (D. Minn. 1985)

Irwin M, Lovitz A, Marder SR, et al: Psychotic patients' understanding of informed consent. Am J Psychiatry 142:1351–1354, 1985

Jaffee R: Informed consent: recall about tardive dyskinesia. Compr Psychiatry 22:434–437, 1981

Jaffee R: Problems of long-term informed consent. Bulletin American Academy Psychiatry Law 14:163–169, 1986

Kalachnik JE: An applied tardive dyskinesia monitoring system (ATDMS). Psychopharmacol Bull 21:327–328, 1985

Kalachnik JE, Slaw KM: Tardive dyskinesia: update for the mental health administrator. J Mental Health Administration 13:1–8, 1986

Kalachnik JE, Sprague RL, Slaw KM: Training clinical personnel to assess for tardive dyskinesia. Prog Neuropsychopharmacol Biol Psychiatry 12:749–762, 1988

Kleinman I, Schacter D, Koritar E: Informed consent and tardive dyskinesia. Am J Psychiatry 146:902–904, 1989

Lidz CW, Meisel A, Osterweis M, et al: Barriers to informed consent. Ann Intern Med 99:539–543, 1983

Lidz CW, Meisel A, Zerubavel E, et al: Informed Consent: A Study of Decisionmaking in Psychiatry. New York, Guilford, 1984

Lidz CW, Appelbaum PS, Meisel A: Two models of implementing informed consent. Arch Intern Med 148:1385–1389, 1988

Mills MJ, Norquist GS, Shelton RC, et al: Consent and liability with neuroleptics: the problem of tardive dyskinesia. International Journal of Law and Psychiatry 8:243–252, 1986

Morrow GR: How readable are subject consent forms? JAMA 244:56–58, 1980

Munetz MR: Overcoming resistance to talking to patients about tardive dyskinesia. Hosp Community Psychiatry 36:283–287, 1985

Munetz MR, Benjamin S: Who should perform the AIMS examination? Hosp Community Psychiatry 41:912–915, 1990

Munetz MR, Roth LH: Informing patients about tardive dyskinesia. Arch Gen Psychiatry 42:866–871, 1985

Rozovsky F: Consent to Treatment: A Practical Guide, 2nd Edition. Boston, MA, Little, Brown, 1990

Slawson P: Psychiatric malpractice: ten years' loss experience. Medicine Law 8:415–427, 1989

Strull WM, Lo B, Charles G: Do patients want to participate in medical decision making? JAMA 252:2990–2994, 1984

Tietz GF: Informed consent in the prescription drug context: the special case. Washington Law Review 61:367–417, 1986

Wettstein RM: Tardive dyskinesia and malpractice. Behavioral Sciences and the Law 1:85–107, 1983

Wettstein RM: Legal aspects of neuroleptic-induced movement disorders, in Legal Medicine 1985. Edited by Wecht CH. New York, Praeger, 1985, pp 117–179

Wettstein RM: Informed consent and tardive dyskinesia. J Clin Psychopharmacol 8 (suppl):65S–70S, 1988

# Chapter 11

# Research Recommendations

## Epidemiology

Although numerous prevalence surveys have been conducted, additional prevalence data in special populations would be helpful. Such samples would include children treated with neuroleptics for a variety of indications, including Tourette's disorder, nonschizophrenic patients receiving neuroleptics, and patients with schizophrenia at the onset of their illness.

Additional prospective studies would be useful in comparing different treatment approaches or specific compounds (e.g., clozapine) that might have a lower risk of producing tardive dyskinesia. Given a resurgence of interest in antipsychotic drug development, we hope that development programs include early studies relevant to neurologic side effects and that prospective studies be established to determine (among those compounds that show promise in this regard) the incidence of associated tardive dyskinesia compared with a reference drug. Although this strategy may seem prohibitively expensive or to require too many patients studied for lengthy intervals, in our view this may not be the case if populations at increased risk are included in such studies. Clearly, the importance of establishing a potential advantage in reducing the risk of tardive dyskinesia would justify such efforts.

## Prevention

In addition to new drug development efforts, further attempts to explore other kinds of treatment research designs should be pursued. To date, the impact of dosage reduction or targeted strategies on the incidence of tardive dyskinesia has not been dramatic, but these strategies may be much more effective when applied to a population of patients at increased risk, rather than a general population, many of whom are not at risk. Further research with plasma-level monitoring directed toward utilizing the lowest-effect blood level might also be of interest. Although several intermittent or targeted treatment studies have been done, we are not aware of a design employing a lengthy fixed-interval drug-withdrawal period. It is our strong view that perfunctory or legalistic drug withdrawal should be avoided and that medication discontinuation, whatever the indication, should take place under appropriate clinical supervision.

In assessing the impact of different treatment strategies on the incidence of tardive dyskinesia, it is important to assess the severity of the disorder and its course and prognosis. It may be that different strategies could influence one of these factors, but not all, or influence them to different degrees, and it would be useful to have this information. In assessing the severity of tardive dyskinesia, it is important not only to consider specific signs but also to assess subjective distress and consequent disability or social dysfunction and to document atypical signs, such as dysphagia, dysarthria, and diaphragmatic involvement.

## Pathophysiology

Much remains to be learned regarding the pathophysiology of tardive dyskinesia. The availability of central nervous system active compounds with more specific and relatively pure effects on particular neurotransmitter receptors may provide new knowledge as to receptor mechanisms.

The study of neuroleptic-induced movement disorders in nonschizophrenic patients may also be helpful from a pathophysiologic standpoint, since individuals with schizophrenia may already have alterations in their dopaminergic (or other relevant neurotransmitter) systems. In addition, it may be particularly valuable to study individuals who are relatively invulnerable to tardive dyskinesia.

The identification and study of identical twins, concordant and discordant for tardive dyskinesia, may be helpful in assessing risk factors and pathophysiology. Other strategies to assess genetic influences on the vulnerability to develop tardive dyskinesia would also be helpful. Further assessment of the extent to which tardive dyskinesia is related to other factors in schizophrenia—such as brain morphology, drug responsiveness, vulnerability to relapse, cognitive dysfunction, and psychopathologic subtype—may also prove to be of value. Although (as reviewed in Chapter 4) there are investigations that have focused on these issues, there are a variety of methodologic challenges remaining in this line of investigation.

Further research on subsyndromes of tardive dyskinesia (and other movement disorders) would be useful with, for example, a focus on pathophysiology, risk factors, pharmacologic response, and long-term outcome.

A variety of research strategies should be brought to bear on the etiology and pathophysiology of tardive dyskinesia, including neuroimaging; neuropathology; and neurochemical, neurophysiologic, and neuroimmunological studies. It would also be useful to study peripheral aspects of involuntary movement disorders, such as functioning at the neuromuscular junction and other aspects of peripheral neuromuscular physiology.

## Treatment

At the present time there are no proven safe and effective treatments for tardive dyskinesia once it develops. We hope that further advances in our understanding of pathophysiology might lead to more effective treatments. In addition, our ability to systematically subtype tardive dyskinesia in terms of onset, phenomenology, course, and response to pharmacologic probes might provide a basis for applying specific treatments to particular patients. Methodologic challenges remain in doing treatment trials in this population: ongoing control or prevention of psychoses may be necessary at the same time the dyskinesia is treated; the longer the treatment trial, the more of an issue this may become; the outcome of untreated tardive dyskinesia is so variable that appropriate controls remain essential. In clinical treatment trials there are various factors that may influence course and outcome besides the treatment being tested, including age, sex, severity and duration of dyskinesia, and concomitant treatments.

When a promising treatment for tardive dyskinesia does emerge, a multicenter clinical trial will, in all likelihood, be necessary to recruit a sufficient number of suitable patients for an appropriately designed study.

## Indications for Neuroleptic Treatment

Perhaps the most striking reminder coming from this review is that a great deal of basic clinical research remains to be done to better establish the appropriate indications and relative efficacy of neuroleptic treatment in a variety of conditions, including but not limited to long-term treatment of bipolar disorder, the treatment of childhood schizophrenia, conduct disorder, behavioral problems associated with mental retardation, agitation and other behavioral problems in elderly patients with dementia or psychoses, and personality disorders.

Chapter 12

# Summary, Conclusions, and Recommendations for the Prevention and Management of Tardive Dyskinesia

The use of antipsychotic medication continues to be an essential component of the acute and long-term treatment of a variety of psychotic disorders, particularly schizophrenia. The therapeutic benefits of these medications have a dramatic impact on the day-to-day lives of hundreds of thousands of patients and their families, frequently making the difference between institutionalization and community living, between working and not working, and between the participation in psychosocial and vocational therapies and the inability to participate. A disease like schizophrenia produces enormous morbidity and mortality, and the availability of effective treatments has produced profound changes in not only our management of these conditions, but also our attitudes toward them. At the same time, the development of late-occurring neurologic side effects associated with the long-term use of these medications continues to be a major concern.

In this report, we have attempted to summarize the progress that has been made during the past decade in our understanding of the differential diagnosis and epidemiology of tardive dyskinesia (and related syndromes), as well as risk factors, course, and treatment. In addition, in order to provide the proper framework for assessing the benefit-to-risk ratio of antipsychotic drug treatment, we have tried to review current knowledge with regard to the indications for and clinical use of these drugs in a variety of psychiatric and neuropsychiatric conditions. In this context we have also reviewed potential alternatives to neuroleptic treatment in specific conditions.

Tardive dyskinesia has served as an important impetus to explore alternative neuroleptic maintenance treatment strategies and to reevaluate minimum dosage requirements in those conditions where neuroleptic drugs are the treatment of choice. The existence of this potentially serious and disabling side effect has also served to stress the importance of the process of informed consent. On a more fundamental level, the problem of tardive dyskinesia has also been one factor that has led to a reevaluation of the benefit-to-risk ratio of neuroleptic drugs in schizophrenia, utilizing a more comprehensive array of measures to better reflect a variety of domains beyond psychopathology, such as subjective well-being, vocational and social adjustment, family interactions, and other more subtle adverse effects. At the same time, enormous efforts have been under way to develop compounds that might have a reduced propensity to produce neurologic side effects while still providing therapeutic benefit. Clearly, the ultimate hope for the real prevention of tardive dyskinesia lies in appropriate research efforts, both preclinical and clinical.

## Differential Diagnosis of Tardive Dyskinesia

Any and all abnormal involuntary movements in a patient on neuroleptic drugs do not constitute tardive dyskinesia. The term *dyskinesia* usually refers to the following kinds of abnormal movements: chorea (rapid, jerky, quasi-purposive, nonrhythmic movements, especially of proximal body parts), athetosis (slow, sinuous, or writhing movements of distal parts of the extremities), and dystonia (slow, sustained muscular contraction or spasms that may produce an involuntary movement).

As discussed in Chapter 2, dyskinesia does not include akathisia, compulsions, continuous partial seizures, mannerisms, myoclonus, stereotypy (repetitive uniform purposeless movements), tics, or tremors.

Neuroleptic drugs are also capable of producing acute dyskinesias that may occur early in the course of treatment. Their prevalence has been reported to be approximately 2–3%. They typically remit quickly after a dose reduction or discontinuation of neuroleptic drugs. Anticholinergic or antihistaminic drugs are also effective treatments. Acute dyskinesia may also be associated with dystonia—that is, intermittent or sustained muscular contraction of the eyes, neck, and throat. These may lead to oculogyric crises, dysarthria, dysphagia, and difficulty breathing. There may be opisthotonos, torticollis, and tortipelvis. The dystonia may only be manifested by cramps, tightening of the jaw, or difficulty speaking. These are very often disturbing and painful, but they respond well to anticholinergic or antihistaminic agents.

Tardive dystonia is considered to be a particular type of involuntary movement associated with long-term neuroleptic treatment. The extent to which this condition should be viewed as a distinct entity or a subtype of tardive dyskinesia remains controversial. The movements evident in tardive dystonia are not dissimilar to those observed in primary torsion dystonia. The face and neck are the most frequently involved body regions. It is important to recognize, however, that some patients with tardive dystonia may have classic orofacial dyskinetic movements at some time during the course of their dystonia or at some time prior to its development. Tardive dystonia has been reported to benefit from anticholinergic medications, whereas, in general, tardive dyskinesia does not respond to this class of pharmacologic agents. Acute dystonic reactions tend to occur in the first 24–48 hours of dopamine antagonist treatment; tardive dystonia, as a rule, occurs much later.

In the differential diagnosis of tardive dyskinesia, it is also important to recognize that other classes of compounds are capable of producing acute dyskinesias and that tardive dyskinesias have been reported to occur with L-dopa, amphetamines, metoclopramide, and a variety of other compounds. In addition, several neurologic disorders are capable of producing abnormal involuntary movements that may be mistaken for tardive dyskinesia, including Huntington's disease, Wilson's disease, Sydenham's chorea, Fahr's syndrome, and Hallervorden-Spatz disease. For a more detailed discussion of these and other conditions that should be considered in the differential diagnosis, see Chapter 2.

There is also evidence that motor disorders may be an inherent feature of the schizophrenic illness, and assumptions should not be made that any abnormal involuntary movements that might occur in the context of neuroleptic treatment are a consequence of such treatment. It is particularly important to examine patients carefully prior to the initiation of neuroleptic treatment in order to establish the presence of any preexisting motoric disorders. This is also of particular concern in elderly patients, for whom the incidence of preexisting involuntary movements associated with a variety of neuromedical conditions may be particularly high.

## Clinical Assessment of a Patient With Movement Disorders

1) If a patient has taken neuroleptics for less than 3 months, he or she does not meet research criteria for tardive dyskinesia. In clinical practice, however, tardive dyskinesia can develop with such a brief exposure to neuroleptics. This is especially true in patients at increased risk for tardive dyskinesia, such as the elderly. 2) Recent use of other drugs that can produce dyskinesia (e.g., L-dopa and amphetamine) should be inquired into. Most non-neuroleptic-induced dyskinesias disappear when those medications are discontinued.) 3) History of a neurologic illness—such as stroke, encephalitis, major head trauma, or symptoms suggestive of a tumor (e.g., headaches)—should lead to a search for a structural lesion affecting the

basal ganglia. 4) A positive family history for a movement disorder should raise a possibility of hereditary disorders, such as Huntington's disease, Wilson's disease, or torsion dystonia. In such cases, details of the disorder in the affected family member should be sought.

### Physical Examination

1) The specific types of abnormal involuntary movements present in a given patient (e.g., tremors, tics, and choreiform movements) should be identified. 2) Presence of signs of dementia may indicate a need to rule out such disorders as Huntington's disease, Wilson's disease, and brain tumor. (Some elderly patients may have both—dementia and neuroleptic-induced tardive dyskinesia. 3) Focal neurologic deficits—such as hemiparesis or gross asymmetry of reflexes—should lead to a search for structural brain lesions. 4) Patients should be examined for signs of metabolic (e.g., jaundice and hepatomegaly secondary to liver disease) and endocrine (e.g., tachycardia, excessive sweating, and goiter due to hyperthyroidism) abnormalities. 5) Specific signs (e.g., Kayser-Fleischer rings in the cornea in Wilson's disease) should be looked for in appropriate cases.

### Laboratory Studies

It is unnecessary and impractical to subject all patients with possible tardive dyskinesia to a large battery of laboratory investigations. There are, however, some pointers in the history and physical examination that would suggest a need for further workup. These include severe or rapidly progressive dyskinesia, a past history suggestive of brain lesion, a family history positive for a movement disorder, presence of dementia, or signs of other neurologic, metabolic, or endocrine abnormalities.

The laboratory workup includes the following: 1) complete blood count—to rule out polycythemia vera and other disorders; 2) serum electrolytes—to exclude abnormalities of sodium and calcium metabolism that may cause movement disorders; 3) liver-function tests—to rule out Wilson's disease and other causes of liver dysfunction; 4) thyroid-function tests—to check for possible hyperthyroidism; 5) serum copper and ceruloplasmin and urinary copper and amino acids in cases of suspected Wilson's disease; 6) connective-tissue disease screen—to assess for systemic lupus erythematous and other vasculitides; 7) computed tomography or magnetic resonance imaging scan of head—this may show atrophy of caudate in Huntington's disease, basal ganglia calcification in Fahr's syndrome or a mass lesion in a brain tumor.

We emphasize that the diagnosis of tardive dyskinesia is a clinical and not a laboratory diagnosis. When the clinician is not certain of the diagnosis, it is advisable to follow the patient closely instead of bringing the diagnostic process to a premature closure.

## Assessment of Tardive Dyskinesia

It is important to recognize that scores on a rating scale cannot be utilized to make a diagnosis of tardive dyskinesia. Assessment techniques are important for identifying possible cases as well as documenting their severity and measuring treatment response or long-term outcome, but a process of clinical evaluation and differential diagnosis is necessary to establish the presence of tardive dyskinesia.

There are various problems in the assessment of tardive dyskinesia, including marked within-patient variation in severity over time and in response to change in medication status or level of arousal. Difficulties also arise where the motor phenomena of tardive dyskinesia need to be distinguished from motor disturbances related to the condition for which the antipsychotic drug was originally prescribed. Although the standard multi-item scales have usually been considered appropriate for most patient populations, scales have also been specifically developed to address this issue. For example, the Rogers Motor Disorder Scale was devised to assess movement disorders in schizophrenia, avoiding the assumptions regarding etiology, and the Dyskinesia Identification System–Coldwater was originally developed for individuals with mental handicaps.

There can be spontaneous intrapatient variability in the site and severity of dyskinesias, posing a problem for the interpretation of ratings based on observations of a patient for a short period of time. Fluctuation in severity may be observed in association with changes in the level of physiologic or emotional arousal, posture, and mobility. A major source of variation in tardive dyskinesia is change in drug treatment. Change in the dosage regimen of antipsychotic drug treatment can influence the severity of the movements. The administration, withdrawal, or change in dose of concomitant anticholinergic medication can also influence the severity of tardive dyskinesia.

Various assessment methods are reviewed in Chapter 3, including instrumentation (electromyography, accelerometers, ultrasound, and electromechanical instruments), frequency counts, and multi-item scales.

The most popular rating method is the multi-item scale, which provides a comprehensive rating of the abnormal involuntary movements in various body sites. Some of these scales incorporate a standard procedure for the examination of patients. Reliability and validity data are available for the most widely used scales, such as the Abnormal Involuntary Movement Scale and the Rockland/Simpson Tardive Dyskinesia Rating Scale. (Examples of widely used multi-item rating scales are provided in the Appendix.)

# Epidemiology, Risk Factors, and Outcome of Tardive Dyskinesia

Although there still remains some debate as to the extent to which antipsychotic drug treatment is either necessary or sufficient to produce abnormal involuntary movements in various psychiatric populations, the consensus of the task force at the present time is that antipsychotic drugs do play a major role in producing, precipitating, or evoking abnormal involuntary movements. This conclusion recognizes that abnormal involuntary movements occurring in schizophrenic patients were described in the preantipsychotic era and have also been observed more recently among chronic schizophrenic patients never treated with antipsychotic drugs. No doubt various predisposing factors play a critical role in determining which individuals are most likely to develop the condition.

Prevalence estimates indicate how many individuals in a given population are affected by a condition at a specified point in time. The precise prevalence rates of tardive dyskinesia are nearly impossible to specify, since these rates vary enormously depending on the patient population studied. It would probably be safe to say that between 15% and 20% of patients receiving chronic neuroleptic treatment will have some evidence of tardive dyskinesia, ranging from a transient form of the condition to those of moderate or extreme severity.

Severe and persistent forms of tardive dyskinesia can occur in all age ranges, including children, and sometimes after relatively brief periods of treatment.

In recent years there has been considerable progress in developing estimates of the incidence of tardive dyskinesia. Here also the rates vary enormously depending on the population studied, with an incidence of 5% per year of neuroleptic exposure seen in young adults and an incidence of 30% seen after 1 year in a population of elderly individuals. The incidence data have also helped to confirm our assumptions that the cumulative incidence of tardive dyskinesia increases with continued neuroleptic exposure.

With regard to risk factors, early observations suggesting that increasing age is associated with an increase in incidence and prevalence has been supported. A relatively stable finding has been that women show a greater prevalence of severe dyskinesia than men, although the available evidence suggests that this is limited to the older age range.

The extent to which psychiatric diagnosis represents a risk factor for the development of abnormal involuntary movements is a complex issue, given the possibility that some patients with schizophrenia, for example, may develop abnormal involuntary movements associated with the disease that only become manifest after several years of illness. At the same time, it is also possible that some conditions, when treated with neuroleptic drugs, are associated with a higher incidence of abnormal involuntary movements than others. The latter appears to be the case, for example, with affective disorders.

The early occurrence of drug-induced parkinsonian side effects appears to indicate increased vulnerability for the subsequent development of tardive dyskinesia.

With regard to drug-treatment variables, the results of dosage-reduction studies provide some encouragement but are also viewed by many as disappointing in their relative impact on the incidence of tardive dyskinesia. The problem here remains one of methodology, however, in that the impact of preventive strategies is difficult to document in a sample of patients, many of whom may not be at particular risk for the development of tardive dyskinesia during the course of the investigation. If studies were focused on individuals at increased risk, then the impact of preventive strategies may be easier to detect and more robust. At present, there are limited data supporting significantly different degrees of risk associated with specific antipsychotic drugs or drug classes; however, sulpiride and clozapine appear to hold some promise in this regard. It is hoped that future studies will allow more definitive conclusions.

The results of recent studies on the long-term outcome of tardive dyskinesia have provided some reassurance that this disorder, in most cases, is nonprogressive and that, even with continued neuroleptic administration, there may be improvement over time (particularly if the lowest effective dosage can be employed). This does not diminish the potential importance of discontinuing neuroleptic drugs when feasible, but for those patients in whom the need and benefit is sufficient to warrant continued administration, clinicians are unlikely to see a significant worsening of the condition. The problem remains, however, that a subgroup of patients does develop a severe and disabling form of tardive dyskinesia, and efforts to identify such patients remain critical.

## Treatment of Tardive Dyskinesia

There remains no proven safe and effective treatment for tardive dyskinesia. The most logical "treatment" remains neuroleptic withdrawal; however, this is frequently not feasible when there is a risk of worsening or relapse of psychotic symptoms. If continued neuroleptic treatment is indicated, an attempt at dose reduction should be considered. Although there is no evidence to show that anticholinergic agents produce tardive dyskinesia, these drugs do sometimes worsen it. Hence, discontinuation of anticholinergics would be advisable. Neuroleptic drugs tend to be potent suppressors of tardive dyskinesia at least in the short term. The suggestion that neuroleptic drugs mask rather than cure tardive dyskinesia is based on the fact that in most cases neuroleptic withdrawal results in a reemergence of tardive dyskinesia; however, systematic long-term studies to address this issue have not been conducted. The extent to which clozapine may be atypical in this regard will require further investigation, but clozapine's apparent reduced propensity to produce tardive dyskinesia is suggestive of a potential role at least in the management of patients who require continued neuroleptic treatment in the presence of moderate or severe tardive dyskinesia.

There are data suggesting that noradrenergic hyperactivity may be present in a subset of patients with tardive dyskinesia, and in some cases such drugs as clonidine or propranolol may be useful. Various catecholamine antagonists have been tried in the treatment of tardive dyskinesia. The overall success rate has been low.

"GABAergic" ($\gamma$-aminobutyric acid) drugs have been given to patients with tardive dyskinesia, with variable success. Commonly used agents with relatively low toxicity (e.g., benzodiazepines) are often of clinical value in the temporary management of moderate or severe tardive dyskinesia. Cholinergic drugs underwent several trials during the 1970s and 1980s; however, more recent studies have somewhat dampened enthusiasm for this class of drugs as a treatment for tardive dyskinesia, although some individual patients may benefit.

Anticholinergic drugs have been shown to be of some value in tardive dystonia; however, in nondystonic tardive dyskinesia, the efficacy of anticholinergic drugs is limited, and in a number of cases they may even worsen the dyskinesia.

Various miscellaneous drugs are reviewed in more detail in Chapter 5. Recently, there have been claims for the efficacy of calcium channel blockers and alpha-tocopherol or vitamin E in the treatment of tardive dyskinesia; however, the general clinical value of these agents needs to be established with large-scale, long-term studies.

It is necessary to stress that in a majority of patients with tardive dyskinesia, the abnormal involuntary movements are mild and may not require any specific treatment, apart from neuroleptic dosage reduction or withdrawal, if feasible. It is important to bear in mind that any pharmacologic agents used to treat tardive dyskinesia will have their own side effects and should be employed only after due consideration of their own risk-to-benefit ratios. The long-term value of most of the drug treatments suggested for tardive dyskinesia have not been established.

# Neuroleptic Drugs: Indications, Efficacy, and Therapeutic Dosages

The task force felt it would be helpful to review this area in order to help establish a framework for developing benefit and risk assessments of neuroleptic treatment in a variety of conditions. The use of antipsychotic or neuroleptic drugs remains a matter of clinical judgment, which must be made on an individual basis; however, it is critical that clinicians weigh the relative indications for alternative treatments when neuroleptics are not the only available treatment. The overall indications for short-term and long-term utilization of neuroleptics have not changed appreciably in the past decade. The primary indications for short-term use include 1) the treatment of an acute episode or exacerbation of a schizophrenic illness, 2) delusional disorder and other psychotic disorders, 3) the manic phase of bipolar disorder when very rapid control is necessary in a highly agitated patient or when lithium treatment is inadequate, 4) the treatment of agitation or psychosis in some organic mental disorders, 5) a major depressive episode with psychotic features, and 6) neurologic or psychiatric manifestations of certain neuropsychiatric conditions, such as Huntington's disease and Tourette's disorder. In addition, a brief therapeutic trial of neuroleptic drugs may be indicated in some severe personality disorders. In children or adolescents, neuroleptics may be indicated in schizophrenia, autism, pervasive developmental disorder, Tourette's disorder, attention-deficit disorder with hyperactivity, conduct disorder, and some cases of aggressive and nonspecific behavioral symptoms associated with mental retardation.

Indications for neuroleptics may be influenced by the relative efficacy of other treatments in a given individual. It is critical that clinicians weigh the relative indications for alternative treatments when neuroleptics are not the only available treatment and document the process of clinical judgment in the medical record (see Chapter 10).

The efficacy of neuroleptic medication is by far the best studied and best confirmed in the acute and long-term treatment of schizophrenia. The long-term efficacy of neuroleptics in the treatment of delusional disorders, bipolar disorder, major depression with psychotic features, organic mental disorders, and chronic characterologic disorders has not been addressed in controlled clinical trials; however, clinical experience would suggest, and the task force agrees, that prolonged neuroleptic therapy may be of benefit in some such individuals.

Although we have seen the development of a variety of different antipsychotic medications during the past 3 decades, there are at present no convincing data that, among those medications currently marketed in the United States, any one is more effective either in schizophrenia in general or in specific subtypes of the disorder, with the exception of clozapine in the treatment of patients who have failed to respond to other antipsychotics. It remains conceivable that other differences do exist but that appropriately designed and executed studies have not been conducted.

Clozapine, however, is associated with a higher incidence of agranulocytosis than that seen with other antipsychotic drugs, limiting the extent of its utilization.

Although we still have insufficient information regarding dose-response curves for antipsychotic drugs, there has been considerable interest in attempting to establish minimum dose requirements for both acute and maintenance treatments. In general, the literature suggests that doses of 400–900 mg/day of chlorpromazine or equivalents should be sufficient for acute treatment in the average patient. There has been a tendency to use particularly large doses of high-potency antipsychotics because, apart from parkinsonian side effects, high doses are generally well tolerated, but this practice should be discouraged unless it is clearly established that such measures are necessary for a specific patient.

Maintenance antipsychotic drug treatment has proven to be of dramatic value in reducing the risk of psychotic relapse and rehospitalization. In the last 10 years we have witnessed the initiation of much more sophisticated, long-term clinical trials that have focused not only on relapse rate and rehospitalization rate but on a variety of other factors that are relevant to assessing the overall benefits and risks of maintenance drug treatment. The efficacy of antipsychotic medication in the long-term management of schizophrenia has been established in more controlled trials than most pharmacologic treatments in other areas of medicine. Despite this, there remain critics of long-term neuroleptic use. To some extent, these criticisms result from the complexity of the schizophrenic illness and the observations that a variety of factors may influence outcome and that, for a given individual, our ability to predict outcome is limited. Despite this, clinical judgments are based on the data available and clinical experience. This body of knowledge has led to a strong consensus that the potential benefits of this treatment outweigh the potential risks. With current knowledge and currently available medication, the development of tardive dyskinesia in some patients is inevitable, even with the most judicious and careful use of these medications. The nature of schizophrenia is such, however, that without neuroleptic treatment many affected individuals remain severely symptomatic and disabled, leading to enormous personal suffering and the suffering of their families and friends.

Antipsychotic drugs are widely used in the treatment of acute mania, particularly during the earlier stages of such treatment. Although lithium is effective in alleviating the signs and symptoms of mania, neuroleptics may work more rapidly and may be more effective in highly agitated or aggressive patients. There are, however, no well-established guidelines for when neuroleptics should be discontinued in this context; most experts would advise relatively short-term use followed by a trial on lithium alone. The relative merits of antipsychotics versus anticonvulsants or other adjuncts to lithium have not been well studied. Neuroleptics may also be indicated in the long-term management of bipolar patients who fail to respond to alternative treatments. Neuroleptics may be efficacious in the treatment of depression with psychotic features, but antidepressants and electroconvulsive therapy may be effective alternatives.

It is impossible to make blanket statements regarding indications for neuroleptic drugs, particularly in areas where few controlled trials have been carried out. It is essential, however, when considering the use of these compounds that, prior to their initiation and again before continuation or long-term maintenance, the clinician should conduct a thorough diagnostic evaluation; a review of alternative treatments and appropriate therapeutic trials if indicated; a careful weighing of potential benefits and risks; a thorough discussion with the patient and the family of the disease, its prognosis and course (both treated and untreated), the potential benefits, and the risks of the treatment; and the methods for assessing outcome. The importance of well-informed clinical judgment regarding the individual patient cannot be overemphasized. This process of judgment and informed consent must be clearly evident in the medical record.

## Alternative Maintenance Treatment Strategies: Clinical Efficacy and Impact on Tardive Dyskinesia

The desire to reduce adverse effects—particularly tardive dyskinesia, akathisia, and akinesia—has led to increasing interest in attempting to identify minimum effective dosage requirements for the long-term treatment of schizophrenia. Two strategies have received considerable attention during the past decade: dosages lower than conventional and intermittent or targeted treatment. Results from dosage-reduction studies suggest that this strategy is feasible for a large subgroup of stable schizophrenic outpatients and can lead to a diminution in adverse effects and improvement in some subjective and nonsubjective measures of well-being. The risk of psychotic exacerbation does increase, however, earlier with very low dosages, and in the second year it increases even with moderately low dosages. Therefore, patients must be monitored clinically with a readiness to increase medication when appropriate and on a temporary basis. This highlights the importance of viewing this approach as a strategy within the context of flexible, observant clinical management. In addition, there may be patients for whom dosage reduction is not feasible, based on past attempts or potential dire consequences of psychotic relapse (e.g., history of serious suicide attempts or violent behavior).

The term *intermittent treatment* has been employed in two ways. The first is to describe fixed medication-administration schedules that incorporate medication-free days, and the second is to refer to the use of medication only during periods of incipient relapse or symptom exacerbation rather than continuous administration. Substantial research efforts during the past decade have focused on the latter strategy. Targeted treatment is based on the assumption that patients require neuroleptic medication only during times of incipient relapse or symptom exacerbation. The use of intermittent or targeted treatment depends heavily on the accurate identification of times at which medication needs to be reinstituted. A second requirement for the use of a targeted medication strategy is the creation of a treatment structure that incorporates an ongoing therapeutic relationship for patient monitoring and support.

The results of recently completed studies suggest that intermittent treatment strategies can be implemented in outpatient maintenance settings and do result in reduced dosage of medication and some reduction of side-effect burden. Particularly during a 2-year period, however, the strategy carries an increased risk of not only the expected prodromal episodes, but also of relapses and rehospitalizations. Further, there are no consistent benefits of intermittent treatment in terms of social functioning.

With regard to the impact of these dosage-reduction strategies on tardive dyskinesia, it appears that the risk of tardive dyskinesia may be influenced by substantial reductions in cumulative neuroleptic exposure; however, the results of the trials to date have not proven to be dramatic. It is possible that these strategies might have more impact in a subgroup of patients selected on the basis of increased risk for developing tardive dyskinesia. For the general population of patients at large, on the basis of the data available, it appears that although medication reduction or discontinuation may be reasonable treatment approaches, they do have significant risks. Indeed, if medication must be started and stopped frequently in order to prevent an exacerbation in psychopathology, the effects on tardive dyskinesia may be worse than simply maintaining the patient on continuous medication. Clearly, more data and, in particular, more data focusing on patients at particular risk would be extremely useful.

## Alternatives to Neuroleptic Therapy

Although neuroleptic drugs clearly play an important role in the treatment of a variety of conditions, their association with tardive dyskinesia and other neurologic side effects remains a limiting factor in their use. As a result, there have been continued efforts to develop alternatives to neuroleptic treatment. Various other drugs, mainly available for other medical indications, have been claimed to have some efficacy in some psychiatric conditions in which neuroleptics are commonly used. None of these to date has shown consistent reliable efficacy when given alone to schizophrenic patients, although occasional patients have shown improvement. A few drugs have limited evidence of efficacy in manic excitement or episodic violence, situations in which neuroleptic drugs are often used; however, none of the widely diverse agents studied in the last 10 years have proven to be safe and effective alone in any other psychiatric condition in which neuroleptics are commonly used. The possible exception is electroconvulsive therapy, where the short-term results in acute psychosis probably equal those achieved by neuroleptics. None of the alternative therapies has been more than tentatively studied as a maintenance treatment.

Although concern about tardive dyskinesia led briefly to a renewed interest in reserpine as an alternative treatment for schizophrenia and mania, the results with this compound are not impressive. Although there are very few reported cases of dyskinesia in reserpine-treated psychiatric patients, if reserpine were widely used in the dosages necessary to treat acute and chronic psychosis, it is impossible to predict whether the risk of tardive dyskinesia in such patients would be less than if they were treated with standard neuroleptic drugs.

Although conventional wisdom suggests that benzodiazepines would not be useful in schizophrenia except perhaps to reduce akathisia, there are several studies, some controlled, that suggest that benzodiazepines sometimes are therapeutically effective in schizophrenia, particularly in higher dosages. There are, however, no data on longer-term administration, and it is impossible to tell whether the effect can be maintained for the prolonged periods often required in chronic psychotic illness. Physical dependence would undoubtedly occur with prolonged, high-dose benzodiazepine therapy. This approach deserves further study but is far from being a generally safe and effective alternative to standard neuroleptic therapy.

After 40 years of clinical experience with the use of lithium in psychotic patients, it is still difficult to make precise statements about the value of lithium therapy in schizophrenia. It appears that lithium alone in chronic schizophrenia is usually not an adequate therapy but may reduce excitement or impulsive, angry outbursts and may improve response in some patients when added to neuroleptics. The extent to which this effect is independent of the schizoaffective versus schizophrenic differentiation remains unclear. Clearly, lithium is the treatment of choice for the long-term prophylaxis of bipolar disorder. A large proportion of bipolar patients, however, experience manic or depressive relapse despite adequate levels of lithium. The use of neuroleptics may be indicated in some such patients, but trials of carbamazepine and other agents may be indicated as well.

There is no direct evidence that carbamazepine alone is effective in the treatment of schizophrenic disorders, although some studies report a good response in a proportion of schizoaffective patients. There is growing evidence that carbamazepine has value as an acute and prophylactic treatment in bipolar patients. Valproic acid may have some efficacy as an acute treatment for mania but is probably not particularly useful as a single therapeutic agent in schizophrenia.

It appears that at present, proven safe and effective alternatives for neuroleptic treatment in the acute and long-term management of schizophrenia have not emerged, despite clinical studies employing a variety of pharmacologic agents. Although subgroups of patients may at times benefit from nonneuroleptic medications, we are unable to identify these individuals prior to appropriate treatment trials. Therefore, neuroleptic drugs continue to remain the treatment of choice for patients with schizophrenia unless there are specific contraindications or clear evidence that such agents are not helpful. The treatment of those patients who fail to benefit adequately from available neuroleptics continues to present a challenge to clinicians, and in this context a variety of experimental treatments might be indicated. Clozapine may hold particular promise in this regard. Alternatives to neuroleptic treatment are, however, well established in a variety of conditions other than schizophrenia, and the use of neuroleptics in that context must be weighed carefully and fully justified.

# Are There Behavioral Analogues of Tardive Dyskinesia?

It has been suggested that prolonged neuroleptic administration might result in neuropharmacologic changes producing alterations in behavior in an analogous fashion to tardive dyskinesia. The general concept has a seductive face validity. Neuroleptic drugs could cause an alteration in dopamine receptors in the limbic area or some other relevant brain area involved in emotion and psychosis, which might parallel the changes in dopamine receptor function in the basal ganglia suspected of causing tardive dyskinesia. If neuroleptics did in fact result in such changes, then one might see some of the varied psychiatric phenomena described in papers on supersensitivity psychosis or tardive dysmentia. The main and unavoidable problem is that tardive dyskinesia is a relatively unique though heterogeneous set of abnormal movements not usually seen as a concomitant of psychosis. If an individual with schizophrenia shows grimacing, tongue protrusion, chewing, and choreoathetoid arm movements, it is relatively unlikely (though possible) that this cluster of dyskinesias is due to the psychosis. If, on the other hand, the same patient shows worsening of psychotic symptoms when coming off of neuroleptic medication or despite increasing doses of neuroleptic drugs, it is impossible to prove that this is an adverse consequence of prolonged antipsychotic drug treatment. The course of psychosis is variable enough to make any outcome or shift in clinical status entirely plausible. Unfortunately, it is equally difficult to prove that any worsening in psychosis is not due to some increase in dopaminergic activity (or other neurotransmitter effect) in the brain.

Given that these phenomena have been described only by a few investigators during the past several years leads to the weak conclusion that the syndromes are either relatively rare or are hard to identify amid the general clinical vagaries of the course of treated psychosis.

## Clinical-Legal Issues

Litigation is a pervasive concern in contemporary American society, both inside and outside medicine. The prescription of psychoactive medication exposes the psychiatrist to significant professional liability claims. Indeed, improper medication was the most common allegation against psychiatrists insured within the American Psychiatric Association professional-liability insurance program from 1973 to 1984. The psychiatrists' prescription liability pertains largely to two areas, negligence and informed consent. Under tort law, a negligence action against the psychiatrist is successful when the plaintiff proves with a preponderance of the evidence that 1) the psychiatrist had a legal duty to care for the patient according to the standard of care; 2) the psychiatrist, in his or her care of the patient, violated that duty through an omission or commission; and 3) the patient suffered a physical or emotional injury as a result of the psychiatrist's violation of the standard of care to the patient.

Prescribing psychiatrists risk negligence liability in a variety of areas when they prescribe psychoactive medication. These include failure to take an adequate history; failure to obtain an adequate physical examination; failure to obtain an adequate laboratory examination; lack of indication for a prescription; contraindication for a prescription; prescription of an improper dosage; prescription for an improper duration; failure to recognize, monitor, and treat medication side effects; failure to abate drug reactions and interactions; and failure to consult with other physicians.

Since the early 1900s, physicians in the United States have been required to obtain the consent of their patient before proceeding with the proposed procedure or treatment. Only in the last 30 years, however, have physicians also been legally required to provide information to the patient about the proposed intervention prior to proceeding. (The elements of informed consent are described in detail in Chapter 10.) The extent of the information to be disclosed is ordinarily governed by state law, whether statute or case law. Two general standards of information disclosure apply, the physician standard and the patient standard. Under the physician standard, the extent of disclosure is dictated by what physicians in the community disclose to their patients about a particular intervention. Under the patient standard, the extent of disclosure is dictated by what information a hypothetical patient, or even the particular patient in question, would need to make the health care decision. There are four general exceptions to the consent and disclosure requirements of informed consent: emergency; waiver; therapeutic privilege; and incompetence. These exceptions vary from state to state, however.

Given the incidence, prevalence, and potential irreversibility of tardive dyskinesia in patients treated with antipsychotic medication for prolonged intervals, it is a sufficiently significant or material risk to merit disclosure to the patient or legal guardian under either the professional medical standard or the patient-centered standard of disclosure. Tardive dyskinesia is neither too infrequent nor too insignificant a risk of treatment to avoid disclosure. Disclosure about the risk of tardive dyskinesia should occur as soon as clinically feasible. Disclosure about tardive dyskinesia is especially important if the patient already has evidence of this condition and the psychiatrist is considering resuming medication. Should the psychiatrist suspect or diagnose tardive dyskinesia in a patient under consultation or treatment, then the patient should be informed of the diagnosis.

Documentation is an important and underappreciated component of health care service. Record keeping is as much a part of providing health care as the underlying care activity itself. Medical records are legal as well as clinical documents. The elements of medical record documentation for informed consent include each of the informed-consent issues noted in Chapter 10. At least in outline form, the psychiatrist should indicate how and what he or she told the patient about his or her condition and its treatment; what the patient said and understood about it, including any questions the patient may have asked; and how they came to a decision about the course of treatment. When possible, the psychiatrist should quote the patient's exact words. When the patient is of questionable capacity to consent to treatment, then data about the patient's decision-making capacities and incapacities should also be included.

Written consent forms for nonexperimental medications are not generally used in medical practice, especially in the chronic-care setting. Given the perceived risks of their use and the uncertain benefits, routine written consent forms for antipsychotic medication are not recommended (see Chapter 10 for further discussion). In some health care facilities and states, written consent forms for antipsychotic medication are required as a matter of policy or law. Clinicians practicing in these settings are obligated to use them, but they should be careful to avoid allowing them to substitute for talking with the patient and the family about the medication and tardive dyskinesia, both before and after the consent form has been signed. Having the patient sign a written consent form does not end the psychiatrist's ethical or legal obligation to obtain and renew a valid consent to treatment.

## Research Recommendations

Although considerable progress has been made in tardive dyskinesia research during the past decade, there are various areas that would benefit from additional research efforts. Prevalence estimates in special populations, such as children treated with neuroleptics for a variety of indications and nonschizophrenic patients receiving neuroleptics, would be specific examples of needed information. Additional prospective studies would be useful in comparing different treatment approaches or specific compounds (e.g., clozapine) that might have a lower risk of producing tardive dyskinesia. With a resurgence of interest in antipsychotic drug development, we hope that development programs will include early studies relevant to neurologic side effects and that prospective studies will be established to determine the incidence of associated tardive dyskinesia compared with a reference drug. Further attempts to explore other kinds of treatment research designs should be pursued. To date, the impact of dosage reduction or targeted strategies on the incidence of tardive dyskinesia has not been dramatic, but these strategies may be much more effective when applied to a population of patients at increased risk, rather than a general population, many of whom are not at risk.

Much remains to be learned regarding the pathophysiology of tardive dyskinesia. The availability of compounds with more specific and relatively pure effects on particular central nervous system neurotransmitter receptors may provide new knowledge as to relevant receptor mechanisms. The study of neuroleptic-induced movement disorders in nonschizophrenic patients may also be helpful from a pathophysiologic viewpoint, since individuals with schizophrenia may already have alterations in their dopaminergic (or other relevant neurotransmitter) systems. In addition, it may be particularly valuable to study individuals who are relatively invulnerable to developing tardive dyskinesia. A variety of research strategies should be brought to bear on the etiology and pathophysiology of tardive dyskinesia, including neuroimaging, neuropathology, neurochemical, neurophysiologic, and neuroimmunological studies.

At the present time, there are no proven safe and effective treatments for tardive dyskinesia. We hope that further advances in our understanding of the pathophysiology might lead to more effective treatments. In addition, our ability to systematically subtype tardive dyskinesia in terms of onset, phenomenology, course, and response to pharmacologic probes might provide a basis for applying specific treatments to particular patients.

Perhaps the most striking reminder coming from this review, however, is that a great deal of basic clinical research remains to be done to better establish the appropriate indications and relative efficacy of neuroleptic treatment in a variety of conditions, including but not limited to long-term treatment of bipolar disorder, the treatment of childhood schizophrenia, conduct disorder, behavioral problems associated with mental retardation, agitation and other behavioral problems in elderly patients with dementia or psychosis, and personality disorders.

## Prevention

In discussing strategies to prevent the development of tardive dyskinesia, it is important to emphasize at the outset that with the treatment options presently available to us and our current state of knowledge, it is impossible to fully prevent the development of tardive dyskinesia. There are strategies that should be employed to reduce the risk and to improve the chances of a more favorable outcome, if and when this disorder develops. The ultimate hope for the real prevention of tardive dyskinesia lies in appropriate research efforts—both preclinical and clinical.

As we discussed in previous chapters, there are several issues that must be considered in the use of neuroleptic drugs. The reliability and validity of the diagnostic process is critical in determining appropriate indications for both short- and long-term treatment. The thoroughness of the diagnostic evaluation has far-reaching implications in illnesses where long-term treatment decisions may be based on phenomenology seen only during a psychotic exacerbation. The diagnostic process must be longitudinal as well as cross-sectional with continual reevaluation, based on new information, pattern and course of symptoms, and so forth.

Although considerable progress has been made in delineating schizophrenia and affective disorders, there remain many cases that are difficult to classify. In addition, the increasing frequency of substance abuse complicating the diagnostic picture presents an enormous challenge to clinicians. All of these factors emphasize the importance of a careful differential diagnosis and avoiding premature closure, which could ultimately lead to a long-term course of neuroleptic medication.

Even in conditions such as schizophrenia, where neuroleptics are clearly indicated, response to treatment is frequently only partial. Clinicians and patients must have a clear understanding of what these drugs can and cannot accomplish. This problem is of particular concern for patients who are poor responders to neuroleptics. It is reasonable for the clinician in this context to institute therapeutic trials of different compounds and different dosages; however, it must be clear that a patient is benefiting from a particular drug or drug combination before it is continued on a long-term basis. This is of particular concern with the use of very high doses.

As we discussed in Chapter 6, there remain enormous areas of uncertainty regarding the indications for neuroleptic drugs in many non-schizophrenic conditions. Clinicians must carefully weigh the indications for acute treatment and then for continuation and maintenance neuroleptic treatment on an individual basis. There are conditions for which neuroleptic drugs may be indicated in one phase of the illness (e.g., severely agitated mania) but can then be replaced with other drugs (e.g., lithium) for long-term maintenance treatment.

There should be clear evidence and documentation of initial and continued therapeutic benefit from neuroleptic drugs. In those conditions or phases of the illness where alternative effective and safe treatments are available, a thorough assessment of the benefits and risks of each alternative should be a matter of course. If neuroleptic drugs are indicated and beneficial, attempts should be made to utilize the minimum effective dose and to consider if and when a trial without medication might be appropriate.

Although the extent to which multiple drugs might influence the risk of tardive dyskinesia (either positively or negatively) remains unclear, there are various clinical reasons to attempt to reduce polypharmacy. With regard to antiparkinsonian medication, although the value of prophylactic antiparkinsonian medication is debated, the critical factor is the careful examination of the patient and the recognition of subtle extrapyramidal side effects that may have an important impact on subjective well-being and social and vocational adjustment. There remains insufficient evidence to determine what role, if any, anticholinergic drugs play in increasing or reducing the risk of tardive dyskinesia, although these compounds can, in some cases, exacerbate the movement disorder once it develops.

It appears that the early occurrence of neuroleptic-induced parkinsonian side effects may indicate an increased vulnerability to the subsequent development of tardive dyskinesia. Therefore, such patients might receive specific consideration for alternative maintenance medication strategies, although the potential value of such strategies in this context remains a hypothesis requiring clinical testing.

## Diagnosis and Management of Tardive Dyskinesia

Patients should be examined regularly, at least every 3–6 months, for early signs of tardive dyskinesia with full appreciation of the varied potential manifestations. If abnormal involuntary movements are observed, a diagnostic evaluation should take place (see Chapter 2) to rule out other neuromedical causes. If the diagnosis remains presumptive tardive dyskinesia,

a careful review of the indications for and evidence of benefit from neuroleptic treatment should take place. In addition, the relative benefit-to-risk
ratio of any potential alternative treatment should be carefully considered.
All of these factors should be discussed with the patient (and family, if appropriate). If the decision is made to continue (or discontinue) neuroleptic drugs, the patient's understanding of this and consent should be
documented in the medical record.

Neuroleptic drugs should be given at the lowest effective dose, and attempts should be made to discontinue any antiparkinsonian medication.
There is no evidence pro or con, with the possible exception of clozapine,
that switching from one class of neuroleptic to another is of potential
value.

The nature and severity of the tardive dyskinesia should be assessed and
documented to provide a baseline for further ongoing evaluation (a standard rating scale may be helpful in this regard; see the Appendix). The
patients should be reevaluated at regular intervals to determine the course
of the movement disorder as well as the ongoing indications and benefit
from the treatment. If the tardive dyskinesia worsens, then new consideration should be given to discontinuing the neuroleptic or switching to an
antipsychotic with possibly lower propensity to exacerbate the tardive dyskinesia (e.g., clozapine). If maintenance antipsychotic treatment is clearly
needed, the addition of an adjunctive treatment specifically for the dyskinesia should be considered as well (e.g., tocopheral and benzodiazepines;
see Chapter 5), keeping in mind that the efficacy of these agents remains
largely unproven.

For patients with moderate to severe tardive dyskinesia who require continued antipsychotic treatment, clozapine may hold some promise; however, further research is necessary to clarify the benefit-to-risk ratio of
clozapine in that context. It is also important to stay alert to new developments in this area.

Frequently, the following question arises: When should a second opinion be sought? It is the task force's feeling that a second opinion is particularly appropriate when the original psychiatric diagnosis is in doubt,
when the diagnosis of the movement disorder is in doubt, or whenever the
movement disorder is severe or disabling. Ideally, the second opinion
should be provided by someone with special expertise in the diagnosis and
management of drug-induced movement disorders.

# Recommendations for the Prevention and Management of Tardive Dyskinesia

1.  Review indications for neuroleptic drugs, and consider alternative
    treatments when available.

2. Educate the patient and his or her family regarding benefits and risks. Obtain informed consent for long-term treatment, and document it in the medical record.
3. Establish objective evidence of the benefit from neuroleptics, and review it periodically (at least every 3–6 months) to determine ongoing need and benefit.
4. Utilize the minimum effective dosage for chronic treatment.
5. Exercise particular caution with children, the elderly, and patients with affective disorders.
6. Examine the patient regularly for early signs of dyskinesia, and note them in the medical record.
7. If dyskinesia does occur, consider an alternative neurologic diagnosis.
8. If presumptive tardive dyskinesia is present, reevaluate the indications for continued neuroleptic treatment and obtain informed consent from the patient regarding continuing or discontinuing neuroleptic treatment.
9. If a neuroleptic is continued, attempt to lower the dosage.
10. If dyskinesia worsens, consider discontinuing the neuroleptic or switching to a new neuroleptic. At present, clozapine may hold some promise in this regard, but it is important to stay alert to new research findings.
11. Many cases of dyskinesia will improve and even remit with neuroleptic discontinuation or dosage reduction. If treatment for tardive dyskinesia is indicated, utilize more benign agents first (e.g., benzodiazepines and tocopheral), but keep abreast of new treatment developments.
12. If movement disorder is severe or disabling, consider obtaining a second opinion.

Appendix

# Sample Rating Scales
# for Tardive Dyskinesia

## Introduction

The rating scales included here are presented as examples of instruments commonly utilized to assess drug-induced movement disorders. There are a variety of other scales available for these purposes and the inclusion of these particular instruments does not signify a specific endorsement or recommendation.

It is also important to emphasize that rating scales cannot and should not be used to make a diagnosis but are intended to classify and quantify a particular sign or symptom. An appropriate process of clinical judgment and differential diagnosis must then be brought to bear.

## A Rating Scale for Tardive Dyskinesia

G. M. Simpson, J. H. Lee, B. Zoubok, and G. Gardos

Patient _____ No. _____

Date _____ Time _____ am pm

Setting_____ Rater _____

### Face

| | Absent | ? | Mild | Moderate | Moderately severe | Very severe |
|---|---|---|---|---|---|---|
| 1. Blinking of eyes | 1 | 2 | 3 | 4 | 5 | 6 |
| 2. Tremor of eyelids | 1 | 2 | 3 | 4 | 5 | 6 |
| 3. Tremor of upper lip (rabbit syndrome) | 1 | 2 | 3 | 4 | 5 | 6 |

Reprinted from Psychopharmacology (Berlin) 64:171–179, 1979, with permission from Springer-Verlag.

| | Absent | ? | Mild | Moderate | Moderately severe | Very severe |
|---|---|---|---|---|---|---|
| 4. Pouting of the (lower) lip | 1 | 2 | 3 | 4 | 5 | 6 |
| 5. Puckering of lips | 1 | 2 | 3 | 4 | 5 | 6 |
| 6. Sucking movements | 1 | 2 | 3 | 4 | 5 | 6 |
| 7. Chewing movements | 1 | 2 | 3 | 4 | 5 | 6 |
| 8. Smacking of lips | 1 | 2 | 3 | 4 | 5 | 6 |
| 9. Bonbon sign | 1 | 2 | 3 | 4 | 5 | 6 |
| 10. Tongue protrusion | 1 | 2 | 3 | 4 | 5 | 6 |
| 11. Tongue tremor | 1 | 2 | 3 | 4 | 5 | 6 |
| 12. Choreoathetoid movements of the tongue | 1 | 2 | 3 | 4 | 5 | 6 |
| 13. Facial tics | 1 | 2 | 3 | 4 | 5 | 6 |
| 14. Grimacing | 1 | 2 | 3 | 4 | 5 | 6 |
| 15. Other (describe)_____ | 1 | 2 | 3 | 4 | 5 | 6 |
| 16. Other (describe)_____ | 1 | 2 | 3 | 4 | 5 | 6 |

**Neck and trunk**

| | Absent | ? | Mild | Moderate | Moderately severe | Very severe |
|---|---|---|---|---|---|---|
| 17. Head nodding | 1 | 2 | 3 | 4 | 5 | 6 |
| 18. Retrocollis | 1 | 2 | 3 | 4 | 5 | 6 |
| 19. Spasmodic torticollis | 1 | 2 | 3 | 4 | 5 | 6 |
| 20. Torsion movements (trunk) | 1 | 2 | 3 | 4 | 5 | 6 |
| 21. Axial hyperkinesia | 1 | 2 | 3 | 4 | 5 | 6 |
| 22. Rocking movement | 1 | 2 | 3 | 4 | 5 | 6 |
| 23. Other (describe)_____ | 1 | 2 | 3 | 4 | 5 | 6 |
| 24. Other (describe)_____ | 1 | 2 | 3 | 4 | 5 | 6 |

**Extremities (upper)**

| | Absent | ? | Mild | Moderate | Moderately severe | Very severe |
|---|---|---|---|---|---|---|
| 25. Ballistic movements | 1 | 2 | 3 | 4 | 5 | 6 |
| 26. Choreoathetoid movements—fingers | 1 | 2 | 3 | 4 | 5 | 6 |
| 27. Choreoathetoid movements—wrists | 1 | 2 | 3 | 4 | 5 | 6 |
| 28. Pill-rolling movements | 1 | 2 | 3 | 4 | 5 | 6 |
| 29. Caressing or rubbing face and hair | 1 | 2 | 3 | 4 | 5 | 6 |
| 30. Rubbing of thighs | 1 | 2 | 3 | 4 | 5 | 6 |
| 31. Other (describe) _____ | 1 | 2 | 3 | 4 | 5 | 6 |
| 32. Other (describe) _____ | 1 | 2 | 3 | 4 | 5 | 6 |

**Extremities (lower)**

| | Absent | ? | Mild | Moderate | Moderately severe | Very severe |
|---|---|---|---|---|---|---|
| 33. Rotation and/or flexion of ankles | 1 | 2 | 3 | 4 | 5 | 6 |
| 34. Toe movements | 1 | 2 | 3 | 4 | 5 | 6 |
| 35. Stamping movements—standing | 1 | 2 | 3 | 4 | 5 | 6 |
| 36. Stamping movements—sitting | 1 | 2 | 3 | 4 | 5 | 6 |

| | Absent | ? | Mild | Moderate | Moderately severe | Very severe |
|---|---|---|---|---|---|---|
| 37. Restless legs | 1 | 2 | 3 | 4 | 5 | 6 |
| 38. Crossing/uncrossing legs—sitting | 1 | 2 | 3 | 4 | 5 | 6 |
| 39. Other (describe) _____ | 1 | 2 | 3 | 4 | 5 | 6 |
| 40. Other (describe) _____ | 1 | 2 | 3 | 4 | 5 | 6 |

**Entire body**

| | Absent | ? | Mild | Moderate | Moderately severe | Very severe |
|---|---|---|---|---|---|---|
| 41. Holokinetic movements | 1 | 2 | 3 | 4 | 5 | 6 |
| 42. Akathisia | 1 | 2 | 3 | 4 | 5 | 6 |
| 43. Other (describe) _____ | 1 | 2 | 3 | 4 | 5 | 6 |

**Comments**

# Tardive Dyskinesia Rating Scale Definitions

## Face

1. Blinking of eyes: Repetitive and more or less continuous or in bursts. To be distinguished from tics, which occur episodically.
2. Tremor of eyelids: Isolated tremor, more frequently bilateral but can occur unilaterally. Usually seen when eyes are closed. Fine in character.
3. Tremor of upper lip (rabbit syndrome): Fine, rapid tremor confined to the upper lip.
4. Pouting of the lower lip: A thrusting out of the lower lip as in solemnness.
5. Puckering of lips: Drawstring or pursing action of the lip.
6. Smacking of lips: Brisk separation of lips, which produces a sharp sound.
7. Sucking movement: Self-explanatory.
8. Chewing movement: Self-explanatory.
9. Bonbon sign: Tongue movement within oral cavity that produces a bulge in the cheek, giving the impression the patient has a hard bonbon pocketed in this cheek. Occasionally a repetitious sweeping movement of the tongue over the buccal lining, which also pushes out the mouth.
10. Tongue protrusion: Clonic—a rhythmic in-and-out movement of the tongue. Tonic—a continuous protrusion of the tongue. Fly-catcher—a

sudden shooting out of the tongue from the mouth at irregular episodes.

11. Tongue tremor: Fine tremor observed with the mouth open and
    tongue within the buccal cavity.

12. Choreoathetoid movements of the tongue: A rolling, wormlike move-
    ment of the tongue muscles without displacement of the tongue from
    the mouth. The tongue may rotate on its longitudinal axis. Observed
    when the mouth is opened.

13. Facial tics: Brief, recurrent, stereotyped movement involving relatively
    small segments of the face.

14. Grimacing: A repetitive, irregularly occurring distortion of the face. A
    complex movement involving large segments of facial muscles.

15. and 16.   Other: Write in items such as unusual buccolingual move-
    ments, blepharospasm, repetitive sounds, etc.

### Neck and Trunk

17. Head nodding: Slower than tremor, may or may not be rhythmic. Can
    occur horizontally or vertically.

18. Retrocollis: Overextension of the neck as a result of which the head is
    bent backwards. Can occur with or without rigidity of the muscles of
    the neck and shoulder.

19. Spasmodic torticollis: Tonic, prolonged contracture of sternocleido-
    mastoides on one side resulting in a downward and lateral fixation of
    the chin. The head may be bent laterally.

20. Torsion movements: Twisting, undulant movements of the upper or
    lower part of the trunk (shoulder or hip girdle) resulting from mobile,
    spastic movements of the axial and proximal muscles. The movements
    are not fast and they involve large portions of the body.

21. Axial hyperkinesia: A front-to-back hip-rocking movement. Resembles
    copulatory movements. Differs from the rocking movement where it is
    the upper torso that has to-and-fro movement.

22. Rocking movements: A rhythmic to-and-fro movement of the upper
    torso that occurs from a repeated bending of the spinal column in the
    lumbar region. Different from axial hyperkinesia, in which the hips
    move to and fro.

23. and 24.   Other: Write in.

### Extremities (Upper)

25. Ballistic movements: Sudden, fast, large amplitude swinging move-
    ments occurring most often in the arms and less frequently in the legs.
    One or both sides may be involved.

26. and 27.   Choreiform movements in fingers, wrists, arms: Variable, pur-

poseless, coarse, quick, and jerky movements that begin suddenly and show no rhythmicity. They vary in distribution and extension.

26. and 27. Athetoid movements in fingers, wrists, arms: Continuous rhythmic, slow, writhing, wormlike movements. They almost invariably appear together with choreiform movements.

28. Finger counting: Rhythmic rubbing of the thumb against the middle and index finger.

29. Caressing face and hair: Gives the impression of an absent-minded or nervous mannerism: has the appearance of being purposeful.

30. Rubbing of thighs: Hands rub the outside or tops of thighs. Sporadic and nonrhythmic.

31. and 32. Other: Write in.

### Extremities (Lower)

33. Rotation and/or flexion of the ankles: Self-explanatory.

34. Toe movements: Slow, rhythmic retroflexion, usually of the big toes although other toes can also be involved.

35. Stamping movements (standing): Weight is shifted back and forth from one foot to the other when patient stands.

36. Stamping movements (sitting): Flapping or tapping of the whole foot on floor when the patient is sitting or may comprise an alternate toe and heel tapping.

37. Restless legs: Constant leg movement; jiggling of legs, of foot when leg is crossed; may involve rapidly moving knees apart and together.

38. Crossing and uncrossing legs: Self-explanatory.

39. and 40. Other: Write in.

### Entire Body

41. Holokinetic movements: Extensive, jerky, rapid, abrupt, awkward, gross movements of large parts or entire body. The movement may appear to be somewhat goal directed and only moderately coordinated. May begin in response to stimulus or spontaneously.

42. Akathisia: An inability to sit or stand still. (The verbal expression of inner restlessness is not required here.)

43. and 44. Other: Write in.

# Abbreviated Dyskinesia Rating Scale (ADRS)

G. M. Simpson, J. H. Lee, B. Zoubok, and G. Gardos

### Abbreviated Dyskinesia Rating Scale

Patient: _____    #  _____

Date: _____  Time: _____  am pm

Setting: _____  Study #: _____

Rating # : _____  Period: _____

### Facial and Oral Movements                     *Rating*

1. Periocular area (blinking of eyes, tremor of eyelids)  1  2  3  4  5  6
2. Movements of the lips (pouting, puckering, smacking)  1  2  3  4  5  6
3. Chewing movements  1  2  3  4  5  6
4. Bonbon sign  1  2  3  4  5  6
5. Tongue protrusion  1  2  3  4  5  6
6. Tremor and/or choreoathetoid movements of the tongue  1  2  3  4  5  6
7. Other (describe) _____  1  2  3  4  5  6

### Neck and Trunk

8. Axial hyperkinesia (patient standing)  1  2  3  4  5  6
9. Rocking movements  1  2  3  4  5  6
10. Torsion movements  1  2  3  4  5  6
11. Other (describe) _____  1  2  3  4  5  6

### Extremities

12. Movements of fingers and wrists  1  2  3  4  5  6
13. Movements of ankles and toes  1  2  3  4  5  6
14. Stamping movements  1  2  3  4  5  6
15. Other (describe) _____  1  2  3  4  5  6

Reprinted from Psychopharmacology (Berlin) 64:171–179, 1979, with permission from Springer-Verlag.

### Entire Body

| | | | | | | |
|---|---|---|---|---|---|---|
| 16. Akathisia | 1 | 2 | 3 | 4 | 5 | 6 |
| 17. Other (describe )_____ | 1 | 2 | 3 | 4 | 5 | 6 |

**Rating:**   1  Absent
              2  Questionable
              3  Mild
              4  Moderate
              5  Moderately severe
              6  Severe
              Total score: _____

# ADRS Examination Procedure

Prior to the examination, observe the patient in the dayroom, waiting room, or while you engage him/her in nonthreatening conversation. Abnormal movements may be more evident if the patient is relaxed. It is helpful for the examiner to demonstrate each of the examination procedures. Movements are rated whether at rest or only after activation.

Seat the patient in a chair that is firm and without armrests.

1. Ask patient to remove:
   a. anything in his or her mouth (food, gum, foreign objects)
   b. loose dentures
   c. shoes and socks
2. Ask patient to lean forward, elbows on thighs, so that hands are hanging over knees or between knees. Observe all body areas.
3. Ask patient if he/she has noticed any movements of fingers, mouth, feet, etc. Do the movements interfere with physical or social function?
4. Ask patient to place hands on thighs, arms relaxed, legs slightly apart, and feet flat on the floor. Observe all body parts.
5. Ask patient to open mouth. Observe tongue within the buccal cavity. Repeat.
6. Ask patient to tap thumb, alternately with each finger, as rapidly as possible for 10 to 15 seconds. Repeat with opposite hand. Observe facial, leg, and truncal movement.
7. Ask patient to open mouth and tap each finger to thumb with both hands simultaneously. Observe tongue and facial movement.
8. Ask patient to stand up. Observe in profile all body areas.
9. Ask patient to extend both arms toward the front (elbows straight) with wrists flexed. Ask patient to open and close mouth rapidly for 10–15 seconds. Observe fingers, wrists, and all other body parts.

10. With patient's arms extended and wrists flexed, ask the patient to open mouth and blink eyes rapidly for 10–15 seconds. Observe tongue and all body areas. (If #7 was negative, repeat #7 with the patient standing.)
11. Have patient walk as fast as possible, with arms at sides, 8–10 paces forward and then back to chair. Repeat. Observe hands and gait.

Note: For patients unable to perform these procedures (i.e., numbers 6, 7, 9, and 10), ask patients to clap hands then slap thighs rapidly for 10–15 seconds, with mouth open. Observe tongue, facial area.

## Sct. Hans Rating Scale for Extrapyramidal Syndromes

Jes Gerlach, M.D., and Soren Korsgaard, M.D., Sct. Hans Hospital, Roskilde, Denmark

| Patient Initials | | Rater | |
|---|---|---|---|
| Hospital | | Hospital | |
| Date of Recording | | Date of Evaluation | |

| Hyperkinesia | Passive | Active | Parkinsonism | |
|---|---|---|---|---|
| Jaw | | | Facial Expression | |
| Tongue | | | Bradykinesia | |
| Lips | | | Tremor | |
| Face | | | Posture | |
| Head | | | Arm Swing | |
| Trunk | | | Gait | |
| Upper Extremities | | | Rigidity | |
| Lower Extremities | | | Salivation | |
| Total | | | Total | |
| Total Mean | | | | |

| Parkinsonism Global | |
|---|---|

| Hyperkinesia Global | |
|---|---|

| Dystonia | |
|---|---|

| Psychic Symptoms | |
|---|---|
| Sedation | |
| Depression | |
| Anxiety | |

| Akathisia | |
|---|---|
| Psychic | |
| Motor | |

**Scoring Code:**  0  Absent
1  Dubious
2  Mild
3  Mild–Moderate
4  Moderate
5  Moderate–Severe
6  Severe

# Sct. Hans Rating Scale for Extrapyramidal Syndromes Scoring Procedure

The Sct. Hans Rating Scale for Extrapyramidal Syndromes is designed to assess some of the more common movement disorders associated with neuroleptic treatment. The primary items to be scored are hyperkinesia (abnormal involuntary movements, e.g., seen in tardive dyskinesia), parkinsonism, dystonia, and akathisia.

The hyperkinesia scores include 8 items that are to be assessed during both passive and active phases. Passive phases are when the patient is just sitting and is relaxed. Active phases are when the patient is speaking or performing motor tasks such as opening and closing the hands, writing, or walking back and forth (use the most intense sequence). The passive and active scores are totalled and then averaged. A global assessment should also be made.

Parkinsonism is scored on 8 items, but there are no distinctions between passive and active phases. A global parkinsonian score is also required.

Dystonia and akathisia (psychic and motor, including stereotypies) are individual syndromes that require only global scores.

All items are scored on a scale of 0 to 6, as follows:

0  Absent/normal
1  Dubious, may be variations of normal
2  Mild
3  Mild to moderate
4  Moderate
5  Moderate to severe
6  Severe

The scale can usually be completed with even the most disturbed patient. Videotaping usually takes from 5 to 7 minutes.

# Sct. Hans Rating Scale for Extrapyramidal Syndromes

### Video Examination Procedure

The examination should be performed in a reproducible sequence and can be easily videotaped for repeated observations and additional review.

1. Invite the patient to sit in a chair which is firm and without arms. Let the patient look towards the camera. Be certain that he/she is comfortable and does not have foreign objects in his/her mouth.
2. For identification, let the patient hold a piece of paper with his/her number, initials, and the date of the recording (5 seconds).
3. The patient is taped in full-length for at least 1 minute. Talk with the patient about some commonly discussed topics to put him/her at ease (e.g., daily activities, energy level, sleep pattern, mood, etc.). Ask specifically about sedation, depression, anxiety, and restlessness (psychic akathisia). Observe orofacial, hand, leg, and truncal movements during speech.
4. Ask the patient to just sit and relax for a minute. Focus on TD. Do not talk with the patient during this time but look away or do some other activities so the patient is passive and at rest. Observe eye blinking rates or count specific movements during a given time, if desired.
5. Ask the patient to open his/her mouth wide so you can see the tongue for approximately 15 seconds. Repeat if desired.
6. Ask the patient to extend the arms straight out from the chest. Ask him/her to rapidly open and close the fingers. Then ask him/her to shake his/her hands at the wrists. If you wish, ask him/her to tap the thumb with each finger. Observe both hyperkinesia and bradykinesia during these tasks.
7. Ask the patient to write his/her name and address on a piece of paper. Observe dyskinesias, particularly orofacial signs, during this activity. Let face and fingers fill up the screen.
8. Ask the patient to stand at rest for 10–15 seconds. Observe for akathisia. The patient is taped in full-length for the rest of the examination. Have him/her walk back and forth across the room (6–10 meters) at his/her normal speed. Repeat once. Observe for movements (especially finger TD) and note bradykinesia, tremor, posture, arm swing, and gait for parkinsonian assessments.
9. Ask the patient to turn around twice.
10. Evaluate the patient's arms and wrists for rigidity. Give your score to the microphone.
11. Ask the patient if he/she has normal, increased, or decreased salivation. Also examine the oral cavity to observe moisture levels. Salivation

is scored only when increased. Give your score to the microphone.
12. Dystonia is scored from the multiple aspects of the evaluation and refers to a sustained abnormal posture.
13. Akathisia documents the patient's feeling of restlessness (psychic akathisia) and increased repetitive or stereotyped motor developments (motor akathisia). The last mentioned is observed when the patient is sitting or standing.

# A Rating Scale for Extrapyramidal Side Effects

G. M. Simpson, M.B., Ch.B., and J. W. S. Angus, F.R.C.P.(C), D.P.M.

1. Gait: The patient is examined as he or she walks into the examining room. Gait, swing of the arms, and general posture all form the basis for overall score for this item. This is rated as follows:
   0 Normal.
   1 Diminution in swing while the patient is walking.
   2 Marked diminution in swing with obvious rigidity in the arm.
   3 Stiff gait with arms held rigidly before the abdomen.
   4 Stooped shuffling gait with propulsion and retropulsion.

2. Arm Dropping: The patient and the examiner both raise their arms to shoulder height and let them fall to their sides. In a normal subject, a stout slap is heard as the arms hit the sides. In the patient with extreme Parkinson's syndrome, the arms fall very slowly:
   0 Normal, free fall with loud slap and rebound.
   1 Fall slowed slightly with less audible contact and little rebound.
   2 Fall slowed, no rebound.
   3 Marked slowing, no slap at all.
   4 Arms fall as though against resistance; as though through glue.

3. Shoulder Shaking: The subject's arms are bent at a right angle at the elbow and are taken one at a time by the examiner who grasps one hand and also clasps the other around the patient's elbow. The subject's upper arm is pushed to and fro and the humerus is externally rotated. The degree of resistance from normal to extreme rigidity is scored as follows:
   0 Normal.
   1 Slight stiffness and resistance.

Reprinted from Simpson GM, Angus JWS: A Rating Scale for Extrapyramidal Side Effects, Acta Psychiatrica Scandinavica 212:11–19, 1970. Copyright 1970 Munksgaard International Publishers, Ltd.

2   Moderate stiffness and resistance.
3   Marked rigidity with difficulty in passive movement.
4   Extreme stiffness and rigidity with almost a frozen shoulder.

4.  Elbow rigidity: The elbow joints are separately bent at right angles and passively extended and flexed, with the subject's biceps observed and simultaneously palpated. The resistance to this procedure is rated. (The presence of cogwheel rigidity is noted separately.) Scoring is from 0 to 4 as in Shoulder Shaking test.
5.  Fixation of position or Wrist Rigidity: The wrist is held in one hand and the fingers held by the examiner's other hand, with the wrist moved to extension, flexion, and both ulnar and radial deviation. The resistance to this procedure is rated as in Items 3 and 4.
6.  Leg Pendulousness: The patient sits on a table with the legs hanging down and swinging free. The ankle is grasped by the examiner and raised until the knee is partially extended. It is then allowed to fall. The resistance to falling and the lack of swinging form the basis for the score on this item:
0   The legs swing freely.
1   Slight diminution in the swing of the legs.
2   Moderate resistance to swing.
3   Marked resistance and damping of swing.
4   Complete absence of swing.

7.  Head Dropping: The patient lies on a well-padded examining table and his or her head is raised by the examiner's hand. The hand is then withdrawn and the head allowed to drop. In the normal subject, the head will fall upon the table. The movement is delayed in extrapyramidal system disorder and in extreme parkinsonism it is absent. The neck muscles are rigid and the head does not reach the examining table. Scoring is as follows:
0   The head falls completely with a good thump as it hits the table.
1   Slight slowing in fall, mainly noted by lack of slap as head meets the table.
2   Moderate slowing in the fall quite noticeable to the eye.
3   Head falls stiffly and slowly.
4   Head does not reach examining table.
8.  Glabella Tap: The patient is told to open eyes wide and not to blink. The glabella region is tapped at a steady, rapid speed. The number of times the patient blinks in succession is noted:
0   0–5 blinks.
1   6–10 blinks.
2   11–15 blinks.

3  16–20 blinks.
4  21 or more blinks.

9. Tremor: Patient is observed walking into the examining room and then is reexamined for this item:
0  Normal.
1  Mild finger tremor, obvious to sight and touch.
2  Tremor of hand or arm occurring spasmodically.
3  Persistent tremor of one or more limbs.
4  Whole body tremor.

10. Salivation: Patient is observed while talking and then asked to open his or her mouth and elevate the tongue. The following ratings are given:
0  Normal.
1  Excess salivation to the extent that pooling takes place if the mouth is open and the tongue is raised.
2  Excess salivation is present and might occasionally result in difficulty in speaking.
3  Speaking is difficult because of excess salivation.
4  Frank drooling.

# Abnormal Involuntary Movement Scale (AIMS)

### Examination Procedure

Either before or after completing the Examination Procedure, observe the patient unobtrusively, at rest (e.g., in waiting room).

The chair to be used in this examination should be a hard, firm one without arms.

1. Ask patient to remove shoes and socks.
2. Ask patient whether there is anything in his/her mouth (i.e., gum, candy, etc.) and if there is, to remove it.
3. Ask patient about the *current* condition of his/her teeth. Ask patient if he/she wears dentures. Do teeth or dentures bother patient *now?*
4. Ask patient whether he/she notices any movements in mouth, face, hands, or feet. If yes, ask to describe and to what extent they *currently* bother patient or interfere with his/her activities.

Source: Department of Health and Human Services; Public Health Service; Alcohol, Drug Abuse, and Mental Health Administration; NIMH Treatment Strategies in Schizophrenia Study; ADM-117, Revised November 1985.

5. Have patient sit in chair with hands on knees, legs slightly apart, and feet flat on floor. (Look at entire body for movements while in this position.)

6. Ask patient to sit with hands hanging unsupported. If male, between legs, if female and wearing a dress, hanging over knees. (Observe hands and other body areas.)

7. Ask patient to open mouth. (Observe tongue at rest within mouth.) Do this twice.

8. Ask patient to protrude tongue. (Observe abnormalities of tongue movement.) Do this twice.

9. Ask patient to tap thumb with each finger as rapidly as possible for 10–15 seconds; separately with right hand, then with left hand. (Observe facial and leg movements.)

10. Flex and extend patient's left and right arms (one at a time). (Note any rigidity.)

11. Ask patient to stand up. (Observe in profile. Observe all body areas again, hips included.)

12. Ask patient to extend both arms outstretched in front with palms down. (Observe trunk, legs, and mouth.)

13. Have patient walk a few paces, turn, and walk back to chair. (Observe hands and gait.) Do this twice.

**Evaluation type** (circle one):

| | | |
|---|---|---|
| 1 Baseline | 5 Major evaluation | 9 Stop open meds |
| 2 2-week minor | 6 Other | 10 Early termination |
| 3 | 7 Start open meds | 11 Study completion |
| 4 Start double-blind | 8 During open meds | |

**Instructions:** Complete examination procedure before making ratings. Rate highest severity observed.

**Code:**
1 None
2 Minimal, may be extreme normal
3 Mild
4 Moderate
5 Severe

### Facial and Oral Movements

1. Muscles of Facial Expression (e.g., movements of forehead, eyebrows, periorbital area, cheeks; include frowning, blinking, smiling, grimacing)

1  2  3  4  5

2. Lips and Perioral Area (e.g., puckering, pouting, smacking)

                                   1    2    3    4    5

3. Jaw (e.g., biting, clenching, chewing, mouth opening, lateral movement)

                                   1    2    3    4    5

4. Tongue (Rate only increase in movement both in and out of mouth, NOT inability to sustain movement.)

                                   1    2    3    4    5

### Extremity Movements

5. Upper (arms, wrists, hands, fingers). Include choreic movements (i.e., rapid, objectively purposeless, irregular, spontaneous), athetoid movements (i.e., slow, irregular, complex, serpentine). Do NOT include tremor (i.e., repetitive, regular, rhythmic).

                                   1    2    3    4    5

6. Lower (legs, knees, ankles, toes). (E.g., lateral knee movement, foot tapping, heel dropping, foot squirming, inversion and eversion of foot.)

                                   1    2    3    4    5

### Trunk Movements

7. Neck, shoulders, hips (e.g., rocking, twisting, squirming, pelvic gyrations)

                                   1    2    3    4    5

### Global Judgments

8. Severity of abnormal movements:
   1  None, normal
   2  Minimal
   3  Mild
   4  Moderate
   5  Severe
9. Incapacitation due to abnormal movements:
   1  None, normal
   2  Minimal
   3  Mild
   4  Moderate
   5  Severe
10. Patient's awareness of abnormal movements (Rate only patient's report)
    1  No awareness

2  Aware, no distress
3  Aware, mild distress
4  Aware, moderate distress
5  Aware, severe distress

## Dental Status

11. Current problems with teeth and/or dentures
    1  No
    2  Yes
12. Does patient usually wear dentures?
    1  No
    2  Yes

# Index

---

Page numbers printed in boldface type refer to tables or figures.